Part I — I

Part II — II

Part III — III

1 Acute kidney injury (AKI) — 1

2 Acute respiratory failure (ARF) – Acute respiratory distress syndrome (ARDS) — 2

3 Acute respiratory failure – Non-ARDS — 3

4 Cardiovascular dynamics — 4

5 Ethics — 5

6 General — 6

7 Health technology — 7

8 Infection — 8

9 Neuro-intensive care — 9

10 Nutrition and metabolism — 10

11 Outcomes — 11

12 Paediatric intensive care — 12

13 Sepsis — 13

14 Trauma and emergency medicine — 14

Part IV — IV

ESICM Systematic Review Group

Clinical Evidence in Intensive Care

Medizinisch Wissenschaftliche Verlagsgesellschaft

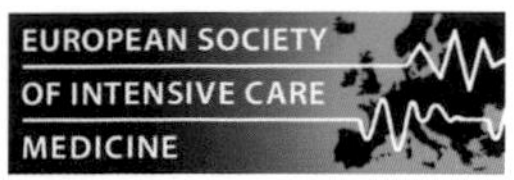

European Society of Intensive Care Medicine
Rue Belliard, 19
1040 Brussels, Belgium
Tel: 0032 2 559 03 50 – Fax: 0032 2 559 03 79
E-mail: administration@esicm.org
www.esicm.org

MWV Medizinisch Wissenschaftliche Verlagsgesellschaft mbH & Co. KG
Zimmerstraße 11
D- 10969 Berlin
www.mwv-berlin.de

ISBN 978-3-941468-61-0

These publications are listed in: Deutsche Nationalbibliothek

Detailed bibliographical information is available via internet http://dnb.d-nb.de.

Project management: Claudia Leonhardt, Berlin
Editorial office: Frauke Budig, Monika Laut-Zimmermann, Berlin
Copy editing: Dr. Michael Kastner, acaman.de, Berlin
Layout and typesetting: eScriptum GmbH & Co KG – Publishing Services, Berlin
Printing: druckhaus köthen GmbH, Köthen

Reply and complaints to:
MWV Medizinisch Wissenschaftliche Verlagsgesellschaft mbH & Co. KG, Zimmerstr. 11, D- 10969 Berlin,
lektorat@mwv-berlin.de

Contents

Part I ix

Foreword xi
Acknowledgments xii
Index of abbreviations xiv
Statistics glossary xvi

Part II xix

How to use this handbook xxi

Part III 1

1 **Acute kidney injury (AKI)** 3
Atrial natriuretic peptide 4
Hydroxyethyl starch (1) 8
Hydroxyethyl starch (2) 14
Sodium bicarbonate 19
AKI in cardiac surgery 25

2 **Acute respiratory failure (ARF) – Acute respiratory distress syndrome (ARDS)** 29
Higher versus lower PEEP 30
Recruitment manoeuvres 34
Inhaled nitric oxide 39
Aerosolized prostacyclin 43
Pharmacological therapies for ARDS 46
Corticosteroids in ARDS 50
ECMO 54

3 **Acute respiratory failure – Non ARDS** 57
Corticosteroids for pneumonia 58
Corticosteroids to prevent and treat post extubation stridor 64
Corticosteroids to prevent extubation failure 70
Protocolized versus non-protocolized weaning 75
NPPV for weaning 82
Heated humidification versus HME 88
Pleural effusions drainage 93

4 **Cardiovascular dynamics** 99
Atrial fibrillation 100
Therapeutic hypothermia 104
Vasopressin for vasodilatory shock 109
Pre-emptive haemodynamic intervention 114

5 **Ethics** 121
Organ donation 122

6 **General** 127
Stress ulcer prophylaxis 128
Critical illness polyneuropathy and polymyopathy 134
Thromboprophylaxis 139
Music therapy 143

7 **Health technology** 151
Chest radiography 152
Oesophageal doppler monitoring 157
Computerised decision support systems 165

8 **Infection** 169
Peripheral venous catheters 170
Procalcitonin 174
Continuous beta-lactam antibiotics 179
Ventilator-associated pneumonia 183
Selective decontamination of the digestive tract 187
Antibiotic prophylaxis for pancreatic necrosis 191

9 **Neuro-intensive care** 195
Haemostatic drugs for TBI 196
Routine ICP monitoring 199
Cooling post stroke 202

10 **Nutrition and metabolism** 207
Early enteral nutrition 208
Nutrition in pancreatitis 212
Enteral versus parenteral nutrition in pancreatitis 216
Glucose-insulin-potassium infusion 223

11 **Outcomes** 227
Off-hours admission and mortality 228
Risk of readmission to ICU 232
Quality of life after ICU 236
Long-term mortality after ICU 241
Health insurance in the USA 245

12 **Paediatric intensive care** 251
Continuous negative extrathoracic pressure 252
Heliox for croup 255
Bacterial meningitis 258
Nutritional support for critically ill children 263
Other relevant reviews 265

13 Sepsis — 267
Early versus late broad spectrum antibiotics — 268
Combination antibiotics — 270
De-escalation of antibiotics — 275
Albumin for fluid resuscitation — 278
Corticosteroids for severe sepsis & septic shock — 283
Granulocyte & granulocyte-macrophage colony stimulating factor — 292

14 Trauma and emergency medicine — 297
Chest-compression-only CPR for out of hospital arrest — 298

Part IV — 303
Appendix A: Review titles — 305
Appendix B: Corresponding authors — 308
Appendix C: The experts — 314
Appendix D: The Systematic Review Group Board — 317
Appendix E: Additional references from the text — 319

Part I

Foreword xi
Acknowledgments xii
Index of abbreviations xiv
Statistics glossary xvi

Foreword

The ESICM Systematic Review Group has committed to provide ESICM members with accurate synthesis of the best evidence in intensive care medicine. The past decade has been characterised by an exponential increase in the number of systematic reviews, such that the CRD database for example, now contains 21,000 reviews. There is no database that is focused purely on intensive care medicine. In addition, the various systematic reviews may not all be of the highest methodological quality. It may be difficult for intensive care physicians to find relevant reviews, therefore ESICM SRG editors have started searching and gathering high quality systematic reviews that are relevant to intensive care physicians. In addition, ESICM SRG will perform systematic reviews for any relevant topic for which accurate synthesis of the literature is lacking. These syntheses of the evidence will be disseminated to ESICM members via a web platform and a handbook. This is the first edition of the ESICM Clinical Evidence in Intensive Care handbook.

I would like to thank all editors and contributors, and more specifically Gihan Abuella for the impressive work they have done these past months allowing the release of the handbook at the annual meeting of ESICM in Berlin. After a systematic search of Pubmed and CENTRAL, we have selected 60 systematic reviews on topics directly relevant for ICU practitioners and published since 2009. Indeed, it is thought that a systematic review remains accurate on average 2 years, and therefore has to be updated at the very least every other year. For each of these SRs, we have provided the readers with an extended summary highlighting the context of the review, its main findings, review authors' conclusions, problems and limitations and advantages. In addition, we analysed the methodological quality of the systematic review on 11 items. For each systematic review, experts in the field highlighted the validity and robustness of the data, whether or not they should translate into changes in routine practice, and what should be the next steps for research. The handbook is organised into 14 sections corresponding to ESICM sections to help the readers searching for specific topics. We selected a pocket format and thumb index to make the book as user friendly as possible. In the near future ESICM will provide its members with the first database of systematic reviews focusing on topics directly relevant to intensive care physicians.

Professor Djillali Annane
Chair of the ESICM Systematic Review Group

Acknowledgments

We are very grateful to all the contributors to the handbook. It would not have been possible to produce this handbook without the work and support received from all those listed below.

We would like to thank all the authors of the systematic reviews and meta-analyses included in this handbook for allowing us to use their publication in this way and for reviewing the summaries to ensure accuracy. We are only able to list the authors with whom we had direct correspondence but we'd like to emphasize that we acknowledge the contribution of every author.

We would particularly like to thank all the experts who took the time and trouble to assess the reviews and provide us with their commentary, some at very short notice.

Original Review Authors

Acute kidney injury (AKI): Sagar U. Nigwekar, Allison B. Dart, Lauralyn McIntyre, Eric Hoste, Chirag Parikh

Acute respiratory failure (ARF) – Acute respiratory distress syndrome (ARDS): Maureen Meade, Carol Hodgson, Arash Afshari, Neill K.J. Adhikari, Benjamin Tang, Anthony S. McLean, Mark E. Mikkelsen

Acute respiratory failure – Non-ARDS: Taixiang Wu, Robinder G. Khemani, John McCaffrey, Anthony P. Delaney, Bronagh Blackwood, Karen E.A. Burns, Margaret Kelly, Donna Gillies, David Todd, Niall Ferguson

Cardiovascular dynamics: Salmaan Kanji, Jasmin Arrich, Djillali Annane, Mark Hamilton

Ethics: Duncan Young

General: Paul E. Marik, Greet Hermans, Greet Van den Berghe, Deborah Cook, Joke Bradt

Health technology: Yugi Oba, Graham Mowatt, Saeid Eslami

Infection: Joan Webster, Petros Kopterides, Jeffrey Lipman, Matthew E. Falagas, Alessandro Liberati, Mike Larvin

Neuro-intensive care: Pablo Perel, Rob J. Forsyth, Heleen M. Den Hertog, Diederik Dippel

Nutrition and metabolism: Gordon S. Doig, Ahmad Al Samaraee, Mohammed Al-Omran, Alan Jones

Outcomes: Paul E. Marik, Steven A. Frost, Sandra G. Oeyen, Bradford D. Winters, Robert A. Fowler

Paediatric intensive care: Matthew E. Falagas, Prakeshkumar S. Shah, Christiane Vorwerk, Tim Coats, Ari Joffe

---

Text and summaries: Gihan Abuella

Major contribution from Pierre Squara for the summary of "Computerised Decision Support Systems"

Peri-operative ICM*: See Cardiovascular dynamics and Health technology

Sepsis: Shahla Siddiqui, Anand Kumar, Brenda Nazaré Gomes Silva, Anthony P. Delaney, John McCaffrey, Djillali Annane, Lulong Bo

Trauma and emergency medicine: Peter Nagele

The Experts

Acute kidney injury (AKI): Eric Hoste, Michael Joannidis, Maria Schetz

Acute respiratory failure (ARF) – Acute respiratory distress syndrome (ARDS): Anders Larsson, Nicola Petrucci, Arthur S. Slutsky, Gianfranco Umberto Meduri, Jeremy Cordingley

Acute respiratory failure – Non-ARDS: John Carlisle, Djillali Annane, Laurent Brochard, Richard Venn, Jonathan Ball

Cardiovascular dynamics: Fernando Clau-Terré, Maurizio Cecconi, Jan Poelaert, Anthony Gordon

Ethics: Jozef Kesecioglu

General: Pedro Navarrete-Navarro, Miguel Tavares, Maurizio Cecconi

Health technology: Pierre Squara, Claudia Spies, Aarne Feldheiser

Infection: George Dimopoulos, Jordi Rello

Neuro-intensive care: Mauro Oddo, Pedro Navarrete-Navarro

Nutrition and metabolism: David Noble, Daren K. Heyland

Outcomes: Maurizia Capuzzo

Paediatric intensive care: Joan Balcells Ramírez

Peri-operative ICM*: See Cardiovascular dynamics and Health technology

Sepsis: Jordi Rello, George Dimopoulos, Richard Ferrer, Christiane Hartog, Charles Sprung

Trauma and emergency medicine: Jacques Duranteau

---

* There is no peri-operative ICM section in this handbook but reviews relevant to this section can be found in the sections on Cardiovascular dynamics and Health technology

Index of abbreviations

ABx antibiotic(s)
ACEi angitensin converting enzyme inhibitor
ADL activity of daily living
AF atrial fibrillation
ALI acute lung injury
AKI Acute kidney injury
AMSTAR 'assessment of multiple systematic reviews' tool
ANP atrial natriuretic peptide
ANZCTR Australian New Zealand Clinical Trials Registry
APACHE acute physiology and chronic health evaluation
ARDS acute respiratory distress syndrome
ARF Acute respiratory failure
BAL bronco-alveolar lavage
BC blood culture
BIOSIS research database for life sciences publications
BNP brain natriurtic peptide
BPD bronchopulmonary dysplasia
BSD brain stem death
CABG coronary artery bypass graft
CBLD Chinese Biomedical Literature Database
CENTRAL Cochrane Central Register of Controlled Trials
c.f. compared with
CI cardiac index
CINHAL Cumulative Index to Nursing and Allied Health Literature
CKD chronic kidney disease
CO cardiac output
CONSORT Consolidated Standards of Reporting Trials
CPAP continuous positive airway pressure
CPB cardiopulmonary bypass
CRD Centre for Reviews and Dissemination
CRP C-reactive protein
CSF cerebrospinal fluid
CVP central venous pressure
CXR chest radiograph
DCCV direct current cardioversion
DM diabetes mellitus
DVT deep vein thrombosis
EMG electromyelogram
ETT endotracheal tube
GCS Glasgow coma scale
GFR glomerular filtration rate
GICU general intensive care unit (mixed)
ICP intracranial pressure
ICU intensive care unit
ISRCTN International Standardised Randomised Controlled Trial Number Register
IWS International Web of Science
LAT latex agglutinin test
LILACS Latin American Caribbean Health Sciences literature
LISS lung Injury Severity Score
LOS length of stay
MA meta-analysis
MAP mean arterial pressure or mean airway pressure (note context)
MICU mixed ICU
MODS multiple organ dysfunction syndrome
MOF multiple organ failure
MPAP mean pulmonary artery pressure
N number of participants
NAC N-acetylcysteine
NAECC North American European Consensus Conference
NCS nerve conduction studies
NICU neurosurgical/neuromedical intensive care unit
NIV non-invasive ventilation
NPPV non-invasive positive pressure ventilation
NSS not statistically significant
PAC pulmonary artery catheter
PEEP positive end-expiratory pressure
PCP pneumoncystis carinii pneumonia (renamed pneumocystis jiroveci)
PCWP pulmonary capillary wedge pressure
PS(V) pressure support (ventilation)

PSB	protected specimen brush
PVR	pulmonary vascular resistance
QTA	quantitative tracheal aspirate
RBF	renal blood flow
RCT	randomized controlled trial
rFVIIa	recombinant factor VIIa
ROSC	return of spontaneous circulation
RRT	renal replacement therapy
RVEF	right ventricular ejection fraction
RVEDV	right ventricular end-diastolic volume
SAH	subarachnoid haemorrhage
SAPS	simplified acute physiology score
SBP	systolic blood pressure
SBT	spontaneous breathing trial
SICU	surgical intensive care unit
SIMV	synchronized intermittent mandatory ventilation
SIRS	systemic inflammatory response syndrome
SOFA	sequential organ failure assessment score
SR	systematic review
SS	statistically significant
STIN	Scientific and Technical Information Network
SVT	supraventricular tachycardia
TBI	traumatic brain injury
TSA	trials sequential analysis
UKNRR	UK National Research Register
USA	United States of America
USS	ultrasound scan
VE	ventricular ectopic
VT	ventricular tachycardia
V/Q	ventilation/perfusion
WCC	white cell count
WHO	World Health Organistaion
WMD	weighted mean difference
WoS	Web of Science

Statistics glossary

Absolute Risk Difference (ARD): A measurement of the amount of difference between two treatments. The ARD indicates how much better one treatment is at reducing an outcome in a population group who usually suffer the outcome, compared to another treatment.

A Priori: Known prior information about a population as opposed to information generated by observation.

Confidence Interval (CI): Measures the precision of the mean value. It is unlikely that the mean calculated from the observed data will be close to the true population due to sampling variation. Therefore, an interval of data distribution is selected in which there is confidence that the sampled data approximates the true mean. This is usually 95%, giving the 95% confidence interval. By generating multiple 95% confidence for multiple data sets, it can be assumed that the 95% CI will include the population mean in 95% of the cases.

Correlation Estimates: An estimate of the relationship existing between at least two variables, for example drugs in a cross-over clinical trial. Two types of correlation tests are used depending on the distribution of the population the data was sampled from: Pearson (Gaussian) and Spearman rank/non-parametric (non-Gaussian). The coefficient of determination, r^2 is commonly used to denote correlation, which ranges from zero to one. The closer to 1, the greater the relationship between two variables.

Exploratory Analysis: Integrates various analytical methods (ranging from simple to sophisticated) to analyse databases of information with a view to generating new hypotheses. This is in contrast to confirmed data analysis, which uses statistical methods to prove hypotheses.

Factor Analysis: A statistical method that describes the variability of a set of observed variables due to the presence of one or more unobserved variables called factors. By identifying factors, the number of variables in a dataset can be reduced, thus simplifying the model. Factor analysis is used widely in psychometrics and behavioural science.

Fixed Effects Model: A statistical model frequently used for meta-analysis. The model assumes that all the studies that comprise the meta-analysis share a common outcome referred to as the true effect. Factors contributing to the true effect are also fixed and therefore any variations in observed true effects between studies are attributed to sampling error.

Random Effects Model: In contrast to the fixed effects model, the random effects model acknowledges that the factors contributing to the true effect vary between the studies that comprise the meta-analysis. Example factors include age, affluence and health status.

Funnel Plot: Scatter-plot of treatment effect vs study size. An inverted symmetrical funnel suggests precise studies and a low publication bias, whereas asymmetrical funnels suggest the opposite. Funnel-plots are one of several methods that can be used to assess publication bias however the Funnel can be significantly affected by sample size, clinical and methodological heterogeneity.

The Statistics glossary was provided by Dr. Davinder Theti BSc PhD, St George's Hospital, London UK

Geometric Mean: Average of the logarithms of a data set, converted to a base 10 number. The geometric mean minimises the impact of large variations in data. For this reason, the geometric mean is useful in studies that wish to define safety standards, such as the amount of bacteria acceptable in drinking water

Intention to Treat (ITT): An analytical approach used in meta-analysis, based on the principle that all participants should be analysed in the groups they were randomised to regardless if they completed the trial, or if they were lost to follow up. This approach ensures the final outcome is not skewed by selection bias, the probability of which is increased if analysis excludes participants unable to complete the trial, for example due to intolerable side effects or resistance.

I^2 Statistic: A model used to calculate the statistical heterogeneity between studies comprising a meta-analysis. On a scale of 0–100%, the higher the number, the greater the heterogeneity. I^2 is often used in conjunction with the Chi^2 statistic, but only the I^2 statistic is quoted in this handbook as it is widely quoted in reviews.

Log transformation: Alters the spread of data by 'squeezing' together larger numbers and spreading out smaller numbers. This reduces skew and data variance.

Meta-Analysis: An important component of the systematic review process in which the common outcome (effect) of many studies are analysed and weighted to give a final average outcome. Consequently, the estimation of the effect size is more powerful compared to the effect derived from a single study. The limitation of meta-analysis is that it is only a statistical analysis of scientific studies and not a scientific study in its own rite.

Meta-Regression: A statistical approach used to analyse the constituent meta-analysis studies, study arms or study arms crossed with an outcome. Meta-regression allows estimation of treatment effect whilst controlling for differences between each study and identification of co-variants that account for statistical heterogeneity. The four regression models used are:

1. Fixed effects model,
2. Random effects model,
3. Control rate model and
4. Bayesian Hierarchical model.

Models 1 and 2 are described separately under their own headings. The reader is referred to the published literature for further information on models 3 and 4.

Nominal Group Techniques (NGT): A decision-making model in which opinions on a given topic are obtained from the entire group. The solutions are ranked and the highest-ranking solution selected as the final decision. This technique ensures each member of the group contributes to the final decision and prevents a single or small group of individuals from dominating and skewing the decision-making process.

Odds Ratio: Defines the odds of a certain outcome in the presence of a certain factor. The odds ratio measures relative risk and therefore determines how much more likely an outcome is in an exposed population compared a control unexposed population. The odds ratio is therefore a mainstay in the interpretation of case-control studies and adjusting for confounding co-variants.

p-Value: The p-value is a measure of significance between two sets of data. It gives the probability of the observed difference between the data sets being due to chance. On a scale of 0–1, a small p-value denotes that the difference between the data is unlikely due to chance. The threshold p-value is commonly set at 5%. Therefore $p < 0.05$ = significant and $p > 0.05$ = non-significant.

Quasi-Randomised Clinical Trial: Uses the Quasi-randomised method of allocating patients to different treatment arms of a trial. The method is not truly random e.g. date of birth, medical record number or the order in which they entered the trial. There is therefore greater chance of selection bias as the allocation is not concealed as well as in a randomised-controlled trial.

Relative Risk (RR): The probability that a member of a group exposed to a certain factor will develop an outcome (e.g. disease) compared to the probability that a member of an unexposed group will develop the same outcome. The odds ratio is a more robust predictor of outcome than relative risk. However, relative risk is closer to how individuals think about risk and therefore of greater value in conveying information to the lay public.

Sample Distribution of the Mean: The sample means will follow a normal distribution only if the sample number is large (even if the underlying data is not normally distributed). The practical importance of this distribution is that the bigger the sample size, the more the centre of the distribution will be equal to the population mean, thus permitting use of a higher confidence interval.

Sensitivity Analysis: A statistical approach that predicts outcome by changing one or more input variables. Sensitivity analysis is widely quoted within this text because if the sensitivity analysis does not alter the results, there is likely to be less uncertainty in the outcome.

Standard Deviation (SD): A measure of data scatter around the mean. The smaller the standard deviation, the closer the data values are to the mean. Increasing sample size does not predictably change SD.

Standard Error of the Mean (SEM): Denotes how close the observed mean is to the true population mean i.e. the precision of the mean. As sample size increases, so does precision and therefore, the SEM approaches the true population mean. The downfall of SEM is that it is based on all the data collected, which inherently decreases precision. This can be corrected for by using a 95% confidence interval.

Weighted Mean Difference (WMD): In meta-analysis, WMD is used to assign weight to a study. For example, with blood pressure monitoring, the weighted mean could be calculated before and after intervention to give the WMD, which is the difference between the pre- and post-intervention values. The greater the WMD, the greater the weight of the study.

References

Campbell MJ, Machin D and Walters SJ. Medical Statistics: A textbook for the health sciences, 4th edition, published by Wiley-Blackwell, 2007.

Peacock J and Peacock P. Oxford Handbook of Medical Statistics, 1st edition, published by OUP Oxford, 2010.

Part II

How to use this handbook xxi

How to use this handbook

It has been estimated that a healthcare professional would need to read 17–20 original articles every day in order to keep up-to-date with their speciality (Davidoff 1995).

The role of systematic reviews in gathering the evidence, informing guidelines and helping professionals keep abreast of their field has been increasingly recognised. A systematic review uses all available empirical evidence to address a specific research question. It employs explicit and systematic methods to minimise bias and select studies that fit pre-defined inclusion criteria. The available evidence is then amalgamated to formulate clinically relevant conclusions (adapted from the Cochrane Collaboration definition). A meta-analysis uses statistical methods to synthesize available data in order to estimate the effect size more accurately. Systematic reviews and meta-analyses should be performed prior to designing any clinical research to ensure that there is justification for further trials.

This handbook is intended as a quick reference guide to facilitate access to some of the most recent systematic reviews and meta-analyses pertaining to critical care. Only reviews published in the last two years and those of high methodological quality were considered. The few exceptions to this represent particularly important topics.

The summaries

The summary format was designed such that at a glance the clinician can assimilate some useful information about the review characteristics and outcomes, bringing the evidence to the bedside. There is no substitute to reading the full review, therefore we would like to encourage the reader to refer to the original article if they find an area of particular interest.

The summaries serve as an abridged version of the reviews which ranged from 6 to over 100 pages long. There is no interpretation, critical appraisal and no further information was requested from the authors. For some reviews we have also included forest plots of primary outcomes or other important results. The only appraisal of the reviews may be found within the expert opinion and the AMSTAR table.

The authors

We were able to contact all the corresponding authors, most of whom kindly reviewed the summaries to ensure their accuracy.

Expert opinions

Sometimes the validity of the data and conclusions represented by the review are unclear particularly to those unfamiliar with statistics. We therefore attempted to ameliorate any confusion by asking the experts how they would use the data. We invited these experts to comment on the reviews with short answers to the following three questions:

1. How valid and robust are the data?
2. Should clinical practice be influenced by this?
3. What's the next step?

Additional information

Interpretation of some reviews was left to the reader. Where appropriate some useful information regarding recently completed trials or other relevant information is provided.

References

References that are not detailed within each section can be found in appendix E.

All the summaries follow this basic format

Condition:
Intervention:
Clinical question:

Review characteristics

- Eligibility criteria:
- Population:
- Number of studies:
- Number of patients:
- Study dates:

Definitions

Results

Primary outcomes +/– Forest plot

Secondary outcomes

Subgroup or sensitivity analysis

Author's conclusion

Problems & limitations

Advantages

The methodological quality is a large determinant of the strength of a systematic review. This is analysed in the AMSTAR section therefore the 'Advantages' component is necessarily short to avoid repetition.

Expert opinion

How valid and robust are the data?

Should clinical practice be influenced by this?

What is the next step?

Citation

+/– Additional information

AMSTAR table: methodological quality of the review

The Methodological Quality of Systematic Reviews

Both the methodological quality of a systematic review and the included studies will determine the validity of the conclusions. It is therefore essential that reviews are appraised on quality. Several tools have been developed to assess the quality of systematic reviews. We chose to use the recently developed AMSTAR (assessment of multiple systematic reviews) tool because it was developed by experts in the field of research methodology, it is comprehensive and user friendly.

It was developed by combining 2 existing assessment tools: the enhanced Overview Quality of Assessment Questionnaire (OQAQ) and the 24-item checklist developed by Sacks; and a further three items were included to address recent methodological developments with regards to language restrictions, publication bias and publication status to give a 37-item questionnaire. This new 37-item questionnaire was used to assess the quality of 151 systematic reviews and meta-analyses then factor analysis was applied to remove items with 'low factor loadings' (or poorly performing items). A panel of 11 experts was used in a nominal group technique to select and label the final 11 items to be included in the checklist.

In addition to this table we added a final table to summarise the quality of included studies as determined by the authors of the review and the overall quality of the review.

- **AMSTAR table** from the paper BMC Medical Research Methodology (2007, 7:10)

1. Was an 'a priori' design provided? The research question and inclusion criteria should be established before the conduct of the review.	☐ Yes ☐ No ☐ Can't answer ☐ Not applicable
2. Was there duplicate study selection and data extraction? There should be at least two independent data extractors and a consensus procedure for disagreements should be in place.	☐ Yes ☐ No ☐ Can't answer ☐ Not applicable
3. Was a comprehensive literature search performed? At least two electronic sources should be searched. The report must include years and databases used (e.g. Central, EMBASE, and MEDLINE). Key words and/or MESH terms must be stated and where feasible the search strategy should be provided. All searches should be supplemented by consulting current contents, reviews, textbooks, specialized registers, or experts in the particular field of study, and by reviewing the references in the studies found.	☐ Yes ☐ No ☐ Can't answer ☐ Not applicable
4. Was the status of publication (i.e. grey literature) used as an inclusion criterion? The authors should state that they searched for reports regardless of their publication type. The authors should state whether or not they excluded any reports (from the systematic review), based on their publication status, language etc.	☐ Yes ☐ No ☐ Can't answer ☐ Not applicable

5. Was a list of studies (included and excluded) provided? A list of included and excluded studies should be provided.	☐ Yes ☐ No ☐ Can't answer ☐ Not applicable
6. Were the characteristics of the included studies provided? In an aggregated form such as a table, data from the original studies should be provided on the participants, interventions and outcomes. The ranges of characteristics in all the studies analyzed e.g. age, race, sex, relevant socioeconomic data, disease status, duration, severity, or other diseases should be reported.	☐ Yes ☐ No ☐ Can't answer ☐ Not applicable
7. Was the scientific quality of the included studies assessed and documented? 'A priori' methods of assessment should be provided (e.g., for effectiveness studies if the author(s) chose to include only randomized, double-blind, placebo controlled studies, or allocation concealment as inclusion criteria); for other types of studies alternative items will be relevant.	☐ Yes ☐ No ☐ Can't answer ☐ Not applicable
8. Was the scientific quality of the included studies used appropriately in formulating conclusions? The results of the methodological rigor and scientific quality should be considered in the analysis and the conclusions of the review, and explicitly stated in formulating recommendations.	☐ Yes ☐ No ☐ Can't answer ☐ Not applicable
9. Were the methods used to combine the findings of studies appropriate? For the pooled results, a test should be done to ensure the studies were combinable, to assess their homogeneity (i.e. Chi-squared test for homogeneity. I^2). If heterogeneity exists a random effects model should be used and/or the clinical appropriateness of combining should be taken into consideration (i.e. is it sensible to combine?).	☐ Yes ☐ No ☐ Can't answer ☐ Not applicable
10. Was the likelihood of publication bias assessed? An assessment of publication bias should include a combination of graphical aids (e.g., funnel plot, other available tests) and/or statistical tests (e.g., Egger regression test).	☐ Yes ☐ No ☐ Can't answer ☐ Not applicable
11. Was the conflict of interest stated? Potential sources of support should be clearly acknowledged in both the systematic review and the included studies.	☐ Yes ☐ No ☐ Can't answer ☐ Not applicable

Shea BJ, Grimshaw JM, Wells A, Boers M, Andersson N, Hamel C, et al. Development of AMSTAR: a measurement tool to assess the methodological quality of systematic reviews. BMC Medical Research Methodology 2007, 7:10 doi:10.1186/1471-2288-7-10

Also accessed online: http://www.biomedcentral.com/1471-2288/7/10

Our own AMSTAR table has been modified slightly

Y = Yes. Methods are fully described

N = No. Not done or not described in the article

U = Unclear

P = Partially performed

NA = Not applicable/not relevant to this review

Review methodology score for the AMSTAR tool

The system that was used to rate the methodological quality of the reviews has not been validated furthermore the reader should be aware that certain components of the AMSTAR tool may have greater impact on the methodology of a review. As an example: assessment of publication bias might affect the outcome of a review more than restricting the search to the English language.

We have used the following simplified system to rate the methodological quality of the reviews:

- **High**: if no more than two "No's" for the AMSTAR tool
- **Moderate**: if 3-4 "No's"
- **Low**: if more than 4 "No's"

Please note that in question 11. "Yes:" means that the authors addressed this component, it does not necessarily mean that there were conflicts of interest.

Useful References

Guidelines for writing Systematic Reviews

- Cochrane Handbook of Systematic Reviews of Interventions

  This is a comprehensive text on all aspects of literature researching, assessing bias, analysing statistics for writing Cochrane intervention systematic reviews.

  Higgins J, Green S. Cochrane Handbook for Systematic Reviews of Interventions. The Cochrane Collaboration and John Wiley & Sons Ltd; 2008

  Also available online: www.cochrane.org/training/cochrane-handbook

- PRISMA (Preferred Reporting Items for Systematic reviews and Meta-Analyses) Guidelines

  This is a revision of the QUOROM (QUality Of Reporting Of Meta-analyses). It provides an evidence-based minimum set of items required for reporting systematic reviews and meta-analyses with a focus on randomized trials but may be used for other types of research particularly evaluations of interventions.

  Moher D, Liberati A, Tetzlaff J, Altman DG, The PRISMA Group (2009). Preferred Reporting Items for Systematic Reviews and Meta-Analyses: The PRISMA Statement. Open Med 2009; 3(3); 123–130

  Also available online: www.prisma-statement.org

- MOOSE Guidelines for Meta-Analyses and Systematic Reviews Of Observational Studies

  Modified from Stroup DF, Berlin JA, Morton SC, Olkin I, Williamson GD, Rennie D, et al. Meta-analyses of observational studies in epidemiology: a proposal for

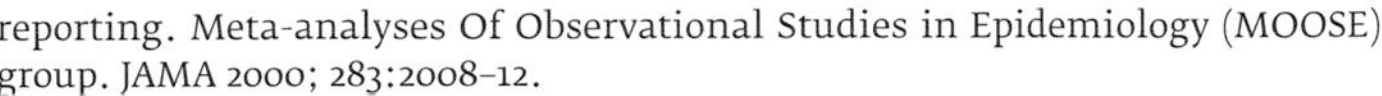

reporting. Meta-analyses Of Observational Studies in Epidemiology (MOOSE) group. JAMA 2000; 283:2008–12.

Assessing the Methodological Quality of Included Studies

Controlled trials

- Cochrane Collabortaion

  Higgins J, Altman DG. Assessing the risk of bias in included studies. Part 1; Chapter 8:188–235. In: Higgins J, Green S. Cochrane Handbook for Systematic Reviews of Interventions. The Cochrane Collaboration and John Wiley & Sons Ltd; 2008

- CONSORT (CONsolidated Standards of Reporting Trials)

  This is a 25-item checklist that focuses on how the trial was designed, analysed and interpreted. An accompanying flow diagram displays the progress of all participants though the trial.

  Schulz KF, Altman DG, Moher D; CONSORT Group. CONSORT 2010 statement: updated guidelines for reporting parallel group randomised trials. BMJ. 2010 Mar 23;340:c332

- Jadad scale

  This is a 3 item questionnaire focused on descriptions randomization, blinding, and withdrawals or dropouts giving a maximum total of 5 points.

  Jadad, AR, Moore RA, Carroll D, Jenkinson C, Reynolds DJM, Gavaghan DJ, McQuay HJ (1996). "Assessing the quality of reports of randomized clinical trials: Is blinding necessary?". Controlled Clinical Trials 17(1): 1–12. doi:10.1016/0197-2456(95)00134-4.

Observational studies

- Newcastle-Ottowa Scale (NOS)

  There is no standardized quality scoring system for observation studies however the NOS is being developed. This was designed for assessment of case-control and cohort studies on three domains: selection of study groups, comparability of groups and ascertainment of outcome.

  Wells GA, Shea B, O'Connell D, Peterson J, Welch V, Losos M, Tugwell P. The Newcastle-Ottawa Scale (NOS) for assessing the quality of nonrandomised studies in meta-analyses.

Part III

1 Acute kidney injury (AKI) 3

2 Acute respiratory failure (ARF) – Acute respiratory distress syndrome (ARDS) 29

3 Acute respiratory failure – Non-ARDS 57

4 Cardiovascular dynamics 99

5 Ethics 121

6 General 127

7 Health technology 151

8 Infection 169

9 Neuro-intensive care 195

10 Nutrition and metabolism 207

11 Outcomes 227

12 Paediatric intensive care 251

13 Sepsis 267

14 Trauma and emergency medicine 297

1

Acute kidney injury (AKI)

Atrial natriuretic peptide 4
Hydroxyethyl starch (1) 8
Hydroxyethyl starch (2) 14
Sodium bicarbonate 19
AKI in cardiac surgery 25

Atrial natriuretic peptide

Condition: acute kidney injury (AKI)
Intervention: atrial natriuretic peptide (ANP)
Clinical question: Does ANP reduce AKI, the need for dialysis or mortality with AKI? Is it safe?

AKI is common, occurring in 30/1000 hospital discharges and 6% of ICU patients and is still associated with high mortality despite advances in treatment. AKI can be defined using the RIFLE criteria which uses absolute or percentage increase in serum creatinine or reduction in urine output. The aetiology of AKI can be pre-renal, intrinsic-renal or post-renal. In the community, pre-renal failure accounts for 70% of AKI whereas in hospital the predominant cause is intrinsic damage such as obstruction to renal tubules, or ischaemia-reperfusion injury. ANP is produced in atrial myocytes. In the early phase of AKI, ANP causes vasodilatation on the pre-glomerular artery, inhibits prostaglandin release and the renin-angiotensin axis, and later it demonstrates a natriuretic effect which may minimise tubular obstruction. ANP is known to improve GFR from animal studies; however human studies have shown conflicting results.

Review characteristics

- **Eligibility criteria:** RCTs or quasi-randomised RCTs comparing any form or dose of ANP with placebo or active treatment
- **Exclusions:** patients on RRT, those with renal transplants, post renal causes of AKI and those on ANP for other reasons
- **Number of studies:** 19 studies – 11 studies of prevention of AKI and 8 studies of treatment of AKI. 14 of these evaluated patients post major surgery (cardiac, aortic, abdominal)
- **Number of patients:** a total of 1861–1818 in prevention studies and 1,043 in treatment studies
- **Population:** patients at risk of or with AKI
- **Study dates:** 1994–2007

Definitions

- **AKI** = Modified Acute Kidney Injury Network criteria. An abrupt (within 48 hours) reduction of kidney function- increase serum creatinine 0.3 mg/dl or more; 50% or more increase from baseline or 50% or more decrease in creatinine clearance that results in RRT
- **At Risk patients:** those undergoing procedures e.g. with radiocontrast or major surgery associated with AKI
- **Intervention:** any dose of ANP given by any route before or immediately after development of AKI
- **High dose ANP:** studies using > 100 ng/kg/min as this is associated with reduction in MAP, RBF and GFR
- **Active control:** use of other intervention such as furosemide or mannitol

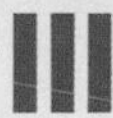

Results

Primary outcomes in studies assessing prevention of AKI

Mortality during hospitalisation or at 30 days: no difference in low-dose ANP group; no mortality events in high-dose ANP study in either intervention group or control.

Need for RRT: lower in low dose but not high-dose ANP group. This effect was not seen when active and placebo controlled groups were analysed separately.

Outcomes	Trials	N	RR	95% CI	I^2
Mortality in low dose ANP group	10	794	0.69	0.21–2.23	0%
RRT in low ANP Group	10	794	0.32	0.14–0.71	0%

Primary outcomes in studies assessing treatment of AKI

Mortality was 35% with no significant difference between ANP and control in low or high dose studies.

Need for RRT: Overall need for RRT was 48% which was lower in the low dose but not high dose ANP group. This effect is also seen with ANP compared to active control but not placebo control.

Outcome	Trials	N	RR	95% CI	I^2
Mortality in low dose ANP group	6	290	0.78	0.41–1.49	36%
RRT in low dose ANP group	6	290	0.54	0.30–0.98	50%

Secondary outcomes in studies

	Studies of prevention of AKI		Studies of treatment of AKI	
Outcome	Trials/N	Results	Trials/N	Results
Hospital LOS	3/201	lower in low dose ANP	NA	NA
ICU LOS	4/219	lower in low dose ANP	1/59	SS in low dose ANP gp
Change in SCr	2/57	No difference	NA	NA
Hypotension	-	No difference	3/813	Higher in high dose ANP gp (I^2 = 72%)
Arrhythmia	1/124	less AF, VE & VT in low dose ANP	2/726	Higher in high dose gp

Subgroup analysis

- **Major surgery**: no difference in mortality; reduction in RRT in prevention but not in treatment studies
- **Radiocontrast nephropathy**: no difference
- **Sensitivity Analysis**: confirmed findings but the reduction in RRT with low-dose ANP was NSS here

Author's conclusion

There aren't enough large, high quality studies to make conclusions regarding the efficacy of ANP however, when used for prevention of AKI in low dose (50–100 ng/kg/min), ANP is well tolerated and may improve some clinical outcomes such as RRT, hospital and ICU LOS. This effect may be most beneficial in patients undergoing major surgery as the time of kidney injury is often known.

Problems & limitations

- The timing of initiation of ANP varied greatly between studies e.g. 2 hours to 7 days in treatment studies
- In most "prevention" studies, definitions of AKI were not given and only severe AKI requiring RRT was reported

Advantages

- Systematic search and methodology

Expert opinion

Eric Hoste

How valid and robust are the data?

This meta-analysis includes 19 studies and 1,861 participants, which would permit strong conclusions if the studies were homogeneous in design. However, there is variation between studies regarding indication for therapy (prevention of AKI and therapy of AKI), study cohorts (cardiac surgery, general ICU etc.), and dose of ANP. Consequently, the results are analysed in several subgroups, such as prevention and therapy of AKI, and high dose and low dose. In addition, there are too few large and high quality studies present.

The data have therefore limited robustness and validity.

Should clinical practice be influenced by this?

No, the data present so far do not permit a change in practice in favour of the use of ANP.

What is the next step?

In contrast to high-dose ANP treatment, low-dose ANP was well tolerated. The data also suggested a beneficial effect of ANP for prevention of development of severe AKI, defined by need for renal replacement therapy (RRT), after cardiac surgery.

Therefore, the potential beneficial effects of ANP should best be further explored in a study aimed at prevention of AKI. This study should be adequately powered and in cardiac surgery patients, comparing a low dose ANP versus placebo. This study should evaluate occurrence of AKI defined by the current sensitive AKI/RIFLE classification, as this is a more sensitive and objective endpoint than initiation of RRT.

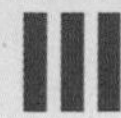

Citation

Nigwekar SU, Navaneethan SD, Parikh CR, Hix JK. Atrial natriuretic peptide for preventing and treating acute kidney injury. Cochrane Database of Systematic Reviews 2009, Issue 4. Art. No.: CD006028. DOI: 10.1002/14651858.CD006028.pub2.

AMSTAR: methodological quality of the review

1.	Was "a priori" design provided?	Y
2.	Was study selection and data extraction adequate?	Y
3.	Was the literature search comprehensive?	Y
4.	Was 'Grey Literature' used?	Y
5.	Was a list of excluded studies provided?	Y
6.	Where the characteristics of included studies provided?	Y
7.	Was the scientific quality of studies assessed & documented?	Y
8.	Was the scientific quality of studies weighted appropriately in forming conclusions?	Y
9.	Were the methods used for data synthesis appropriate?	Y
10.	Was the potential for publication bias assessed?	Y
11.	Were any conflicts of interest stated?	Y

Overall quality of trials included	Mostly low
Overall quality of the review	High

1

Hydroxyethyl starch (1)

Condition: acute kidney injury (AKI)

Intervention: hydroxyethyl starch (HES) solutions

Clinical questions: Does HES have a detrimental effect on renal function compared with other fluid therapies when used in the prevention and treatment of relative intravascular depletion?

Does HES have different renal effects in different ICU populations?

Do the molecular characteristics or amount of HES make any difference?

AKI occurs in up to 30% of critically ill patients and is associated with increases in mortality proportional to the degree of kidney injury. The aetiology of renal damage is often multifactorial although volume depletion leading to hypo-perfusion is a common cause. Intravenous volume replacement remains the main therapy to restore renal perfusion and prevent kidney injury. Starch solutions have duration of action and efficacy as volume expanders, that surpass that of other synthetic colloids except for some dextrans: however they have a tendency to accumulate in the tissues. Starch solutions have been associated with renal damage although the mechanism by which this occurs is poorly understood and a definite survival disadvantage has not been demonstrated.

Review characteristics

- **Eligibility:** RCTs and Quasi-randomised trials comparing HES to another intravenous (iv) fluid
- **Exclusions:** crossover studies & cluster RCTs. Healthy volunteers or euvolaemic patients
- **Number of studies:** 34
- **Number of patients:** 2,577 (median 56, only 1 study had more than 150)
- **Population:** all ages, in a variety of peri-operative and critical care settings, most without pre-existing kidney disease
- **Study dates:** 1982–2008

Definitions

- **HES:** all types; mostly 6% 130/0.4, 200/0.5 and 200/0.6
- **IV fluids:** all types including blood products (but not synthetic blood products)
- **Renal failure:** author defined
- **RIFLE:** Criteria were worked out from individual patient serum creatinine levels where provided by the study authors

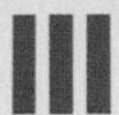

Results

Primary outcomes: effects according to various definitions of AKI and various populations

Outcome	Trials	N	RR	95% CI	GRADE
RRT – overall	12	1236	1.38	0.89–2.16	-
RRT in sepsis group	3	702	1.59	1.2–2.1	High
RRT in non-sepsis group	8	487	0.44	0.14–1.38	Moderate
Renal failure – overall	9	1199	1.5	1.2–1.87	
Renal failure in sepsis group	4	832	1.55	1.22–1.96	Moderate
Renal failure in non-sepsis gp	5	367	1.13	0.57–2.25	Low

Sepsis Group	Trials	N	RR	95% CI	GRADE
RIFLE: risk	2	140	1.28	0.81–2.02	High
RIFLE: injury	2	140	1.39	0.84–2.3	High
RIFLE: failure	2	140	1.45	0.8–2.64	High

Non-sepsis group	Trials	N	RR	95% CI	GRADE
RIFLE: risk	2	185	0.88	0.27–2.85	Moderate
RIFLE: injury	2	185	0.81	0.12–5.4	Moderate
RIFLE: failure	2	185	0.49	0.07–3.73	Moderate

Secondary outcomes

Mean serum creatinine and creatinine clearance showed no significant difference.

No difference was found between different MW HES solutions however these studies were underpowered and generally lacked outcome data.

Author's conclusion

This review shows an overall increased risk of renal failure (as defined by original study authors) in the HES group, as well as a non-significant risk of requiring RRT. Subgroup analysis showed that septic patients treated with HES had a 55% increased risk of developing renal failure and 59% increased risk of requiring dialysis. In non-septic (trauma/surgery) patients there were no significant differences however these studies lacked statistical power due to small participant numbers and low event rates.

There were insufficient data to fully evaluate different HES products.

Fig. 1 Comparison 1 HES versus other fluid, Outcome 1 Renal replacement therapy [from Dart AB, Mutter TC, Ruth CA, Taback SP. Hydroxyethyl starch (HES) versus other fluid therapies: effects on kidney function. Cochrane Database of Systematic Reviews 2010, Issue 1. Art. No.: CD007594, © Cochrane Collaboration, reproduced with permission]

Review: Hydroxyethyl starch (HES) versus other fluid therapies: effects on kidney function
Comparison: 1 HES versus other fluid
Outcome: 1 Renal replacement therapy

Study or subgroup		HES n/N	Other fluid n/N	Risk Ratio M-H, Random, 95% CI
1 Non-sepsis	Kumle 1999	0/40	0/20	0.0 [0.0, 0.0]
	Boldt 2007a	0/25	0/25	0.0 [0.0, 0.0]
	Boldt 2003	0/20	0/20	0.0 [0.0, 0.0]
	Boldt 2006	0/25	0/25	0.0 [0.0, 0.0]
	Mahmood 2007	2/42	3/20	0.32 [0.06, 1.75]
	Godet 2008	0/32	1/33	0.34 [0.01, 8.13]
	Boldt 2008	1/30	2/30	0.50 [0.05, 5.22]
	London 1989	1/50	1/50	1.00 [0.06, 15.55]
	Subtotal (95% CI)	**264**	**223**	**0.44 [0.14, 1.38]**
	Total events: 4 (HES), 7 (Other fluid)			
	Heterogeneity: $Tau^2 = 0.0$; $Chi^2 = 0.52$, df = 3 (P = 0.91); $I^2 = 0.0\%$			
	Test for overall effect: Z = 1.41 (P = 0.16)			
2 Sepsis	Schortgen 2001	13/65	11/64	1.16 [0.56, 2.40]
	Brunkhorst 2008	81/261	51/272	1.66 [1.22, 2.25]
	McIntyre 2008	3/19	1/21	3.32 [0.38, 29.23]
	Subtotal (95% CI)	**345**	**357**	**1.59 [1.20, 2.10]**

Risk Ratio M-H, Random, 95% CI: 0.01 0.1 1 10 100
Favours HES Favours other fluid

(Continued ...)

(... *Continued*)

Study or subgroup	HES n/N	Other fluid n/N	Risk Ratio M-H, Random, 95% CI	Risk Ratio M-H, Random, 95% CI
Total events: 97 (HES), 63 (Other fluid)				
Heterogeneity: $Tau^2 = 0.0$[illegible]; $Chi^2 = 1.22$, df = 2 (P = 0.54); I^2 = [illegible]0%				
Test for overall effect: Z = 3.24 (P = 0.00[illegible]2)				
3 Deceased organ donor				
Cittanova 1996	9/27	1/20		6.67 [0.92, 48.45]
Subtotal (95% CI)	**27**	**20**		**6.67 [0.92, 48.45]**
Total events: 9 (HES), 1 (Other fluid)				
Heterogeneity: not applicable				
Test for overall effect: Z = 1.87 (P = 0.0[illegible]1)				
Total (95% CI)	**636**	**600**		**1.38 [0.89, 2.16]**
Total events: 110 (HES), 71 (Other fluid)				
Heterogeneity: $Tau^2 = 0.0$[illegible]; $Chi^2 = 8.4$[illegible], df = [illegible] (P = 0.29); I^2 = 17%				
Test for overall effect: Z = 1.43 (P = 0.[illegible]5)				

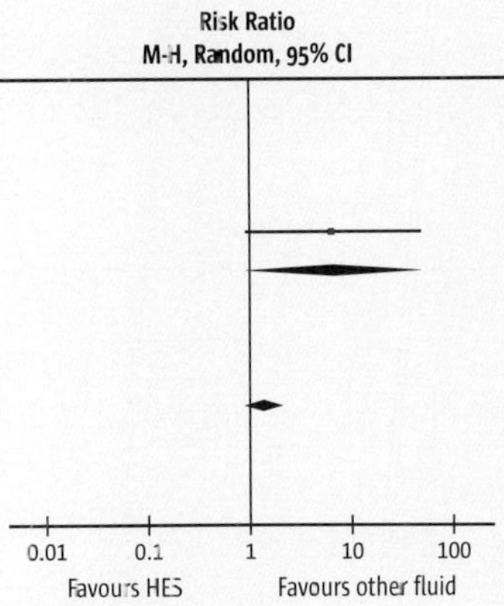

Problems & limitations

- There was significant clinical heterogeneity due to different populations, fluid regimes and duration
- Mortality data was not consistently available. Renal problems may develop later than the follow-up period in the studies (1 day for many)
- No published studies used the RIFLE format instead used various definitions of acute kidney injury/failure. Use of RIFLE format would have ensured consistency and is validated at predicting outcomes. Varying definitions of kidney failure
- Some studies included peri-operative patients that weren't critically ill. Many of these studies are old and almost none used the more recent starch solutions
- There were problems with reliability of some trials (Boldt)
- One large study of septic patients was responsible for the majority of outcomes (Brunkhorst 2008)

Advantages

- A comprehensive review that even identified studies that had renal complications as secondary outcomes
- Conclusion of this review agrees with previous analyses in that HES may adversely affect renal function particularly in septic patients

Expert opinion

Michael Joannidis

How valid and robust are the data?

The review detected 34 randomized and quasi randomized controlled trials published since 1982. The analysis indicates an increased risk of author defined acute kidney injury and a trend toward increased requirement of RRT by HES, which turned out significant in the predefined subgroup of septic patients. However, findings are compromised by heterogeneity in trial design as well in the HES products investigated. Consequently no statement can be made about differences in effects by different HES products showing various molecular weights.

Should clinical practice be influenced by this?

HES products may have the potential of kidney damage especially in patients with sepsis. Consequently the use of HES cannot be recommended for this patient group. The studies showing the most pronounced detrimental effects for the kidneys, however, used older generation large molecular weight HES.

What's the next step?

Colloids are often necessary in cases of true hypovolaemia. Since newer HES products with lower molecular weight and degree of substitution are claimed to have a better safety profile further randomized controlled trials are urgently warranted to clarify whether this class of HES can be used safely.

Citation

Dart AB, Mutter TC, Ruth CA, Taback SP. Hydroxyethyl starch (HES) versus other fluid therapies: effects on kidney function. Cochrane Database of Systematic Reviews 2010, Issue 1. Art. No.: CD007594. DOI: 10.1002/14651858.CD007594.pub2.

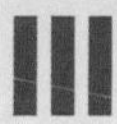

AMSTAR: methodological quality of the review

1.	Was "a priori" design provided?	Y
2.	Was study selection and data extraction adequate?	Y
3.	Was the literature search comprehensive?	Y
4.	Was 'Grey Literature' used?	Y
5.	Was a list of excluded studies provided?	Y
6.	Where the characteristics of included studies provided?	Y
7.	Was the scientific quality of studies assessed & documented?	Y
8.	Was the scientific quality of studies weighted appropriately in forming conclusions?	Y
9.	Were the methods used for data synthesis appropriate?	Y
10.	Was the potential for publication bias assessed?	Y
11.	Were any conflicts of interest stated?	Y

Overall quality of trials included	Moderate
Overall quality of the review	High

Hydroxyethyl starch (2)

Condition: acute kidney injury (AKI)
Intervention: hydroxyethyl starch (HES) solutions
Clinical question: Does the use of HES for volume resuscitation in critically ill patients adversely affect renal outcomes or mortality?

1

The pathophysiology of kidney damage associated with the use of HES is poorly understood but may be related to histological changes related to variation in osmotic pressure, "osmotic nephrosis-like lesions". Critically ill patients with sepsis, appear to be particularly vulnerable to the adverse effects of HES on renal function. AKI has been validated as an independent risk factor for long-term morbidity, impaired QOL and mortality.

Review characteristics

- **Eligibility criteria:** RCTs of acute volume resuscitation in critically ill patients comparing HES to other fluids
- **Exclusions:** crossover trials, trials using blood, HES for elective surgery or normovolaemic haemodilation
- **Number of studies:** 22 trials (only 6 are the same as in review by Dart et al.)
- **Number of patients:** 1,865 (range 12–537, median 48)
- **Population:** adult patients admitted to ICU or ED who had an indication for acute fluid resuscitation e.g. hypotension, hypovolaemia (8 trials: severe sepsis or septic shock only, 5 others include septic + trauma patients)
- **Study dates:** 1982–2008

Definitions

- **HES:** all types (6 different molecular weights [MW])
- **Control Fluids:** crystalloids, albumin, gelatines, dextrans
- **AKI:** here is defined by the use of RRT
- **Need for urgent fluid resuscitation varied between trials:** low SBP/MAP, lactate, CVP, PCWP or CI
- **Severe sepsis and septic shock:** not specified

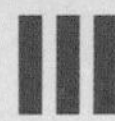

Results

Primary outcome: AKI – RRT or the doubling of serum creatinine

Population	Trials	N	OR	95% CI	I^2
Trials reporting RRT	4	749	1.90	1.22–2.96	9.5
Severe sepsis & Septic shock (SS & SS)	3	702	1.82	1.27–2.61	0
Severe sepsis **OR** Septic shock (SS or SS)	2	662	1.91	1.36–2.68	0
Kidney transplant (from BSD patients)	1	47	9.5	1.09–82.72	-

Secondary outcomes

Outcome	Trials	N	Result
Mortality	17	1657	No difference even in different populations, types of HES, or comparator fluid
Mechanical ventilation	3	876	No difference
ICU LOS in (SS or SS)	4	749	No difference
ICU LOS in trauma patients	1	59	Significantly shorter in HES group
Complications/allergy	4	234	No reactions/anaphylaxis/complications reported
Allergy & bleeding	1	535	No difference

Author's conclusion

The use of HES is associated with a significant risk of requiring RRT in patients with severe sepsis or septic shock and in recipients of renal transplants from BSD donors resuscitated with HES. Overall there was no difference in mortality however, in trials enrolling patient with severe sepsis and septic shock and high quality or multicentre trials there was a trend towards higher mortality in the HES group.

Problems & limitations

- 4 of the included trials received funding from the manufacturers of HES
- Huge variation in the duration of study protocol (2 hours to 21 days), variation in total volume of HES given (364 ml – 5,350 mls)
- Only 4 trials reported RRT, 5 trials reported creatinine but these results weren't pooled because timing of measurements varied. Some studies didn't report baseline creatinine and in others the HES group had higher creatinines (9 studies excluded those with abnormal renal function). None of the trials used RIFLE criteria

Fig. 2 Renal replacement therapy associated with hydroxyethyl starch (HES) [from Renal outcomes and mortality following hydroxyethyl starch resuscitation of critically ill patients: systematic review and meta-analysis of randomized trials. Ryan Zarychanski, Alexis F Turgeon, Dean A Fergusson, Deborah J Cook, Paul Hébert, Sean M Bagshaw, Danny Monsour, Lauralyn McIntyre. Open Medicine 2009;3(4):e196–209]

Study	Studies n	No. of events HES	No. of participants Control	Odds Ratio (95% CI)
All studies				
Brunkhorst		81/261	51/272	1.95 (1.30–2.91)
McIntyre		3/21	1/19	3.00 (0.28–31.63)
Schortgen		13/65	11/64	1.20 (0.49–2.93)
Cittanova		9/27	1/20	9.50 (1.09–82.72)
Overall	**4**	**106/374**	**64/375**	**1.90 (1.22–2.96)**
Subgroup analyses				
Patient population				
Severe sepsis/septic shock	3	97/347	53/355	1.82 (1.27–2.61)
Organ	1	9/27	1/20	9.50 (1.09–82.72)
Type of comparator				
Gelatin	2	22/92	12/84	2.64 (0.37–18.96)
Crystalloid	2	84/282	52/291	1.98 (1.33–2.94)

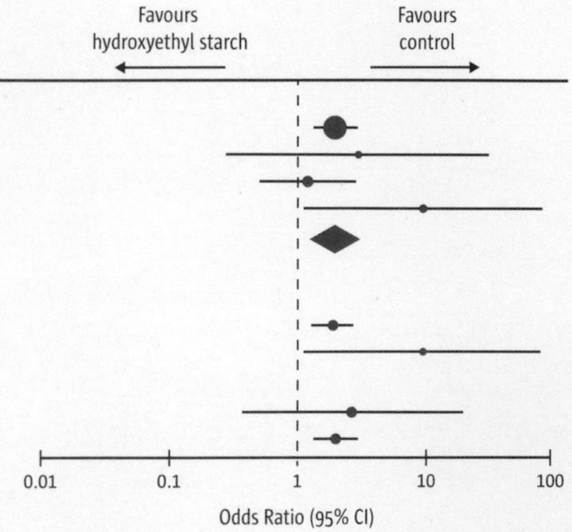

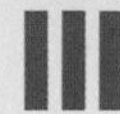

Advantages

- Adequate literature search
- Trials reporting RRT as outcome were more recent (1996–2008)

Expert opinion

Michael Joannidis

How valid and robust are the data?
The review detected 22 randomized controlled trials, over the last 29 years. There was significant heterogeneity in trial design as well in the HES products investigated. Control consisted of both crystalloids and various colloids i.e. gelatine, dextrans and human serum albumin. Several trials showing no detrimental effect of HES are currently under investigation with respect to scientific validity. Exclusion of these trials would likely result in a even more pronounced trend towards a higher mortality associated with HES. The major finding of an increased rate of RRT was predominantly influenced by one large trial with several protocol violations as well as using higher dose of HES than recommended. Despite these limitations the data can be considered quite valid.

Should clinical practice be influenced by this?
HES products, especially those with higher molecular weight should be used with caution in critically ill patients. In sepsis HES should be avoided.

What's the next step?
I believe that unrestricted use of HES may be hazardous to our critically ill patients. Further randomized trials investigating the effects and safety profile of newer HES products with lower molecular weight and grade of substitution are highly warranted.

1

Citation

Zarychanski R, Turgeon AF, Fergusson DA, Cook DJ, Hébert P, Bagshaw SM, Monsour D, McIntyre L. Renal outcomes and mortality following hydroxyethyl starch resuscitation of critically ill patients: systematic review and meta-analysis of randomized trials. Open Medicine 2009;3(4):e196–209

AMSTAR: methodological quality of the review

1.	Was "a priori" design provided?	Y
2.	Was study selection and data extraction adequate?	Y
3.	Was the literature search comprehensive?	Y
4.	Was 'Grey Literature' used?	Y
5.	Was a list of excluded studies provided?	Y
6.	Where the characteristics of included studies provided?	Y
7.	Was the scientific quality of studies assessed & documented?	Y
8.	Was the scientific quality of studies weighted appropriately in forming conclusions?	Y
9.	Were the methods used for data synthesis appropriate?	Y
10.	Was the potential for publication bias assessed?	Y
11.	Were any conflicts of interest stated?	Y

Overall quality of trials included	Mostly low, 4 high quality
Overall quality of the review	High

Sodium bicarbonate

Condition: contrast-induced acute kidney injury (CI-AKI)

Intervention: sodium bicarbonate

Clinical question: Does the use of sodium bicarbonate before and after radiocontrast protect from AKI?

CI-AKI is third most common cause of hospital-acquired AKI accounting for 11% of all cases. Several studies have found an association between AKI and increased hospital length of stay and mortality. Numerous pharmacological interventions, volume therapy and choice of contrast media have been evaluated for the prevention of AKI. The role of sodium bicarbonate remains unclear particularly as the largest study to-date found an increased incidence of CI-AKI with its use.

Review characteristics

- **Eligibility criteria:** prospective randomised studies, published in a peer reviewed journal that used intravenous sodium bicarbonate for prevention of CI-AKI, that had data on AKI as defined below
- **Number of studies:** 18 studies (9 only in abstract form)
- **Number of patients:** 3,055 (range 27–502)
- **Population:** patients that received intravenous or intra arterial iodinated contrast (1 paediatric study)
- **Study dates:** 2004–2008

Definitions

- **AKI:** an increase of serum creatinine of 25% or more, OR 0.5 mg/dl or more within 48 or 7 hours after contrast administration
- **Sodium bicarbonate:** protocol as described by Merten et al. used in 11/18 studies
- **Merten protocol:** 3 ml/kg of $NaHCO_3$ in a glucose solution containing 154 mmol/l of $NaHCO_3$, during 1 hour preceding contrast; then 1 ml/kg of the same solution for 6 hours post contrast
- **Control:** isotonic saline in all but 2 studies

Results

Primary occurrence of AKI

Highest incidence = 34.5% in 1 study control arm of patients undergoing coronary procedures

Overall incidence was 11.6% (355/3055 patients)

Pooled data: showed a decrease in the risk of AKI in bicarbonate group (RR 0.66, 95% CI 0.45–0.95)

Fig. 3 Effect of sodium bicarbonate on the occurrence of contrast-induced acute kidney injury. Prospective studies on the use of sodium bicarbonate for prevention of CI-AKI [from Eric AJ Hoste, Jan J. De Waele, Sofie A. Gevaert, Shigehiko Uchino and John A Kellum. Sodium Bicarbonate for the prevention of contrast-induced acute kidney injury. Nephrol Dial Transplant (2010) 25: 747–758, by permission of Oxford University Press]

	Bicarbonate		Control			Risk Ratio	
Study or subgroup	**Events**	**Total**	**Events**	**Total**	**Weight**	**M-H, Random, 95% CI**	**Year**
1.1.1 coronary procedures only							
Saidin 2006	9	29	4	28	6.4%	2.17 [0.75, 6.25]	2006
Shaikh 2007	14	159	19	161	9.5%	0.75 [0.39, 1.44]	2007
Masuda 2007	2	30	10	29	4.5%	0.19 [0.05, 0.81]	2007
Recio-Mayoral 2007	1	56	12	55	2.7%	0.08 [0.01, 0.61]	2007
Ozcan 2007	4	88	23	176	6.6%	0.35 [0.12, 0.97]	2007
Kim 2007	10	56	8	44	8.0%	0.98 [0.42, 2.28]	2007
Tamura 2008	1	72	9	72	2.7%	0.11 [0.01, 0.85]	2008
Brar 2008	26	158	30	165	11.0%	0.91 [0.56, 1.46]	2008
Shavit 2008	5	51	3	36	4.8%	1.18 [0.30, 4.61]	2008
Maioli 2008	25	250	38	252	11.1%	0.66 [0.41, 1.06]	2008
Subtotal (95% CI)		**949**		**1018**	**67.2%**	**0.65 [0.42, 1.00]**	
Total events	97		156				

Heterogeneity: $Tau^2 = 0.22$; $Chi^2 = 19.86$, $df = 9$ ($P = 0.02$); $I^2 = 55\%$

Test for overall effect: $Z = 1.96$ ($P = 0.05$)

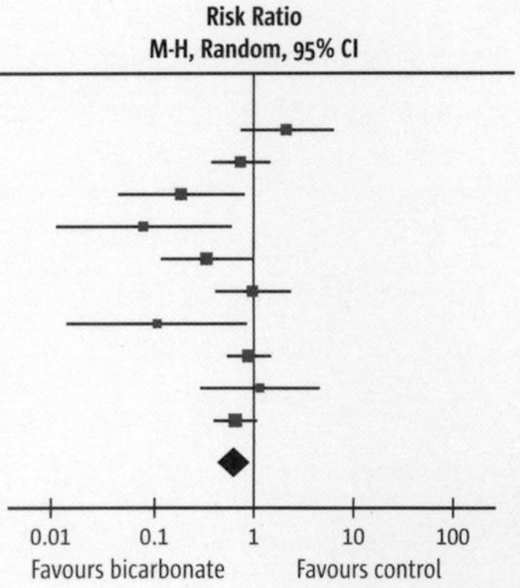

(*Continued* ...)

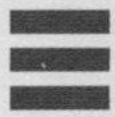

(... *Continued*)

Study or subgroup	Bicarbonate Events	Bicarbonate Total	Control Events	Control Total	Weight	Risk Ratio M-H, Random, 95% CI	Year
1.1.2 coronary and non-coronary procedures							
Merten 2004	1	60	8	59	2.6%	0.12 [0.02, 0.95]	2004
Assadi 2006	4	45	0	50	1.5%	9.77 [0.54, 175.56]	2006
Addad 2006	24	140	13	70	9.9%	0.92 [0.50, 1.70]	2006
Chen 2007	1	55	7	50	2.6%	0.13 [0.02, 1.02]	2007
Briguori 2007	2	108	21	218	4.5%	0.19 [0.05, 0.80]	2007
Heguilen 2007	6	18	1	9	2.8%	3.00 [0.42, 21.30]	2007
Adolph 2008	3	71	2	74	3.3%	1.55 [0.27, 9.08]	2008
Lin 2008	4	30	5	30	5.5%	0.80 [0.24, 2.69]	2008
Subtotal (95% CI)		**528**		**560**	**32.8%**	**0.68 [0.30, 1.52]**	
Total events	45		57				
Heterogeneity: $Tau^2 = 0.66$; $Chi^2 = 15.66$, df = 7 (P = 0.03); $I^2 = 55\%$							
Test for overall effect: Z = 0.94 (P = 0.35)							
Total (95% CI)		**1477**		**1578**	**100.0%**	**0.66 [0.45, 0.95]**	
Total events	142		213				
Heterogeneity: $Tau^2 = 0.26$; $Chi^2 = 35.52$, df = 17 (P = 0.005), $I^2 = 52\%$							
Test for overall effect: Z = 2.23 (P = 0.03)							

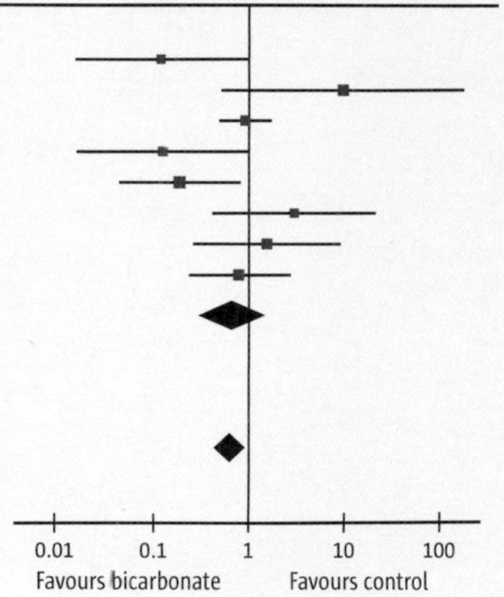

Risk Ratio M-H, Random, 95% CI

0.01 0.1 1 10 100

Favours bicarbonate Favours control

1

Subgroup analysis:

- Borderline significant effect in patients undergoing coronary procedures
- No benefit in studies that included mixed cohort of coronary & non-coronary procedures
- Studies that include patients with DM were inconclusive; those with CKD had borderline benefit

Secondary outcomes

Outcome	Trials/n	Result
RRT	11/2203	Overall only 26 patients required RRT. There was only a trend to less RRT in NaHCO group.
Mortality	5/1388	No difference

Author's conclusion

The preventative effect of CI-AKI of sodium bicarbonate is borderline, heterogeneity and low quality studies mean that only a limited recommendation can be made. The greatest benefit appears to be in patients undergoing emergency coronary procedures and in patients with CKD. 6 studies showed benefit from sodium bicarbonate whereas 12 studies did not however the patients in these trials had a lower risk profile: lower baseline creatinine, younger age or less contrast used. The term contrast associated AKI is proposed because recent studies suggest that in-patients not exposed to contrast have a similar incidence of AKI therefore aetiology is likely to be multifactorial.

Problems & limitations

- 4 studies didn't report the type of contrast used
- There was significant heterogeneity in the total volume of contrast used
- Considerable clinical heterogeneity in patients with DM or CKD
- Marked publication bias, studies published as abstracts had aggregates that were NSS whereas those published in full reported significant effects
- The Mayo Clinic study that showed a detrimental effect of sodium bicarbonate is not included/did not meet criteria

Advantages

- 13 studies use low or iso-osmolar contrast and 16 studies used isotonic saline as control intervention and most studies used Merten protocol for administering sodium bicarbonate
- Included studies were recent

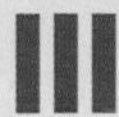

Expert opinion

Maria Schetz

A meta-analysis summarizing randomized controlled trials that compared hydration with sodium bicarbonate versus saline for the prevention of contrast nephropathy found a pooled relative risk of 0.66 (0,45–0.95) suggesting a protective effect of sodium bicarbonate.

How valid and robust are the data?

The meta-analysis included 18 studies and 3055 patients. The effect appeared most pronounced in coronary procedures, especially when emergent, and in patients with chronic kidney disease (CKD) However the individual studies had relatively low quality, there was considerable heterogeneity in treatment effect and evidence of publication bias, confirming the results of other recent meta-analysis on this subject. In general no significant effect was found in unpublished studies and in the largest published manuscripts. Older, small and poor-quality studies were more likely to show benefit Mortality and need for renal replacement therapy were not affected.

Should clinical practice be influenced by this?

The use of bicarbonate for the prevention of contrast nephropathy has possible but inconsistent benefit. Strongly recommending the routine use of bicarbonate for prophylaxis of contrast nephropathy might therefore be premature. Ensuring adequate hydration might be more important than the composition of the fluid.

What's the next step?

The next step should be a well-performed sufficiently powered prospective randomized controlled trial comparing the effect of hydration with sodium bicarbonate and normal saline on the incidence of contrast nephropathy in patients at risk (CKD, congestive heart failure, diabetes). Preferably this trial should also evaluate hard clinical endpoints such as need for renal replacement therapy or mortality. However, in view of the low incidence of these outcomes, the execution of such a trial will be hampered by the need for a very large study population.

1

Citation

Eric AJ Hoste, Jan J. De Waele, Sofie A. Gevaert, Shigehiko Uchino and John A Kellum. Sodium Bicarbonate for the prevention of contrast-induced acute kidney injury. Nephrol Dial Transplant (2010) 25: 747–758 Doi: 10.1093/ndt/gfp389

1

AMSTAR: methodological quality of the review

1.	Was "a priori" design provided?	Y
2.	Was study selection and data extraction adequate?	Y
3.	Was the literature search comprehensive?	Y
4.	Was 'Grey Literature' used?	Y
5.	Was a list of excluded studies provided?	Y
6.	Where the characteristics of included studies provided?	Y
7.	Was the scientific quality of studies assessed & documented?	Y
8.	Was the scientific quality of studies weighted appropriately in forming conclusions?	Y
9.	Were the methods used for data synthesis appropriate?	Y
10.	Was the potential for publication bias assessed?	Y
11.	Were any conflicts of interest stated?	Y

Overall quality of trials included	Low
Overall quality of the review	High

AKI in cardiac surgery

Condition: acute kidney injury (AKI) in patients undergoing cardiac surgery
Interventions: pharmacological therapies
Clinical question: Are there any interventions to prevent or treat AKI in this population?

The incidence of AKI is particularly high (up to 50%) in patients undergoing cardiac surgery, with mortality up to 24% for those requiring RRT. The aetiology of AKI in these patients is relatively homogenous: hypoperfusion and inflammation due to cardiopulmonary bypass, and the timing of injury is known. CPB with non-pulsatile flow leads to vasoconstriction and ischaemic injury, yet patients undergoing "off-pump" procedures are still at risk of AKI implying alternative mechanisms for injury.

Review characteristics

- **Eligibility criteria:** RCTs that assessed kidney injury with serum creatinine, creatinine clearance/GFR; any intervention administered before, during or after surgery; comparison with no therapy, placebo or standard care
- **Exclusions:** healthcare service interventions such as level of care; patients on RRT before surgery or those with kidney transplants
- **Number of studies:** 70 studies (66 prevention studies and 4 treatment studies)
- **Number of patients:** 5,554 (range 14–388; 9 trials < 20 pts; 17 trials > 100 pts, 6 trials > 200 pts)
- **Population:** adults aged 19 years and above undergoing cardiac surgery
- **Study dates:** 1990–2008

Intervention definitions

- **Vasodilators:** dopamine, dopexamine, fenoldopam, ACEi, diltiazem, prostacyclin, nifedipine, PGE-1, nitroprusside, theophylline
- **Induced natriuresis or diuresis:** ANP, BNP, urodilutin, loop diuretics, mannitol
- **Anti-inflammatory agents:** NAC, aspirin, glutathione, corticosteroids & leukodepletin
- **Others:** clonidine, albumin, isotonic saline, insulin therapy, CVVH, pulsatile CPB, off-pump surgery

Results

Primary outcome: incidence of AKI

Intervention	Trials	N	Associated with reduction in AKI
Vasodilators	29	1766	Fenoldopam and ACEi in 6 trials/496 patients
Natri/diuretics	12	837	ANP, BNP and urodilutin
Anti-inflammatory	14	1347	No effect
Others	15	1560	No effect

Secondary outcomes

Outcome	Trials	N	Results
Acute RRT	21	2172	No difference*
Mortality	18	2227	No difference*

* Trials were not powered adequately to show these outcomes

1

Author's conclusion

The review demonstrates the large number of studies in this category although the vast majority were small single centre trials. In general, strategies to prevent AKI were effective if administered pre and intraoperatively. Exploratory analysis showed that most types of prophylaxis were protective from AKI especially fenoldopam, ANP/nesiritide and Off-Pump CABG. No conclusions can be drawn about treatment of AKI as these studies were too few.

Problems & limitations

- Definitions of AKI and criteria for initiation of RRT were not standardised across studies. Heterogeneity and study quality were significant limitations
- Frequency of kidney function assessment varied widely from every 8 hours in the high quality studies to days 1, 5 and 15

Advantages

- Encompassed all interventions for prevention of AKI

Expert opinion

Eric Hoste

How valid and robust are the data?

This review highlights that much work has been done in this field, but also that despite all these efforts many questions remain unsolved.

The review considers 70 studies including 5,554 patients. The number of patients included per study is therefore relatively low. Further, there was considerable heterogeneity, low methodological quality, and variation in definitions for AKI.

This systematic review does not include a meta-analysis and therefore, also does not report Risk Ratio's or Odds Ratio's for specific interventions, which makes it more difficult to evaluate the effect of specific interventions.

Should clinical practice be influenced by this?

Given the quality of study data, we cannot recommend changing practice based on data from this systematic review.

What is the next step?

Cardiac surgery is a common procedure, and AKI can occur in up to 50% of patients. Further, many studies demonstrated that AKI is associated with worse outcomes. Therefore, this calls for properly designed and adequately powered multicentre studies on specific therapies for prevention and treatment of AKI, defined by the sensitive AKI/RIFLE classification.

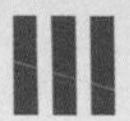

Citation

Park M, Coca SG, Nigwekar SU, Garg AX, Garwood S, Parikh CR. Prevention and Treatment of Acute Kidney Injury in Patients Undergoing Cardiac Surgery: A Systematic Review. Am J Nephrol 2010;31:408–418, DOI: 10.1159/000296277

AMSTAR: methodological quality of the review

1.	Was "a priori" design provided?	Y
2.	Was study selection and data extraction adequate?	Y
3.	Was the literature search comprehensive?	Y
4.	Was 'Grey Literature' used? English & full manuscripts only	N
5.	Was a list of excluded studies provided?	N
6.	Where the characteristics of included studies provided?	Y
7.	Was the scientific quality of studies assessed & documented?	Y
8.	Was the scientific quality of studies weighted appropriately in forming conclusions?	Y
9.	Were the methods used for data synthesis appropriate?	Y
10.	Was the potential for publication bias assessed? Due to high heterogeneity	NA
11.	Were any conflicts of interest stated?	Y

Overall quality of included studies	50% low quality, 26% high quality
Overall quality of the review	High

2

Acute respiratory failure (ARF) – Acute respiratory distress syndrome (ARDS)

Higher versus lower PEEP ____ 30
Recruitment manoeuvres ____ 34
Inhaled nitric oxide ____ 39
Aerosolized prostacyclin ____ 43
Pharmacological therapies for ARDS ____ 46
Corticosteroids in ARDS ____ 50
ECMO ____ 54

Also see:

Section 4: Cardiovascular dynamics
Therapeutic hypothermia

Section 9: Neuro-intensive care
Haemostatic drugs for TBI

Higher versus lower PEEP

Condition: acute lung injury (ALI) and acute respiratory distress syndrome (ARDS)
Intervention: positive end-expiratory pressure (PEEP)
Clinical question: Is higher or lower PEEP better for patients with ALI and ARDS?

Lung protective ventilation with low tidal volumes and low plateau pressures is now an established principle to minimise ventilator induced lung injury and mortality. PEEP is applied to keep alveoli open, without which the cyclical opening and closing of lung units would promote atelectrauma. Traditional levels of PEEP are values between 5–12 cmH_2O however experimental data suggest that higher PEEP levels are required to prevent cyclical alveolar collapse in patients with significant alveolar oedema and collapse. In patients with milder lung injury, higher PEEP may result in over distension and potential harm.

2

Hypotheses: All patients with ALI/ARDS would benefit from a higher PEEP. Patients with more severe lung disease as defined by lower compliance, lower PaO_2:FiO_2 and higher oxygenation index would have more recruitable lung units therefore were more likely to benefit from higher PEEP. Less benefit would be observed in patients with high BMI because of fewer recruitable lung units.

Review characteristics

- **Eligibility criteria:** RCTs that compared higher versus lower PEEP that used tidal volume < 8 ml/kg of predicted body weight
- **Number of studies:** 3 RCTs (ALVEOLI, LOVS, EXPRESS)
- **Number of patients:** 2,299 patients
- **Population:** adults (over 16 years) with ALI or ARDS
- **Study dates:** 2004–2008 (recruitment period 1999–2005)

Definitions

- **ALI & ARDS:** according to the NAECC definition
- **Higher versus lower PEEP:** mean difference of at least 3 cm H_2O between groups during the first 3 days after randomisation
- **Rescue therapy for refractory hypoxaemia:** not standardized (varied between centres)

Results

Primary outcome: hospital mortality

Group	N	Higher PEEP mortality	Lower PEEP mortality	RR	95% CI	*p*	Result
All	2299	32.9%	35.2%	0.94	0.86–1.04	0.25	NSS
ARDS	1892	34.1%	39.1%	0.90	0.81–1.00	0.049	SS
Non-ARDS	404	27.2%	19.4%	1.37	0.98–1.92	0.07	NSS

Fig. 1 Time to Death in Hospital and Time to Unassisted Breathing for Higher and Lower Positive End-Expiratory Pressure (PEEP) Stratified by Presence of Acute Respiratory Distress Syndrome (ARDS) at Baseline [from M. Briel, M. Meade, A. Mercat, RG. Brower, D. Talmor, SD. Walter, AS. Slutsky, E. Pullenayegum, Q. Zhou, D. Cook, L. Brochard, JM. Richard, F. Lamontagne, N. Bhatnagar, TE. Stewart, G. Guyatt. Higher vs Lower Positive End-Expiratory Pressure in Patients With Acute Lung Injury and Acute Respiratory Distress Syndrome: Systematic Review and Meta-analysis. JAMA. 2010;303(9):865–873.]

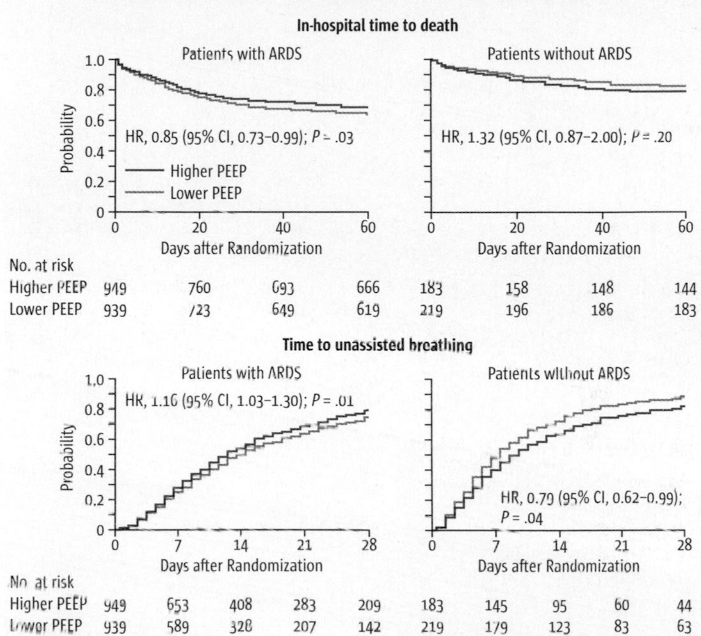

Cox regression models adjusting for age, probability of death in hospital derived from prognostic scores at baseline, severe sepsis at baseline, and trial. For the analysis of time to unassisted breathing, data were censored at the time of death because time to death was modeled separately and a sensitivity analysis without censoring at death yielded very similar results. Additionally including the Esophageal Pressure Directed Ventilation trial (n = 61) revealed adjusted hazard ratios (HRs) for hospital mortality of 0.83 (95% confidence interval [CI], 0.71–0.96; *P* = .01; 33.9 % vs 39.0%) for patients with ARDS (n = 1941) and 1.26 (95% CI, 0.84–1.88; *P* = .27; 26.5% vs 19.4%) for patients without ARDS (n = 416). Corresponding hazard ratios for time to unassisted breathing were 1.14 (95% CI, 1.02–1.28; *P* = .02; proportions at 28 days, 64.2% vs 58.0%) for patients with ARDS (n = 1941) and 0.80 (95% CI, 0.64–1.01; *P* = .06; proportions at 28 days, 70.4% vs 79.7%) for patients without ARDS (n = 416).

2

Secondary outcomes

Outcome	Result
ICU death	SS reduction in ICU death for patients allocated to higher PEEP
Pneumonthorax	No difference
Px deaths	No difference
Vasopressors	No difference (65% overall)
Neuromuscular blockers	No difference (45% overall)
Corticosteroids	No difference (45% overall)
Unassisted breathing days	ARDS patients with higher PEEP achieved unassisted breathing earlier

Sensitivity analysis with 1 additional trial (EPVENT) included did not change results.

Author's conclusion

This meta-analysis showed that overall there was no difference in mortality or secondary outcomes but a subgroup with ARDS ventilated with high PEEP had a relative mortality reduction of about 10%. Patients without ARDS did not benefit and may even be harmed by higher PEEP. ARDS patients were at a slightly higher risk of pneumothoraces (absolute risk difference 1.6%) but no other adverse consequences. In ALVEOLI and LOVS PEEP was titrated to oxygenation whereas in EXPRESS it was titrated to inspiratory plateau pressure therefore no recommendations can be made with regards to optimal PEEP setting.

Problems & limitations

- Results for ARDS patients receiving higher PEEP were obtained as a result of a pre-specified subgroup analysis and achieved borderline statistical significance
- 2 studies were terminated early for perceived futility
- Plateau pressures were significantly higher in the higher PEEP groups in all studies but were still, on average, below 30 cmH_2O

Advantages

- All studies used tidal volume of approximately 6mls/kg
- This was a meta-analysis of individual patient data which has several advantages over conventional meta-analyses therefore outcome definitions and data analysis was standardized

Expert opinion

Anders Larsson

How valid and robust are the data?
This is a carefully performed and valid meta-analysis. I doubt that we ever will get better data regarding the effects of low and high PEEP in an ALI/ARDS population. The data are fairly robust, but still the power was only 72% in main analysis with a $p < 0.05$.

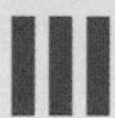

Should clinical practise be influenced by this?
This study supports the (common) clinical practice, where PEEP is individualized and higher PEEP is used in the more severe cases. However, high PEEP is probably not indicated in the less severe cases.

What's the next step?
To develop and validate bedside methods that predict whether PEEP (and which PEEP level) would be beneficial in the individual patient. Thereafter an RCT might be performed where an individualized PEEP setting is compared with a protocol-based PEEP setting, e.g., the ARDS net approach.

Citation

Briel M, Meade M, Mercat A, Brower RG, Talmor D, Walter SD, Slutsky AS, Pullenayegum E, Zhou Q, Cook D, Brochard L, Richard JM, Lamontagne F, Bhatnagar N, Stewart TE, Guyatt G. Higher vs Lower Positive End-Expiratory Pressure in Patients With Acute Lung Injury and Acute Respiratory Distress Syndrome: Systematic Review and Meta-analysis. JAMA. 2010;303(9):865–873

AMSTAR: methodological quality of the review

1.	Was "a priori" design provided?	Y
2.	Was study selection and data extraction adequate?	Y
3.	Was the literature search comprehensive?	Y
4.	Was 'Grey Literature' used?	Y
5.	Was a list of excluded studies provided?	Y
6.	Were the characteristics of included studies provided?	Y
7.	Was the scientific quality of studies assessed & documented?	Y
8.	Was the scientific quality of studies weighted appropriately in forming conclusions?	Y
9.	Were the methods used for data synthesis appropriate?	Y
10.	Was the potential for publication bias assessed?	Y
11.	Were any conflicts of interest stated?	Y

Overall quality of trials included	High
Overall quality of the review	High

Recruitment manoeuvres

Condition: acute lung injury (ALI) and acute respiratory distress syndrome (ARDS)
Intervention: recruitment manoeuvres (RMs)
Clinical question: How do RMs affect patient outcomes such as duration of mechanical ventilation (MV) and mortality?

Patients with ALI and ARDS are susceptible to lung injury by excessive alveolar distension, cyclical opening and closing of lung units; and failure to open collapsed alveolar units. Protective lung ventilation that improves survival in patients includes small tidal volumes and low plateau pressures. Recruitment manoeuvres and higher PEEP are also associated with better survival in some studies, however outcomes have been variable. The aim of RMs is to open collapsed lung units and therefore improve oxygenation. Recruitment involves increasing transpulmonary pressure above the normal ventilatory level, for a prolonged time which can potentially cause barotrauma or reduce venous return and cardiac output; thus their use has been controversial. Application of recruitment manoeuvres can vary in maximum pressure, end-expiratory pressure and duration which may account for the inconsistent outcomes.

Review characteristics

- **Eligibility criteria:** RCTs comparing recruitment manoeuvres to standard care
- **Number of studies:** 7 RCTs
- **Number of patients:** 1,170 (range: 8 in a cross-over trial to 983 in a multicentre RCT)
- **Population:** adults (above 18 years) with ALI or ARDS who were intubated and mechanically ventilated for at least 24 hours
- **Study dates:** 1998–2008

Definitions

- **Recruitment manoeuvre:** any technique that transiently increased alveolar pressure (plateau, peak or end-expiratory pressure) above normal tidal ventilation, sustained beyond the normal time. These varied between studies: Peak pressure range 35–50 cmH_2O; Time range 20–40 seconds; Mean PEEP range 10–16.4 cmH_2O
- **ALI & ARDS:** with the lung injury severity score (LISS) or N. American-European consensus conference (NAECC)

Results

Primary outcomes

Outcome	Trials	N	RR	95% CI	I^2	Result
28 day mortality	2	1036	0.73	0.46–1.17	67%	NSS
ICU mortality	2	1036	0.73	0.46–1.16	66%	NSS
In-hospital mortality	2	1036	0.81	0.59–1.12	48%	NSS

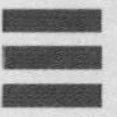

Fig. 2 Comparison 1 Recruitment manoeuvres versus no recruitment manoeuvres, Outcome 1 28 day mortality [from Hodgson C, Keating JL, Holland AE, Davies AR, Smirneos L, Bradley SJ, Tuxen D. Recruitment manoeuvres for adults with acute lung injury receiving mechanical ventilation. Cochrane Database of Systematic Reviews 2009, Issue 2. Art. No.: CD006667, © Cochrane Collaboration, reproduced with permission]

Review: Recruitment manoeuvres for adults with acute lung injury receiving mechanical ventilation
Comparison: 1 Recruitment manoeuvres versus no recruitment manoeuvres
Outcome: 1 28 day mortality

Study or subgroup	Treatment n/N	Control n/N	Risk Ratio M-H, Random, 95% CI	Weight	Risk Ratio M-H, Random, 95% CI
Amato 1998	11/29	17/24		37.1%	0.54 [0.31, 0.91]
Meade 2008	135/475	164/508		62.9%	0.88 [0.73, 1.06]
Total (95% CI)	**504**	**532**		**100.0%**	**0.73 [0.46, 1.17]**

Total events: 146 (Treatment), 181 (Control)
Heterogeneity: $Tau^2 = 0.08$; $Chi^2 = 3.00$, $df = 1$ ($P = 0.08$); $I^2 = 67\%$
Test for overall effect: $Z = 1.29$ ($P = 0.20$)

Outcome	Trials	N	Results
Duration of MV	1	53	62% of study group weaned by day 28 c.f. 29% of controls
Duration of MV	1	983	No difference between the two groups
Hospital LOS	1	983	No difference

Secondary outcomes

Outcome	Trials	N	Results
Barotrauma	3	1108	No significant difference
Oxygenation	5	1108	General improvement that was only maintained in the short term, except for 1 trial (n = 983) which used a ventilation package where benefit was maintained for 3 days
Blood Pressure	4	125	No significant difference in MAP in 3 studies. 1 study terminated RM early due to hypotension in 3/72 patients
Heart Rate (HR)	3	110	No difference in 2 studies. Higher HR with suction & RM c.f. suction alone in 1 study (n = 8)

Author's conclusion

No study examined the effect of recruitment manoeuvres alone, these were assessed as part of a ventilator package with differences in PEEP and plateau pressure, therefore any benefit or harm may be due to any one of the ventilation strategies or the combination. Overall there was no difference in mortality, duration of mechanical ventilation, LOS or adverse effects; however, there isn't enough evidence to support or refute RMs. Recent CT evidence suggests that response to recruitment is heterogeneous and may lead to over distension in some cases, therefore RMs may benefit some or may be harmful to others.

Problems & limitations

- 1 study included patients aged 15–18 years which contravened the protocol (because it was one of only two studies that looked at long-term outcomes)
- Four cross-over studies were included. RMs in the 2 main RCTs were applied inconsistently and associated with ventilator disconnections, the cause of which may have a more profound impact on results
- 1 RCT used higher tidal volumes (12 mls/kg) in the control group which we know is associated with worse outcome

Advantages

- Most trials demonstrated improvements in oxygenation following RM however this was not sustained in any except 1 study. This may assist future researches to apply the more successful ventilator package in this respect

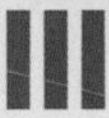

Expert opinion

Anders Larsson

How valid and robust are the data?

This study tried to examine the effect of lung recruitment manoeuvres per se, but in reality examined the effects of lung recruitment manoeuvre combined with other interventions. Therefore, in strict terms the study is not valid. However, the study still indicates that lung recruitment manoeuvres may not change outcome in patients with ALI/ARDS, but is underpowered (not robust enough) to exclude such possibility. In addition, it is not possible from this meta-analysis to assess whether lung recruitment manoeuvres are associated with a survival benefit in patients with lungs that have a recruitment potential.

Should clinical practise be influenced by this?

The data do not support the use of lung recruitment manoeuvres in all patients with ALI/ARDS.

What's the next step?

To develop and validate bedside methods for determination of lung recruitability, i.e., methods that predict whether lung recruitment manoeuvres would recruit collapsed lung regions in the individual patient. Thereafter an RCT could be performed in ARDS patients with recruitable lungs, where a ventilation protocol with lung recruitment manoeuvres is compared with the same protocol but without lung recruitment manoeuvres.

2

Citation

Hodgson C, Keating JL, Holland AE, Davies AR, Smirneos L, Bradley SJ, Tuxen D. Recruitment manoeuvres for adults with acute lung injury receiving mechanical ventilation. Cochrane Database of Systematic Reviews 2009, Issue 2. Art. No.: CD006667. DOI: 10.1002/14651858.CD006667.pub2.

Additional information from the author

This review will be updated in the near future as there are two further RCTs to include.

2

AMSTAR: methodological quality of the review

1.	Was "a priori" design provided?	Y
2.	Was study selection and data extraction adequate?	Y
3.	Was the literature search comprehensive?	Y
4.	Was 'Grey Literature' used?	Y
5.	Was a list of excluded studies provided?	Y
6.	Were the characteristics of included studies provided?	Y
7.	Was the scientific quality of studies assessed & documented?	Y
8.	Was the scientific quality of studies weighted appropriately in forming conclusions?	Y
9.	Were the methods used for data synthesis appropriate?	Y
10.	Was the potential for publication bias assessed?	Y
11.	Were any conflicts of interest stated?	Y

Overall quality of trials included	Only 1 high quality
Overall quality of the review	High

Inhaled nitric oxide

Condition: acute hypoxaemic respiratory failure (AHRF)
Intervention: nitric oxide (NO)
Clinical question: Does the use of inhaled nitric oxide confer any clinical or mortality benefit in patients with ALI or ARDS? Is there any risk involved with its use?

Recent figures suggest that the incidence of ARDS in adults is 10.6 and in children is 13 per 100,000 population, with mortality between 24–60% and 18–23% respectively. Mortality is greatest amongst patients with sepsis, MOF, the immuno-compromised and those whose oxygenation doesn't improve after 6 days. Hypoxaemia in ARDS results from intrapulmonary shunting and pulmonary hypertension. Nitric oxide is a potent vasodilator, when inhaled can provide selective vasodilatation in the well ventilated lung units, improving V/Q mismatch and PVR within 40 minutes of treatment. Subsequently RVEF improves, whereas RVEDV decreases and prevents acute cor pulmonale. NO has oxidative and immune protective properties, it has a short half-life but inhaled nitric oxide (INO) is a cytotoxic free radical and its metabolites may accumulate and cause tissue damage. INO is widely used as rescue therapy in ARDS; however, previous reviews suggest that its benefits are transient and that it may be associated with renal dysfunction.

2

Review characteristics

- **Eligibility:** RCTs comparing INO with placebo or no intervention
- **Exclusion:** quasi-randomised and observational studies; neonates with BPD or chronic lung disease
- **Number of studies:** 14 trials
- **Number of patients:** 1,303 (trial range 14–385)
- **Population:** adults or children
- **Study dates:** 1997–2007

Definitions

- **ALI & ARDS:** European-American consensus definition
- **INO:** any dose, any duration of treatment
- **Mortality:** at longest follow up. Overall 28-day mortality (range: 25–30 days)
- **"Standard treatment" and "critically ill":** accepted (author definitions)

2

Results

Primary outcome: including subgroup analyses

Mortality Outcome	Trials	N	Deaths study versus control	RR	95% CI	I^2	GRADE
Mortality at longest FU	14	1250	40.2%/38.6%	1.06	0.93–1.22	0	Low
28-day mortality	9	1082	36%/32.7%	1.12	0.95–1.31	0	Low
Paediatric mortality	3	162	40%/41.5%	0.97	0.67–1.38	0	Low
Median INO Rx for > 1 week	8	826	–	1.07	0.90–1.29	0	Low

Secondary outcomes*

Outcome	Trials/n	Results	GRADE
Mechanical ventilation	9/1147	No difference	–
Oxygenation measure	10 / 615	Improved at 24 hours, no difference thereafter	Low-Mod
Renal impairment	4/765	RR 1.59 95% CI 1.17–2.16 I^2 = 0%	Low
Other adverse events	Variable	NSS	–
ICU LOS & MOF	1/385	No difference	–
QOL/ADL	1/368	NSS	–

* Too many analyses therefore overall results given only

Sensitivity analyses showed the same results

Author's conclusion

In adults, the use of INO in AHRF has no proven long term benefit. There is a transient improvement in oxygenation; however, trials reported this using different measures, therefore results weren't pooled adequately. INO increased the risk of renal injury but although there was no difference in mortality, these data were sparse.

Problems & limitations

- Duration of MV varied from 24 hours to one year
- Varying doses and duration of INO therapy
- 5 trials applied co-interventions e.g. recruitment manoeuvres, prone positioning and corticosteroids
- 6 trials funded by industry, trials were generally underpowered
- Many trials were conducted before the recommendations for lung protective ventilation was introduced

Advantages

- The funnel plot showed no indication of publication bias
- Various statistical methods such as trial sequential analysis were applied to minimise the influence of bias

Expert opinion

Nicola Petrucci

How valid and robust are the data?
This review found 14 RCTs for a total of 1,303 participants. The retrieved trials were assessed for quality, and only 4 RCTs were classified as good quality trials. The Authors concluded that inhaled NO cannot be recommended for patients with AHRF. Subgroup analysis and sensitivity analysis were consistent with that conclusion, heterogeneity was not significant. Thus, data are robust and valid.

Should clinical practise be influence by this?
This review showed that inhaled NO improved oxygenation at short-term, without decreasing mortality at longer follow up. Therefore, apart from transient effects, this intervention does not affect the outcome of patients with ARDS and should not change clinical practice among children and adults.

What's the next step?
A very moderate effect of inhaled NO cannot be completely excluded, unless a very large RCT is performed (more than 36,000 patients for a relative risk reduction of about 4%). This will be challenging, since decrease in mortality in ARDS can be achieved by other different interventions.

Citation

Afshari A, Brok J, Møller AM, Wetterslev J. Inhaled nitric oxide for acute respiratory distress syndrome (ARDS) and acute lung injury in children and adults. Cochrane Database of Systematic Reviews 2010, Issue 7. Art. No.: CD002787. DOI: 10.1002/14651858.CD002787.pub2.

AMSTAR: methodological quality of the review

1.	Was "a priori" design provided?	Y
2.	Was study selection and data extraction adequate?	Y
3.	Was the literature search comprehensive?	Y
4.	Was 'Grey Literature' used?	Y
5.	Was a list of excluded studies provided?	Y
6.	Were the characteristics of included studies provided?	Y
7.	Was the scientific quality of studies assessed & documented?	Y
8.	Was the scientific quality of studies weighted appropriately in forming conclusions?	Y
9.	Were the methods used for data synthesis appropriate?	Y
10.	Was the potential for publication bias assessed?	Y
11.	Were any conflicts of interest stated?	Y

Overall quality of trials included	Low. Only 4 were high quality
Overall quality of the review	High

Aerosolized prostacyclin

Condition: acute lung injury (ALI) and acute respiratory distress syndrome (ARDS)

Intervention: aerosolized prostacyclin

Clinical question: Is there any benefit or harm from using aerosolized prostacyclin in these conditions?

ARDS is an inflammatory process involving the lungs, which results in non-cardiogenic pulmonary oedema and severe hypoxaemia. The initial exudative phase is characterised by disruption of the alveolar-capillary membrane leading to neutrophil invasion, alveolar oedema and collapse. The initiation of lung repair and increased surfactant production that occur at days 7–21 mark the proliferative phase when life-threatening hypoxaemia may occur. ALI is at the milder end of the spectrum and hypoxaemia is less severe. ARDS is associated with significant morbidity and although mortality has decreased over the last decade, it remains high at 44% in adults and 23% in children.

2

Prostaglandins have anti-inflammatory properties (inhibit platelet aggregation and neutrophil adhesion); and they relax smooth muscle thereby producing significant vasodilation of pulmonary and systemic vasculature. Inhaled prostaglandins lower pulmonary arterial pressures, redistribute blood flow to ventilated areas and therefore reduce shunting. The lower PVR and MPAP improve right heart afterload and function. Inflammation modulating effects and antithrombic properties also appear to improve the microcirculation in ALI/ARDS. They have been used to improve oxygenation but their efficacy remains unproven.

Review characteristics

- **Eligibility criteria:** RCTs that compared aerosolized prostacyclin with placebo (saline) or no treatment
- **Exclusions:** quasi randomisation and observational studies; neonates with bronchopulmonary dysplasia or chronic lung disease
- **Number of studies:** 1 paediatric RCT (2 on-going trials have been identified: 1 adult, 1 paediatric)
- **Number of patients:** 14
- **Population:** children or adults with ALI or ARDS
- **Study date:** 2004

Definitions

- **ALI/ARDS:** the review allowed various definitions according to the literature but the included study used European-American consensus definition
- **Standard Treatment:** as defined by authors (no protocol). Standard ventilation and aerosolized saline in the included trial

Results

Primary outcome: all-cause 28-day mortality

Trial	N	Prostacyclin: deaths	Control: deaths	RR	95% CI	GRADE
1	14	2 out of 8	1 out of 6	1.5	0.17–12.94	Low

Secondary outcomes

No secondary outcomes were reported by this study.

Author's conclusion

There are insufficient data to draw any conclusions about benefits or harms. There was a significant improvement in oxygenation index (as indicated by case reports and observational studies) however this does not necessarily translate into other clinical benefits.

Problems & limitations

- Extremely small number of patients
- The intervention was only administered for 24 hours
- Original protocol was not available and reviewers were unable to examine selective outcome reporting
- Results from a paediatric population cannot be extrapolated to an adult population

Advantages

- This review has highlighted the lack of evidence for or against the use of aerosolized prostacyclin, however 2 on-going trials have been identified

Expert opinion

Nicola Petrucci

How valid and robust are the data?
This review found only 1 paediatric randomized trial that included 14 participants. The retrieved trial was classified with low risk of bias. The trial did not show any benefit on 28-day mortality in the intervention group, despite a transient effect on oxygenation. The small sample size challenges the robustness of the results.

Should clinical practise be influenced by this?
Due to insufficient evidence, we cannot exclude benefit or harm till a large randomized trial will be performed testing aerosolized prostacyclin for ALI/ARDS. Current clinical practice should not change.

What's the next step?
There is a need for large randomized trials with low risk of bias. However, data from two ongoing studies could shed more light on this matter.

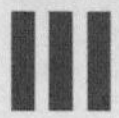

Citation

Afshari A, Brok J, Møller AM, Wetterslev J. Aerosolized prostacyclin for acute lung injury (ALI) and acute respiratory distress syndrome (ARDS). Cochrane Database of Systematic Reviews 2010, Issue 8. Art. No.: CD007733. DOI: 10.1002/14651858.CD007733.pub2.

AMSTAR: methodological quality of the review

1.	Was "a priori" design provided?	Y
2.	Was study selection and data extraction adequate?	Y
3.	Was the literature search comprehensive?	Y
4.	Was 'Grey Literature' used?	Y
5.	Was a list of excluded studies provided?	Y
6.	Were the characteristics of included studies provided?	Y
7.	Was the scientific quality of studies assessed & documented?	Y
8.	Was the scientific quality of studies weighted appropriately in forming conclusions?	Y
9.	Were the methods used for data synthesis appropriate?	NA
10.	Was the potential for publication bias assessed?	Y
11.	Were any conflicts of interest stated?	Y

Overall quality of trials included	Low
Overall quality of the review	High

Pharmacological therapies for ARDS

Condition: acute lung injury (ALI) and acute respiratory distress syndrome (ARDS)
Interventions: various pharmacotherapies
Clinical question: Do any of the pharmacologic therapies investigated improve outcomes from ALI/ARDS?

ALI and ARDS can occur as a result of direct lung injury e.g. pneumonia, aspiration or indirect injury e.g. sepsis, trauma, pancreatitis. Regardless of the aetiology, the pathophysiology consists of damage to the alveolar-capillary membrane with resultant leakage of proteinaceous fluid into the alveolar space. As injury involves the epithelial basement membrane and type I and II alveolar cells, surfactant production is compromised leading to increased alveolar surface tension, atelectasis and reduced lung compliance. The inflammatory reaction involves neutrophil and mesenchymal cell recruitment; microvascular thrombosis as a result of coagulation system activation; and production of oxygen free radicals and inflammatory mediators. The plethora of pharmacologic therapies investigated reflects attempts to target each of these processes.

Review characteristics

- Eligibility criteria: RCTs comparing any pharmacological intervention with placebo or no therapy, published in full or abstract form
- Exclusions: quasi-randomised trials or use of data from which ALI/ARDS patients were subgroups in larger trials e.g. for sepsis; nutritional interventions, INO, and strategies combined with fluid management or ventilation techniques e.g. partial liquid ventilation
- Number of studies: 33 RCTs
- Number of patients: 3,272 (range 9–25)
- Population: adults with ALI and ARDS admitted to ICU
- Study dates: 1985–2002

Definition

- **All-cause mortality**: at or before 3 months from randomisation
- **ALI/ARDS**: NAECC for some studies

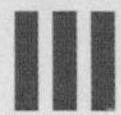

Results

Primary outcome: all-cause mortality

Intervention	Trials	N	Pooled analysis	I^2
Prostaglandin E_1	7	693	No statistically significant difference	21.3%
N-acetylcysteine	5	239	No statistically significant difference	0%
Corticosteroids – high dose	2	180	No statistically significant difference	50.1%
Corticosteroids – low dose	1	24	Statistically significant reduction in mortality	
Surfactant	9	1416	No statistically significant difference	18.7%
Pentoxifylline	1	30	Statistically significant reduction mortality in patients with metastatic cancer	NA

2

Secondary outcomes: adverse events

Intervention	Result
Prostaglandin E_1	5 trials reported adverse events leading to drug discontinuation: hypotension, dysrhythmias, hypoxia and agitation
N-acetylcysteine	1 patient got a rash so NAC was stopped
Corticosteroids	More infectious complications in high dose steroid group
Surfactant	Reported as: 'some respiratory events and haemodynamic instability'
Pentoxifylline	No adverse events reported

Subgroup analysis: no difference in outcomes between patients with ALI versus ARDS with NAC or corticosteroids steroids

Sensitivity Analysis: no difference with studies reporting adequate allocation concealment

Author's conclusion

None of the pharmacologic therapies included in this review convincingly reduced mortality in patients with ALI and ARDS therefore clinical application of these cannot be recommended. With regards to adverse events, all PGE_1, high dose steroids and 4 out of 5 surfactant trials reported more adverse events with active therapy.

Problems & limitations

- There were significant differences between trials in study population, severity of illness, and drug regimens

- The number of trials and patients for each intervention were very small
- Some trials may have been conducted before optimal dosing and durations in terms of drug pharmacokinetics and pharmacodynamics have been fully understood

Advantages

- Results between trials for each intervention were consistent
- Two potential therapies were identified for further research: prolonged corticosteroids and pentoxifylline; although these outcomes need to be interpreted with caution

Expert opinion

Arthur S. Slutsky

2

How valid and robust are the data?
This was a methodologically rigorous review of the literature; the authors examined 33 studies with almost 3,300 patients. Most studies were relatively small, and likely underpowered to address mortality as the primary end-point. The major limitation of applying this study relates to the fact that the review was limited to studies published until early 2004. Nonetheless, the conclusion that "effective pharmacotherapy for ALI and ARDS is extremely limited" remains valid in 2011.

Should clinical practise be influenced by this?
The review is useful, but it is incumbent upon clinicians to read the key articles to better understand the nuances, controversies and implications for their individual patients for the various therapies. In addition, because the last study reviewed was published in 2004, it is important to review more recent studies. For example, a study in 2006 (1) demonstrated that corticosteroids do not decrease mortality in patients with persistent ARDS, but may be useful in other clinically important end-points, and a recent intriguing study in 2010 (2) suggests that a neuromuscular blocking agent may decrease mortality when given early in patients with ARDS.

What's the next step?
We need a better understanding of the underlying biology of ARDS, a more precise definition of ARDS, better surrogate end-points, further thoughtful clinical studies, and replication of key studies.

References

(1) The Acute Respiratory Distress Syndrome Network. Efficacy and safety of corticosteroids for persistent acute respiratory distress syndrome. N Engl J Med 2006;354:1671–84

(2) Papazian L, Forel JM, Gacouin A, Penot-Ragon C, Perrin G, Loundou A, et al. for the ACURASYS Study Investigators. Neuromuscular Blockers in Early Acute Respiratory Distress Syndrome. N Engl J Med 2010;3631107–16

Citation

Adhikari NKJ, Burns KEA, Meade MO, Ratnapalan M. Pharmacologic therapies for adults with acute lung injury and acute respiratory distress syndrome. Cochrane Database of Systematic Reviews 2004, Issue 4. Art. No.: CD004477. DOI:10.1002/14651858.CD004477.pub2.

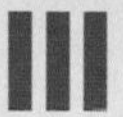

Additional information from the review's author

This review needs to be up-dated as there are potentially 15 or more new studies to include.

AMSTAR: methodological quality of the review

1.	Was "a priori" design provided?	Y
2.	Was study selection and data extraction adequate?	Y
3.	Was the literature search comprehensive?	Y
4.	Was 'Grey literature' used?	Y
5.	Was a list of excluded studies provided?	Y
6.	Were the characteristics of included studies provided?	Y
7.	Was the scientific quality of studies assessed & documented?	Y
8.	Was the scientific quality of studies weighted appropriately in forming conclusions?	Y
9.	Were the methods used for data synthesis appropriate?	Y
10.	Was the potential for publication bias assessed?	Y
11.	Were any conflicts of interest stated?	Y

Overall quality of trials included	Variable but mostly low
Overall quality of the review	High

2

Corticosteroids in ARDS

Condition: Acute lung injury (ALI) and acute respiratory distress syndrome (ARDS)
Intervention: corticosteroids
Clinical question: Does the use of prolonged low to moderate dose corticosteroid reduce morbidity and mortality in ALI and ARDS?

ALI and ARDS are characterised by intense host inflammatory responses against pulmonary parenchyma. Consequently corticosteroids have been investigated as potential therapy in view of their anti-inflammatory properties. Earlier trials using high dose corticosteroids failed to show any benefit, but more recent trials using longer courses of lower dose regimes have been promising. However results have been conflicting, and concerns about the potential adverse effects of corticosteroids such as infectious and neuromyopathic complications have not been addressed satisfactorily. This meta-analysis aimed to resolve issues regarding timing, duration and dose of therapy.

Review characteristics

- **Eligibility criteria:** randomised and non-randomised studies and cohort studies that used low dose corticosteroid
- **Exclusions:** studies that did not use a control group; used high dose corticosteroids or included inflammatory conditions other than ALI or ARDS such as PCP
- **Number of studies:** 4 RCTs and 5 cohort studies
- **Number of patients:** 341 in RCTs and 307 in cohort studies
- **Population:** adults over 18 years who had ALI or ARDS
- **Studies dates:** 1998–2005

Definition

- **Low dose corticosteroid:** 0.5–2.5 mg/kg/day of methylprednisolone or equivalent
- **High dose corticosteroid:** 30 mg/kg/day of methylprednisolone or equivalent
- **ALI/ARDS:** NAECC definition

Results

Primary outcome: mortality

All studies showed a trend towards reduced mortality but the effect was only statistically significant when all studies were pooled.

Trials	N	RR	95% CI	*p*	Results
4 RCTs	341	0.51	0.24–1.09	0.08	NSS
5 Cohort	307	0.66	0.43–1.02	0.06	NSS
All 9	648	0.62	0.43–0.91	0.01	SS

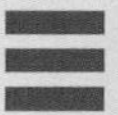

Fig. 3 Effect of steroid on mortality. Size of data markers is proportional to the weight of each study in the forest plot. RCT, randomized controlled trial; CI, confidence interval [from Tang BMP, Craig JC, Eslick GD, Seppelt I, McLean AS. Use of corticosteroids in acute lung injury and acute respiratory distress syndrome: A systematic review and meta-analysis. Crit Care Med 2009 Vol. 37, No. 5]

Group by Study Design		Events/Total Treated	Events/Total Control	Risk Ratio and 95% CI	Relative weight (%)	Risk Ratio	Lower limit	Upper limit	p-Value
Cohort	Keel	5/13	12/18		19.39	0.58	0.27	1.24	0.16
Cohort	Varpula	3/16	3/15		7.56	0.94	0.22	3.94	0.93
Cohort	Huh	6/14	25/34		23.70	0.58	0.31	1.10	0.10
Cohort	Lee	1/12	7/8		4.65	0.10	0.01	0.63	0.02
Cohort	Annane	54/85	67/92		44.69	0.87	0.71	1.07	0.19
	Subtotal	**140**	**167**			**0.66**	**0.43**	**1.02**	**0.06**
RCT	Meduri 1	[illegible]/16	5/8		18.05	0.20	0.05	0.81	0.02
RCT	Confalonieri	[illegible]/23	7/23		6.40	0.07	0.00	1.10	0.06
RCT	ARDSNet	28/89	29/91		40.13	0.99	0.64	1.52	0.95
RCT	Meduri 2	15/63	12/28		35.42	0.56	0.30	1.03	0.06
	Subtotal	**191**	**150**			**0.51**	**0.24**	**1.09**	**0.08**
	Total	**331**	**317**			**0.62**	**0.43**	**0.91**	**0.01**

Test for overall effect: $Z = -2.88$, $p = 0.004$
Test for heterogeneity: $p = 0.039$, $I^2 = 51\%$

0.01 0.1 1 10 100
Favours treatment Favours control

2

Secondary outcomes: morbidity outcomes

These results were in favour of corticosteroid in all summary estimates with over half reaching statistical significance.

Outcome	Result
Duration of mechanical ventilation	Reduced by > 4 days
ICU LOS	Reduced by > 4 days
Ventilator free days	Reduced (4.8 versus 4.4)
MODS score	Reduced by 32%
Lung injury score	Reduced by 18%
Oxygenation (PaO_2/FiO_2)	Improved by more than half a SD

Subgroup analysis: No statistically significant difference with regards to timing, formulation or tapering of therapy.

Adverse events: No increase in infections, neuromyopathy or other major complications

Author's conclusion

Morbidity and mortality were reduced with low dose corticosteroid therapy; there was no increase in adverse events, and neither timing nor discontinuation policy (tapering versus abrupt) made any difference. As a result of the small number of RCTs, these had to be combined with non-randomised studies. A significant effect was found in terms of mortality reduction with NNT = 4. The cohort studies carried more weight with mortality outcomes.

Problems & limitations

- 5 cohort studies are included and morbidity outcome data were different to those in RCTS but the RCTs contributed more weight
- Treatment regimens varied considerably between trials (dose range 40–250 mg/d; duration 7–32 days; initiation of treatment – within 1 week in 4 studies and later in 5)
- There was moderate to large heterogeneity in the mortality (51%) and morbidity (> 75%) outcomes respectively; therefore subgroup and metaregression analysis was performed
- Not all studies closely monitored for adverse events therefore these may have been under-reported

Advantages

- Findings suggest that the treatment effect of steroids did not differ between studies conducted before 2000 and after 2000 when ARDS network study on low tidal volume ventilation was published and lung protective strategies were propagated

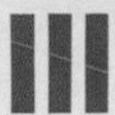

Expert opinion

Gianfranco Umberto Meduri

How valid and robust are the data?

This review identified 5 RCTs and 4 cohort studies (n = 648) of fair methodological quality conducted over a 17 years period. The use of prolonged (7–28 days) low-dose corticosteroids was associated with improved mortality and morbidity without increased adverse reactions. While heterogeneity was observed, subgroup and metaregression analyses showed that heterogeneity had minimal effect on treatment efficacy. The sizable increase in mechanical ventilation-free days (6.5 days; $p < 0.001$) and ICU-free days (7.0 days; $p < 0.001$) by day 28 is superior to any investigated intervention in ARDS.

Should clinical practice be influenced by this?

While evidence for mortality benefit is weak (grade 1B), evidence for increased mortality is lacking. The strong level of evidence (grade 1B) for improvement in patient-centred outcomes without increased adverse reactions makes low-dose corticosteroid treatment an essential aspect of treatment for ALI-ARDS. Secondary prevention and prolonged tapering to prevent rebound inflammation are essential to maximize benefits.

What is the next step?

A trial in paediatric ALI, and one in adults with severe pneumonia are in progress. A confirmatory trial in adult with early ALI-ARDS with mortality as a primary end-point is urgently needed.

2

Citation

Tang BMP, Craig JC, Eslick GD, Seppelt I, McLean AS. Use of corticosteroids in acute lung injury and acute respiratory distress syndrome: A systematic review and meta-analysis. Crit Care Med 2009 Vol. 37, No. 5 DOI: 10.1097/CCM.0b013e31819fb507

AMSTAR: methodological quality of the review

1.	Was "a priori" design provided?	Y
2.	Was study selection and data extraction adequate?	Y
3.	Was the literature search comprehensive?	Y
4.	Was 'Grey Literature' used?	Y
5.	Was a list of excluded studies provided?	P
6.	Were the characteristics of included studies provided?	Y
7.	Was the scientific quality of studies assessed & documented?	Y
8.	Was the scientific quality of studies weighted appropriately in forming conclusions?	Y
9.	Were the methods used for data synthesis appropriate?	Y
10.	Was the potential for publication bias assessed?	Y
11.	Were any conflicts of interest stated?	Y

Overall quality of trials included	Moderate
Overall quality of the review	High

ECMO

Condition: acute respiratory failure

Intervention: extra-corporeal membrane oxygenation (ECMO)

Clinical question: Does the use of ECMO improve survival in adults with acute respiratory failure?

Experience with the recent Influenza A (H1N1 subtype) pandemic has demonstrated that patients who require mechanical ventilation often develop severe respiratory failure with refractory hypoxaemia. ECMO has emerged as a potential rescue therapy; however, it is a specialised therapy which few centres can offer. There are currently no evidence-based clinical guidelines to inform institutions which patients are likely to benefit or about the optimal timing for transfer to ECMO centres.

Review characteristics

- **Eligibility criteria:** any study that reported on the use of ECMO in patients with influenza and any controlled trials or cohort studies comparing the management of acute respiratory failure (ARF) with and without ECMO: that had > 10 patients and reported mortality
- **Population:** adults with ARF due to H1N1 or any cause
- **Number of studies:** 3 RCTs of ECMO in ARF, 3 comparison studies of ECMO in ARF.
- **Only 1 case series of ECMO in patients with H1N1 influenza:** Australia, New Zealand ECMO influenza investigators. JAMA 2009; 302: 1888–1895
- **Number of patients:** RCTs + cohort n = 827 patients, case series n = 68
- **Study dates:** 1979–2009

Definitions

- For case series only: Severe hypoxaemia = median lowest PaO_2/FiO_2 of 56
- For other studies: ARDS not defined

Results

Primary outcome: mortality

Study type	Publication date	N (ECMO)	N (non- ECMO)	% H1N1	ECMO Mortality	Non-ECMO Mortality	p
RCT	2009	90	90	0	37%	50%	0.07
RCT	1994	21	19	0	67%	58%	0.8
RCT	1979	48*	42	0	90%	92%	0.84
Cohort	2006	32	118	0	47%	29%	0.06
Cohort	2000	62	183	0	45%	39%	NS
Cohort	1997	49	73	0	45	11	< 0.0001

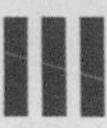

Study type	Publication date	N (ECMO)	N (non- ECMO)	% H1N1	ECMO Mortality	Non-ECMO Mortality	p
Case Series	2009	68	133	100%	23	13	0.06

* This included patients with other reasons for mechanical ventilation (MV)

Secondary outcomes

No secondary outcomes were reported.

Authors' conclusion

There is insufficient evidence to recommend ECMO for rescue therapy either in patients with H1N1 or other causes of severe acute respiratory failure. In the cohort studies and case series, it was the patients with the most severe respiratory failure that were in the ECMO group, thus mortality figures cannot be attributed to the use of ECMO.

2

Problems & limitations

- Few trials and small numbers
- RCT heterogeneity was statistically significant (I^2 = 58%)
- Trials were conducted over a 30-year period
- ECMO technology and expertise have improved over the last decade so how valid are the older studies?

Advantages

- This review has highlighted the lack of evidence as opposed to evidence against the use of ECMO

Expert opinion

Jeremy Cordingley

How valid and robust are the data?

This systematic review identified and conducted a meta-analysis of 3 RCTs of adult ECMO for severe acute respiratory failure of heterogeneous aetiology and reported no benefit associated with ECMO in the combined analysis. The included studies were conducted over a timescale of over 30 years using such widely varying ECMO techniques and equipment and thus meta-analysis is not valid. The review reports that there is very little evidence available to assess the benefit of ECMO versus conventional care in adult patients with influenza related ARDS.

Should clinical practice be influenced by this?

No new insights are described. The most relevant RCT of respiratory ECMO (CESAR trial) to modern practice, of patients with severe acute respiratory failure, found improved survival without severe disability at 6 months in patients transferred to an ECMO capable centre. The Australian and New Zealand case series showing good survival rates in patient with severe H1N1 influenza related ARDS treated with ECMO.

What's the next step?
The next step should be development of patient management guidelines that include discussion with an ECMO capable centre early enough in the course of severe acute respiratory failure for ECMO to be effective. Further RCTs will be difficult because of potential lack of equipoise in ECMO centres and the need for ECMO as a 'rescue' therapy in patients randomised to conventional management.

Citation

Mitchell MD, Mikkelsen ME, Umsheid CA, Lee I, Fuchs BD, Halpern SD. A systematic review to inform institutional decisions about the use of extracorporeal membrane oxygenation during the H1N1 influenza pandemic. Crit Care Med 2010; 38(6): 1398–1404

Additional information

This is the only recent RCT of ECMO in adults. From the Leicester Group (UK)

Efficacy and economic assessment of conventional ventilatory support versus extracorporeal membrane oxygenation for severe adult respiratory failure (CESAR): a multicentre randomised controlled trial.

Peek GJ, Mugford M, Tiruvoipati R, Wilson A, Allen E, Thalanany MM, Hibbert CL, Truesdale A, Clemens F, Cooper N, Firmin RK, Elbourne D, CESAR trial collaboration. Lancet. 2009 Oct 17;374(9698):1351–63. Epub 2009 Sep 15.

Useful editorial from the Brompton group (UK)

Finney SJ, Cordingley JJ, Griffiths MJD, Evans TW. ECMO in adults for severe respiratory failure finally comes of age: just in time? Thorax 2010;65:194–195

AMSTAR: methodological quality of the review

1.	Was "a priori" design provided?	Y
2.	Was study selection and data extraction adequate?	Y
3.	Was the literature search comprehensive?	Y
4.	Was 'Grey Literature' used?	Y
5.	Was a list of excluded studies provided?	NA
6.	Were the characteristics of included studies provided?	Y
7.	Was the scientific quality of studies assessed & documented?	Y
8.	Was the scientific quality of studies weighted appropriately in forming conclusions?	Y
9.	Were the methods used for data synthesis appropriate?	Y
10.	Was the potential for publication bias assessed?	N
11.	Were any conflicts of interest stated?	Y

Overall quality of trials included	Low
Overall quality of the review	High

3

Acute respiratory failure – Non-ARDS

Corticosteroids for pneumonia ____ 58
Corticosteroids to prevent and treat post extubation stridor ____ 64
Corticosteroids to prevent extubation failure ____ 70
Protocolized versus non-protocolized weaning ____ 75
NPPV for weaning ____ 82
Heated humidification versus HME ____ 88
Pleural effusions drainage ____ 93

Corticosteroids for pneumonia

Condition: pneumonia
Intervention: corticosteroids
Clinical question: Does the use of corticosteroids reduce mortality or influence the course of the illness in patients with pneumonia?

Pneumonia can be classified into three types: community acquired (CAP); hospital acquired (HAP) or aspiration pneumonitis. CAP and HAP can be caused by bacterial, viral, fungal or parasitic infections, and can cause a wide range of symptoms and signs from a mild cough to a severe life-threatening critical illness. Pneumonia is a common condition; the annual incidence in Europe & N. America is 34–40 per 1,000 in children and those over 60. Corticosteroids are anti-inflammatory, alter immune regulation and the stress response. Carbohydrate metabolism, protein catabolism, and fluid and electrolyte balance are all affected. They are used in a variety of inflammatory conditions but their benefit in pneumonia remains unclear. Short term side effects of steroids include hyperglycaemia and hypertension but these are reversible upon discontinuation. Most other complications are related to dose and duration of therapy, these include: immunosuppression, disturbance of metabolism, impaired wound healing, Cushing's, diabetes, hirsutism, osteoporosis and growth retardation in children.

3

Review characteristics

- **Eligibility criteria:** RCTs comparing corticosteroids with no steroids or corticosteroids of different doses in patient receiving appropriate treatment such as antibiotics
- **Exclusions:** cases associated with immunosuppression, HIV, TB, fungal or parasitic infections, chemotherapy or radiotherapy induced lung changes
- **Population:** patients of any age with pneumonia. In 1 paediatric study (n = 120) conducted in China all children had *mycoplasma pneumonia*, in the other paediatric study (n = 82) half the participants had bronchiolitis
- **Number of studies:** 6 RCTs. 2 trials in children, 4 trials in adults
- **Number of patients:** 437 in total. children n = 202, adults/elderly n= 235
- **Study dates:** 1 study from 1972, 1 study from 1993. The rest were between 2003–2007

Definitions

- **Pneumonia:** diagnosis based on history, examination and CXR +/– sputum cultures or CT scan
- **Pneumonia resolution:** improvement in CXR, normalisation of body temperature, WCC and CRP
- **Adverse events:** any event that might require intervention or jeopardise the patient
- **Corticosteroids:** hydrocortisone and prednisolone in the adult studies. Budesonide and dexamethasone in the paediatric studies

Fig. 1 Comparison 1 Hydrocortisone versus placebo, Outcome 1 Mortality [from Chen Y, Li K, Pu H, Wu T. Corticosteroids for pneumonia. Cochrane Database of Systematic Reviews 2011, Issue 3. Art. No.: CD007720, © Cochrane Collaboration, reproduced with permission]

Review: Corticosteroids for pneumonia
Comparison: 1 Hydrocortisone versus placebo
Outcome: 1 Mortality

Study or subgroup	Experimental n/N	Control n/N	Peto Odds Ratio Peto, Fixed, 95% CI	Weight	Peto Odds Ratio Peto, Fixed, 95% CI
Confalonieri 2005	0/23	2/23		35.4%	0.13 [0.01, 2.13]
Marik 1993	1/14	3/16		64.6%	0.38 [0.05, 3.01]
Total (95% CI)	**37**	**39**		**100.0%**	**0.26 [0.05, 1.37]**

Total events: 1 (Experimental), 5 (Control)
Heterogeneity: $Chi^2 = 0.36$, df = 1 (P = 0.55); $I^2 = 0.0\%$
Test for overall effect: Z = 1.59 (P = 0.11)

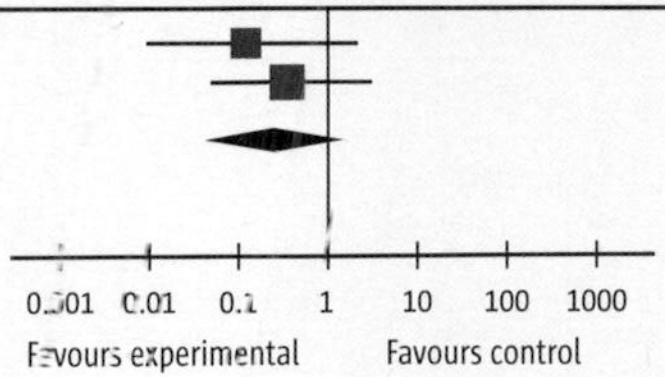

3

Results

Primary outcome: mortality

There was no statistically significant differences compared with placebo in 3 studies that used hydrocortisone or prednisolone (OR 0.26, 95% CI 0.05 to 1.37). There was 1 death in the corticosteroid group compared to 5 in the placebo group.

Secondary outcomes

Oxygenation

In 1 high quality study (n = 46) there was a significant improvement in PaO_2:FiO_2. Another low quality study (n = 31) reported no difference in the number of days that it took for the saturations to normalise

Time to pneumonia resolution

3 studies showed faster resolution in symptoms and signs with corticosteroids and 1 study showed no difference

Relapse of illness

In 1 paediatric study, 30 patients receiving budesonide had a lower rate of relapse

Ventilatory and/or inotropic support

2 adult studies (n = 76) there was less need for mechanical ventilation in the hydrocortisone group

In 1 high quality paediatric study (n = 82) the dexamethasone group had significantly longer duration of mechanical ventilation and supplemental oxygen

Time to discharge

In 2 studies there was no difference in ICU LOS

Adverse events

Adult studies: 1 episode of arrhythmia, and 1 GI bleed

Paediatric studies: 1 patient developed malignant hypertension after 3 days of corticosteroids

Author's conclusion

Corticosteroids did not significantly reduce mortality but there was some benefit. Corticosteroids can improve oxygenation, accelerate the resolution of symptoms and signs, and reduce relapse rate. This effect was observed in the study that included severe cases and not the study that excluded them so it may be that corticosteroid are only beneficial in cases of severe pneumonia. Subgroup analysis in paediatric studies showed that those with bronchiolitis and mycoplasma pneumonia are likely to benefit most.

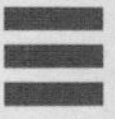

Fig. 2 Comparison 2 Prednisolone plus antibiotics versus antibiotics alone, Outcome 1 Death [from Chen Y, Li K, Pu H, Wu T. Corticosteroids for pneumonia. Cochrane Database of Systematic Reviews 2011, Issue 3. Art. No.: CD007720, © Cochrane Collaboration, reproduced with permission]

Review: Corticosteroids for pneumonia
Comparison: 2 Prednisolone plus antibiotics versus antibiotics alone
Outcome: 1 Death

Study or subgroup	Experimental n/N	Control n/N	Peto Odds Ratio Peto, Fixed, 95% CI	Weight	Peto Odds Ratio Peto, Fixed, 95% CI
1 Ampicillin (1g daily) vs ampicillin (1g daily) with prednisolone (20mg daily)					
McHardy 1972	7/43	1/20		65.1%	2.72 [0.56, 13.22]
Subtotal (95% CI)	**43**	**20**		**65.1%**	**2.72 [0.56, 13.22]**
Total events: 7 (Experimental), 1 (Control)					
Heterogeneity: not applicable					
Test for overall effect: Z = 1.24 (P = 0.21)					
2 Ampicillin (2g daily) vs ampicillin (2g daily) with prednisolone (20mg daily)					
McHardy 1972	2/43	2/20		34.9%	0.41 [0.05, 3.57]
Subtotal (95% CI)	**43**	**20**		**34.9%**	**0.41 [0.05,3.57]**
Total events: 2 (Experimental), 2 (Control)					
Heterogeneity: not applicable					
Test for overall effect: Z = 0.80 (P = 0.42)					
Total (95% CI)	**86**	**40**		**100.0%**	**1.41 [0.39, 5.04]**
Total events: 9 (Experimental), 3 (Control)					
Heterogeneity: $Chi^2 = 1.91$, df = 1 (P = 0.17); $I^2 = 48\%$					
Test for overall effect: Z = 0.53 (P = 0.60)					
Test for subgroup differences: $Chi^2 = 1.91$, df = 1 (P = 0.17); $I^2 = 48\%$					

0.01 0.1 1 10 100
Favours experimental Favours control

3

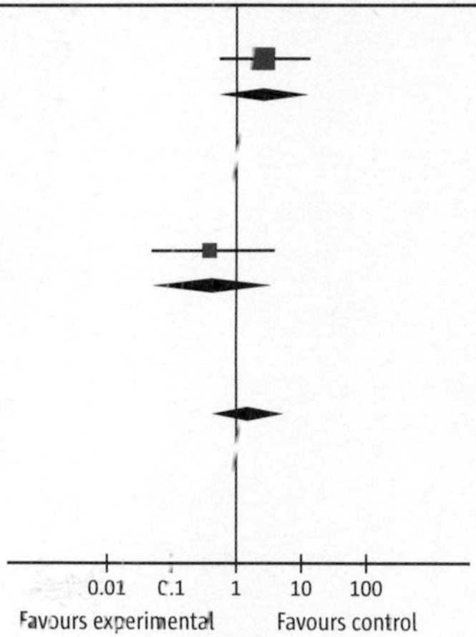

Problems & limitations

- 10 trials were excluded due to difficulty retrieving the article or contacting authors but will be include in the review update and may alter the results
- Mostly low quality trials with a small number of participants
- Results were inconsistent between studies

Advantages

- This has highlighted the need for better quality and larger clinical trials in this area

Expert opinion

John Carlisle

3

How valid and robust are the data?
13 studies still await assessment, 11 of which might be RCTs (can only be determined by retrieving full text). Only one or two RCTs contributed meagre data to each outcome. Therefore retrieval and analysis of these 11 studies might considerably change the results. The results of this systematic review cannot therefore be considered a robust reflection of current evidence.

There are a few minor discrepancies within the systematic review that are however a little unsettling, for instance the authors intended to analyse dichotomous outcomes with a random-effects model, reported as relative risk, but they reported mortality as an odds ratio using a fixed-effect model. Both models produce non-significant differences, yet the casual reader might be more encouraged to consider using corticosteroid by reading the odds ratio with fixed-effect model rather than the relative risk with random-effects model, the latter of which produces a smaller difference with wider confidence intervals.

Should clinical practice be influenced by this?
Yes, to the extent that enthusiastic users of steroids should consider the paucity of evidence, which at the moment cannot be considered to support corticosteroids as a standard treatment for pneumonia.

What's the next step?
The evidence for harm was not significant, with the proviso that study analysis was incomplete and rare severe complications will not be identified by even large RCTs. Clinical use of steroids for pneumonia is not a standard, yet it is probably sufficiently widespread that a multinational RCT should be planned to determine whether the practice harms patients with pneumonia, benefits them or makes no difference.

Citation

Chen Y, Li K, Pu H,Wu T. Corticosteroids for pneumonia. Cochrane Database of Systematic Reviews 2011, Issue 3. Art. No.: CD007720. DOI: 10.1002/14651858.CD007720.pub2.

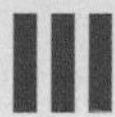

AMSTAR: methodological quality of the review

1.	Was "a priori" design provided?	Y
2.	Was study selection and data extraction adequate?	Y
3.	Was the literature search comprehensive?	Y
4.	Was 'Grey Literature' used?	Y
5.	Was a list of excluded studies provided?	Y
6.	Were the characteristics of included studies provided?	Y
7.	Was the scientific quality of studies assessed & documented?	Y
8.	Was the scientific quality of studies weighted appropriately in forming conclusions?	Y
9.	Were the methods used for data synthesis appropriate?	P
10.	Was the potential for publication bias assessed?	Y
11.	Were any conflicts of interest stated?	Y

Overall quality of trials included	Only 2 were high quality
Overall quality of the review	High

Corticosteroids to prevent and treat post extubation stridor

Condition: post extubation stridor
Intervention: corticosteroids
Clinical question: Does the use of corticosteroids before elective extubation reduce the incidence of stridor and re-intubation?

Following intubation the pressure or irritation from the endotracheal tube (ETT) may cause glottic or sub-glottic reactive oedema. This is thought to occur in up to 37% of critically ill children. Airway anatomy in neonates, infants and children is considerably different to that in adults; their airways are narrower therefore any oedema would represent a relatively larger proportion of the airway diameter. In infants and children the narrowest part of the airway is at the level of the cricoid therefore subglottic obstruction is more likely whereas in adults laryngeal oedema is more likely. Post extubation airway obstruction causing stridor or respiratory distress may result in reintubation, prolonging ICU stay and associated complications. The anti-inflammatory action of corticosteroids steroids may prevent or reduce oedema; however steroids are associated with a range of side effects including hypertension and hyperglycaemia.

Review characteristics

- **Eligibility criteria:** RCTs comparing parenteral corticosteroids (intravenous, intramuscular or inhaled) with placebo in the 24 hours prior to and following extubation
- **Exclusions:** trials that did not assess laryngeal oedema or stridor
- **Population:** infants, children and adults in medical or surgical intensive care units
- **A priori:** to analyse data from studies on infants, children, and neonates separately; to analyse data from trials assessing prevention and treatment separately
- **Number of studies:** 11 RCTs: 2 studies on neonates; 3 studies on paediatric patients; 6 studies on adults. (10 studies of prophylactic corticosteroids, 1 study of dexamethasone given to neonates already re-intubated for stridor)
- **Number of patients:** neonates n = 109; non-neonate paediatric n = 242, adults n = 1959
- **Study dates:** 1989–2007

Definitions

- **Corticosteroid:** varies between studies. 7 used dexamethasone (0.25–0.5 mg/kg or 5–8 mg); 3 studies used methylprednisolone 20–40 mg; 1 study used hydrocortisone 100 mg

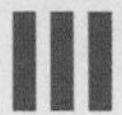

Results

Corticosteroids for prevention of post-extubation airway obstruction

Neonates

Overall there was no significant difference in the incidence of stridor between steroid and placebo groups (RR 0.42, 95% CI 0.07–2.32). There were too few re-intubations to make meaningful conclusions regarding the re-intubation rate

In 1 study: high risk patients treated with multiple doses of steroid who had traumatic or multiple intubations had a lower incidence of stridor

Children

There was a trend towards less post-extubation stridor (RR 0.53, 95% CI 0.36–0.97, I^2 = 53%) with steroids but the studies were too heterogeneous to make meaningful conclusions

One study demonstrated a trend towards reduction in re-intubation in patients with airway anomalies but NSS

Adults

The adult studies were very heterogeneous with a trend toward less stridor

(RR 0.47, 95% CI 0.22–0.99, I^2 = 81%) and

A trend towards less re intubation in the treatment group (RR 0.48, 95% CI 0.19–1.22, I^2 = 50%)

This potential benefit of steroids were due to the 3 most recent trials (2006–2007), 2 of which only recruited patients with < 24% cuff leak volume, possibly representing a higher risk group.

Post-hoc subgroup analysis

Multiple doses of steroid given 12–24 hours before extubation versus single dose

There was a statistically significant reduction in stridor with multiple doses compared to single doses (Ratio of Relative Risk (RRR) 0.23, 95% CI 0.11–0.48)

No significant difference in re-intubation risk with multiple doses compared to a single dose (RRR 0.26, 95% CI 0.07–1.04)

Corticosteroids for the treatment of airway obstruction

1 study (n = 33) in children already re-intubated for airway obstruction

No significant difference in stridor score after the second extubation between those given steroids prior to the second extubation and those who were not.

Adverse events

Variable reporting, overall incidence was low

Included glycosuria in children; GI bleed and hypertension

Fig. 3 Forest plot of comparison: Treated versus Controls; all, outcome: Re-intubation Rate [from Khemani RG, Randolph A, Markovitz B. Corticosteroids for the prevention and treatment of post-extubation stridor in neonates, children and adults. Cochrane Database of Systematic Reviews 2009, Issue 3. Art. No.: CD001000, © Cochrane Collaboration, reproduced with permission]

Study or subgroup		Treatment Events	Treatment Total	Control Events	Control Total	Weight	Risk Ratio M-H, Random, 95% CI
1.1.1 Neonates	Couser 1992	0	27	4	23	100.0%	0.10 [0.01, 1.68]
	Ferrara 1998	0	30	0	29		Not estimable
	Subtotal (95% CI)		**57**		**52**	**100.0%**	**0.10 [0.01, 1.68]**
	Total events	0		4			
	Heterogeneity: Not applicable						
	Test for overall effect: Z = 1.61 (P = 0.11)						
1.1.2 Children	Anene 1996	0	31	7	32	28.6%	0.07 [0.00, 1.15]
	Tellez 1991	9	76	4	77	71.4%	2.28 [0.73, 7.09]
	Subtotal (95% CI)		**107**		**109**	**100.0%**	**0.49 [0.01, 19.65]**
	Total events	9		11			
	Heterogeneity: $Tau^2 = 6.00$, $Chi^2 = 5.99$, df = 1 (P = 0.01); $I^2 = 83\%$						
	Test for overall effect: Z = 0.38 (P = 0.70)						
1.1.3 Adults	Cheng 2006	5	85	8	43	25.3%	0.32 [0.11, 0.91]
	Darmon 1992	18	343	20	351	30.4%	0.92 [0.50, 1.71]
	Francois 2007	1	355	14	343	14.9%	0.07 [0.01, 0.52]]
	Gaussorgues 1987	2	138	0	138	8.8%	5.00 [0.24, 103.20]
	Ho 1996	0	39	1	38	8.2%	0.33 [0.01, 7.74]
	Lee 2007	1	40	2	40	12.4%	0.50 [0.05, 5.30]
	Subtotal (95% CI)		**1000**		**953**	**100.0%**	**0.48 [0.19, 1.22]**
	Total events	27		45			
	Heterogeneity: $Tau^2 = 0.57$, $Chi^2 = 9.95$, df = 5 (P = 0.08); $I^2 = 50\%$						
	Test for overall effect: Z = 1.55 (P = 0.12)						

Fig. 4 Forest plot of comparison. Post hoc subgroup analysis: adults, multiple doses, 12–24 hours prior to extubation, outcome: Re-intubation Rate [from Khemani RG, Randolph A, Markovitz B. Corticosteroids for the prevention and treatment of post-extubation stridor in neonates, children and adults. Cochrane Database of Systematic Reviews 2009, Issue 3. Art. No.: CD001000, © Cochrane Collaboration, reproduced with permission]

Study or subgroup	Treated Events	Treated Total	Control Events	Control Total	Weight	Risk Ratio M-H, Random, 95% CI
3.1.1 Multiple Doses, 12–24 h prior to extubation						
Cheng 2006	3	42	4	21	45.3%	0.38 [0.09, 1.52]
Francois 2007	1	355	14	343	29.6%	0.07 [0.01, 0.52]
Lee 2007	1	40	2	40	23.6%	0.50 [0.05, 5.30]
Subtotal (95% CI)		**437**		**404**	**100.0%**	**0.25 [0.07, 0.83]**
Total events	5		20			
Heterogeneity: $Tau^2 = 0.27$; $Chi^2 = 2.57$, df = 2 (P = 0.28); $I^2 = 22\%$						
Test for overall effect: Z = 2.27 (P = 0.02)						
3.1.2. Single dose, within 12 hours of extubation						
Darmon 1992	18	343	20	351	72.9%	0.92 [0.50, 1.71]
Gaussorgues 1987	2	133	0	138	14.1%	5.00 [0.24, 103.20]
Ho 1996	0	39	1	38	13.0%	0.33 [0.01, 7.74]
Subtotal (95% CI)		**520**		**527**	**100.0%**	**0.05 [0.52, 1.72]**
Total events	20		21			
Heterogeneity: $Tau^2 = 0.00$, $Chi^2 = 1.61$, df = 2 (P = 0.45); $I^2 = 0\%$						
Test for overall effect: Z = 0.18 (P = 0.86)						
3.1.3. Single dose, 24 hours prior to extubation						
Cheng 2006	[illegible]	43	4	22	100.0%	0.26 [0.05, 1.29]
Subtotal (95% CI)		**43**		**22**	**100.0%**	**0.26 [0.05, 1.29]**
Total events	2		4			
Heterogeneity: Not applicable						
Test for overall effect: Z = 1.65 (P = 0.10)						

3

Author's conclusion

Routine use of corticosteroids in all patients is not recommended, however corticosteroids may be beneficial in certain high risk neonates and in high risk adults if administered as multiple doses 12–24 hours before extubation. There is insufficient evidence to conclude that prophylactic intervention with corticosteroids is beneficial for children.

Problems & limitations

- Clinical and statistical heterogeneity between all trials $I^2 > 50\%$ regardless of age
- Some studies in neonates and children excluded high risk groups such as those with known airway abnormalities or infections and some studies included them.
- In neonates the duration of intubation ranged from 48 hours to 14 days
- In adults corticosteroid treatment ranged from a single dose not long before extubation to multiple doses commencing 24 hours prior to extubation
- Most studies in adults excluded high risk patients: those with airway disease or surgery
- Duration of corticosteroids varied greatly from 24 hours to 30 minutes before extubation
- Small number of patients in neonate and paediatric trials

Advantages

- Outcome in neonates is similar to that of a previous review on the same topic
- Acceptable overall number of patients in the adults trials

Expert opinion

Djillali Annane

How valid and robust are the data?
This review met high standard for methodological quality. There are very few studies in neonates and children, and available studies are small sized. In adults, there are sufficient data favouring the beneficial effects of multiple-doses of corticosteroids initiated 12 to 24 hours prior extubation. The authors' conclusions are fair and valid.

Should clinical practice be influenced by this?
The current incidence of significant post extubation stridor is too low to warrant the systematic use of corticosteroids before extubation. This treatment should be considered only in patients at high risk of post extubation stridor as identified by the cuff leak test.

What is the next step?
Additional trials are needed in neonates and children to evaluate the benefit to risk ratio of multiple-doses corticosteroids given 12 to 24 hours before extubation. Additional studies are needed to optimise the identification of high risk patients.

Citation

Khemani RG, Randolph A, Markovitz B. Corticosteroids for the prevention and treatment of post-extubation stridor in neonates, children and adults. Cochrane Database of Systematic Reviews 2009, Issue 3. Art. No.: CD001000. DOI: 10.1002/14651858.CD001000.pub3

Additional information

Also see next review summary on "Corticosteroids to prevent extubation failure" which included all 11 studies here and a further 3.

AMSTAR: methodological quality of the review

1.	Was "a priori" design provided?	Y
2.	Was study selection and data extraction adequate?	Y
3.	Was the literature search comprehensive?	Y
4.	Was 'Grey Literature' used?	Y
5.	Was a list of excluded studies provided?	Y
6.	Were the characteristics of included studies provided?	Y
7.	Was the scientific quality of studies assessed & documented?	Y
8.	Was the scientific quality of studies weighted appropriately in forming conclusions?	Y
9.	Were the methods used for data synthesis appropriate?	Y
10.	Was the potential for publication bias assessed?	N
11.	Were any conflicts of interest stated?	Y

Overall quality of trials included	Moderate to high on Jadad scale
Overall quality of the review	High

Corticosteroids to prevent extubation failure

Condition: extubation failure

Intervention: corticosteroids

Clinical question: Does the use of corticosteroids prior to extubation reduce the incidence of extubation failure?

Laryngeal oedema is a common complication of prolonged intubation and may contribution to extubation failure. Re-intubation is associated with increased duration of mechanical ventilation, higher risk of nosocomial pneumonia, prolonged ICU and hospital length of stay and increased mortality. Some studies have shown reductions in the subjective signs of laryngeal oedema with the use of corticosteroids prior to intubation however these were not powered to determine whether clinically relevant outcomes such as extubation failure were altered.

Review characteristics

- **Eligibility criteria:** RCTs that compared any corticosteroid with placebo or standard care
- **Population:** neonates, children and adults on critical care units
- **Number of studies:** total of 14 RCTs. 3 neonatal studies (in 2 studies mean gestational age was 33 weeks), 4 paediatric (age 19 months to 2.5 years) and 7 adult
- **Number of patients:** 2,600
- **Study dates:** 1987–2007

Definitions

- **Corticosteroid:** dexamethasone 0.25–0.5 mg/kg; methylprednisolone 20–80 mg; prednisolone 1 mg/kg; and hydrocortisone
- **Standard care:** not specified

Results

Outcomes	GRADE
Mean duration of days of mechanical ventilation Neonate studies: 6–20 days Paediatric studies: 3.3–21 days Adult studies: 5.3–14 days (except 1 study < 36 hours)	–
13 studies (1 study had no re-intubations): There was a significant reduction in the rate of re-intubation with the use of corticosteroids (OR 0.56, 95% CI 0.41–0.77, $p < 0.0005$) NNT to prevent 1 re-intubation is 29 or 35 re-intubations prevented per 1,000 extubations Heterogeneity was low ($I^2 = 38\%$)	High

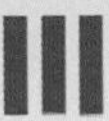

Outcomes	GRADE
Sensitivity analysis There tended to be a greater effect of corticosteroids and less heterogeneity with duration of therapy for more than 12 hours, and in studies with adequate allocation concealment	–
9 studies reported subjective assessment: these showed a significant reduction in subjective manifestations of laryngeal oedema (OR 0.36, 95% CI 0.27–0.49, $p < 0.0005$) but there was significant heterogeneity ($I^2 = 72\%$)	High
Adverse events were infrequently reported These included hyperglycaemia and glycosuria	–

Author's conclusion

Corticosteroids significantly reduce the rate of reintubation for mechanically ventilated intensive care patients, and this effect may have been more pronounced when therapy is commenced 12 hours or more before extubation. The patients in these studies were ventilated for prolonged periods therefore the results of this review cannot be extrapolated to patients who require a short duration of intubation.

The optimal regimen of treatment remains to be defined, but should be commenced at least 12 hours before extubation. Studies in neonates and children used 0.25–0.5 mg/kg of dexamethasone. The dose and type of steroid varied more in the adult studies therefore it would be reasonable to use the same regimen as the largest high quality RCT which used 20 mg of methylprednisolone.

Steroids may have prevented re-intubation by mechanisms other than that related to laryngeal oedema alone.

3

Problems & limitations

- Different corticosteroid types, doses and regimens use in the trials
- Pooling of results from paediatric and adult populations
- High heterogeneity in the studies of subjective assessment of laryngeal oedema
- Subjective assessment cannot be reliable without clear criteria: only 6 studies included a cuff leak test; 8 studies had criteria for extubation and only 5 studies defined criteria for re-intubation

Advantages

- There was no suggestion of bias on the funnel plot
- Results were consistent across all populations
- Results agreed with those of the largest high quality RCT

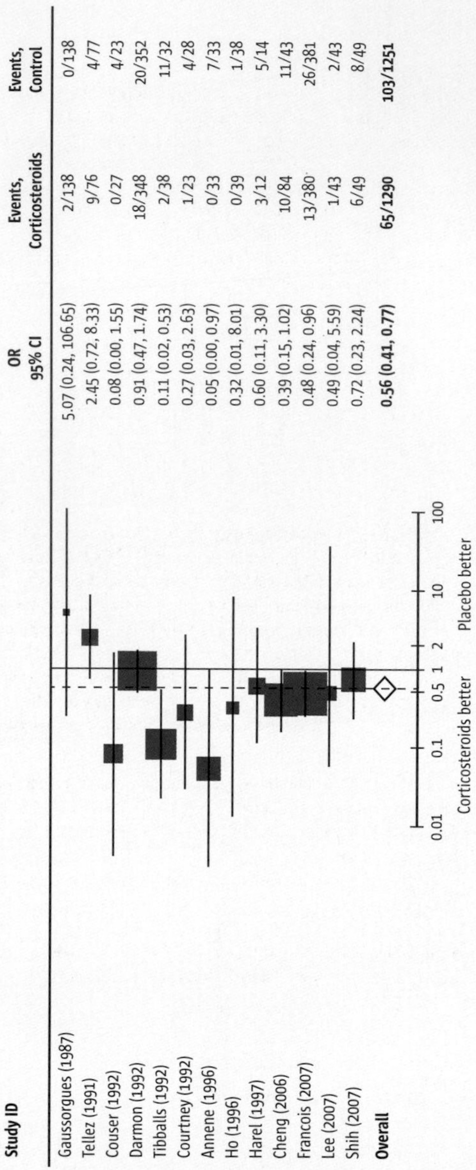

Fig. 5 The effect of corticosteroids on reintubation [With kind permission from Springer Science+Business Media: Corticosteroids to prevent extubation failure: a systematic review and meta-analysis. Intensive Care Med (2009) 35:977–986, John McCaffrey, Clare Farrell, Paul Whiting, Arina Dan, Sean M. Bagshaw, Anthony P. Delaney, figure 2]

Study ID	OR 95% CI	Events, Corticosteroids	Events, Control
Gaussorgues (1987)	5.07 (0.24, 106.65)	2/138	0/138
Tellez (1991)	2.45 (0.72, 8.33)	9/76	4/77
Couser (1992)	0.08 (0.00, 1.55)	0/27	4/23
Darmon (1992)	0.91 (0.47, 1.74)	18/348	20/352
Tibballs (1992)	0.11 (0.02, 0.53)	2/38	11/32
Courtney (1992)	0.27 (0.03, 2.63)	1/23	4/28
Annene (1996)	0.05 (0.00, 0.97)	0/33	7/33
Ho (1996)	0.32 (0.01, 8.01)	0/39	1/38
Harel (1997)	0.60 (0.11, 3.30)	3/12	5/14
Cheng (2006)	0.39 (0.15, 1.02)	10/84	11/43
Francois (2007)	0.48 (0.24, 0.96)	13/380	26/381
Lee (2007)	0.49 (0.04, 5.59)	1/43	2/43
Shih (2007)	0.72 (0.23, 2.24)	6/49	8/49
Overall	**0.56 (0.41, 0.77)**	**65/1290**	**103/1251**

0.01 0.1 0.5 1 2 10 100

Corticosteroids better Placebo better

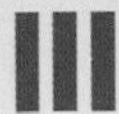

Expert opinion

Laurent Brochard

How valid and robust are the data?

This nice systematic review found 14 RCTs meeting their criteria and including 2,600 patients. All causes of reintubation were examined, which is a clinically relevant outcome. Neonates, infants and adults were included. Although it seems there is no statistical heterogeneity, there was indeed some heterogeneity on important clinical issues: timing of administration, e.g. right before extubation versus 12 to 24 hours before extubation, type of patients and underlying respiratory disease, e.g. inclusion of children with viral croup, and whether or not a selection of high risk patients was performed, including the use of cuff-leak test. Overall, the study strongly suggests that there is a beneficial signal regarding steroids for preventing reintubation, coming from all these studies, and this result has a strong biological plausibility.

Should clinical practice be influenced by this?

As mentioned above, the major clinical heterogeneity of several important clinical factors does not allow to determine us exactly what should be done in clinical practice and for which patients. This has to be also confronted with several other systematic reviews on the same topic, some suggesting that the benefit exist only in high risk patients (Effects of steroids on reintubation and post-extubation stridor in adults: meta-analysis of randomised controlled trials. Jaber S, Jung B, Chanques G, Bonnet F, Marret E. Crit Care. 2009;13(2):R49), some suggesting that the conclusion cannot be extended to neonates, or only to high risk patients (Steroids for post extubation stridor: pediatric evidence is still inconclusive. Khemani RG, Randolph A, Markovitz B. Intensive Care Med. 2010 Jul;36(7):1276–7; Corticosteroids for the prevention and treatment of post-extubation stridor in neonates, children and adults. Khemani RG, Randolph A, Markovitz B. Cochrane Database Syst Rev. 2009 Jul 8;(3):CD001000). This is important because the number needed to treat may vary widely depending on the category of patients selected and treated. Therefore, regarding clinical practice, once one can identify high risk patients (for reintubation or stridor), this study is reassuring about the preventive effect of previous steroid administration. It does not allow defining a more precise strategy. As an example, administration of steroids 12 or 24 h before extubation requires a weaning strategy which predicts extubation attempts 12 or 24 h in advance, otherwise it will delay extubation for many patients.

What is the next step?

Better characterize the high risk groups and the place of the cuff leak test. One possibility could be that performing the cuff-leak test either in high risk selected patients or systematically in all patients, followed by steroids in case of negative leaks could be an interesting pragmatic strategy which needs to be tested

Citation

McCaffrey J, Farrell C, Whiting C, Dan A, Bagshaw SM, Delaney AP. Corticosteroids to prevent extubation failure: a systematic review and meta-analysis. Intensive Care Med (2009) 35:977–986 DOI 10.1007/s00134-009-1473-9

Additional information

Go to preview review summary on "Corticosteroids for the prevention of extubation stridor"

Compared to the previous review, this review had 3 more trials and used all cause re-intubation not just reintubation due to stridor. In this review assessment of stridor was felt to be prone to ascertainment bias and all-cause reintubation was felt to be a more clinically relevant outcome.

3

AMSTAR: methodological quality of the review

1.	Was "a priori" design provided?	Y
2.	Was study selection and data extraction adequate?	Y
3.	Was the literature search comprehensive?	Y
4.	Was 'Grey Literature' used?	Y
5.	Was a list of excluded studies provided?	P
6.	Were the characteristics of included studies provided?	Y
7.	Was the scientific quality of studies assessed & documented?	Y
8.	Was the scientific quality of studies weighted appropriately in forming conclusions?	Y
9.	Were the methods used for data synthesis appropriate?	Y
10.	Was the potential for publication bias assessed?	Y
11.	Were any conflicts of interest stated?	Y

Overall quality of trials included	Moderate to high
Overall quality of the review	High

Protocolized versus non-protocolized weaning

Condition: mechanical ventilation

Intervention: protocolized weaning

Clinical question: Does protocolized weaning reduce the duration of mechanical ventilation or improve clinically important outcomes?

The majority (75%) of intensive care patients can be weaned easily form mechanical ventilation. The remaining 25% in whom weaning is difficult, experience greater morbidity including ventilator associated pneumonia and ventilator associated lung injury; required longer ICU and hospital lengths of stay and have higher mortality. Several weaning strategies exist amongst critical care clinicians: gradual weaning from initiation of mechanical ventilation; full support initially and gradual weaning with early signs of improvement; or weaning only when the condition has significantly resolved. There is evidence (Levine 2008) that marked atrophy of diaphragmatic myofibrils occurs within three days of mechanical ventilation which suggest that some early spontaneous breathing would be beneficial. 3

Weaning strategy often depends upon the experience and judgement of the attending physician, however predictions based on judgement alone have low sensitivity and specificity and physicians tend to underestimate the probability of successful weaning. Ventilation techniques that have been used to assist weaning include: gradual reduction of pressure support; spontaneous breathing with CPAP, intermittent T piece or newer ventilation modes such as BIPAP. These all seem to be equally successful however evidence suggests that SIMV is the least effective.

Weaning protocols take advantage of collective knowledge, maximise consistency and objectivity. They are based on three components: "readiness to wean" criteria; reducing ventilator support; and finally extubation. Protocols can be presented as algorithms for healthcare professional to make manual adjustments to ventilation or the newer automated weaning modes such as adaptive support ventilation (ADV) can be used which titrate support according to patient interactions with the ventilator. Weaning protocols have been shown to be safe and effective however the evidence supporting their use in clinical practice has been inconsistent.

Review characteristics

- **Eligibility criteria:** randomised and quasi randomised trials comparing a standardized weaning protocol to usual weaning practice
- **Exclusions:** trials of NIV as a weaning strategy and trials of tracheostomized patients only
- **A priori:** sensitivity analysis to examine effect of excluding trials with high risk of bias on total duration of mechanical ventilation and weaning duration. Subgroup analysis on the impact of the type of ICU and type of protocol
- **Population:** adults from medical/surgical/trauma and mixed ICUs
- **Number of studies:** 11 studies, 2 of which were quasi randomised. Europe (3 studies), N. America (6 studies), Brazil (1 study) and Australia (1 study)
- **Number of patients:** 1971 (range 15–357)
- **Study dates:** 1996–2009

Definitions

- **Usual weaning practice:** varied between trials. Defined as physician's discretion in 7 studies. 4 studies used reductions in the following: SIMV & PSV, PSV alone, PEEP & PSV
- **Weaning protocol:** had to have criteria to initiate weaning; structured guidelines for reducing ventilator support; and may have had extubation criteria
- **Protocol delivery:** professional (physician, respiratory nurse or therapist) in 6 studies or computerised in 3 studies, unclear in 2 studies
- **Discontinuation from MV:** when mechanical ventilation support was stopped and the patient was breathing spontaneously through a T-piece or following extubation
- **End of weaning:** the patient should be extubated and breathing spontaneously without the need for ventilator support or re-intubation for 48–72 hours

Results

Primary outcome: total duration of mechanical ventilation

Outcome/Analysis	Results
Total duration of MV	Pooled analysis of 10 studies (n = 1973) showed a significant reduction with protocolized weaning of 19.5 hours* (MD −19.5, 95% CI −35.91 to −3.10, $p = 0.02$)
Subgroup analysis according to ICU type on duration of MV	Mixed ICUs, medical ICUs and neurosurgical showed a non-significant reduction in the protocolized group Surgical ICUs showed a significant reduction in the protocolized group
Subgroup analysis according to protocol delivery on duration of MV	8 studies that used professional led weaning showed a significant reduction favouring protocolized weaning 2 studies using computerized weaning showed a non-significant reduction favouring protocolized methods

* GRADE = low

The outcome data were skewed and therefore log-transformation was use to represent the primary analysis. Data are reported in terms of log mean and geometric mean (refer to original article).

Fig. 6 Forest plot of comparison: 1 Primary Analysis: Protocolized versus non-protocolized weaning, outcome: 1.1 Total duration of MV by type of unit [reproduced from Bronagh Blackwood, Fiona Alderdice, Karen Burns, Chris Cardwell, 3 Gavin Lavery, Peter O'Halloran. Protocolized versus non-prtocolized weaning for reducing the duration of mechanical ventilation in critically ill patients. Cochrane database of systematic reviews 2010, Issue 5. Art NO.: CD006904, with permission from BMJ Publishing Group Ltd]

	Experimental			Control				Mean Differnce
Study or subgroup	Mean [log hours]	SD [log hours]	Total	Mean [log hours]	SD [log hours]	Total	Weight	IV, Random, 95% CI [log hours]
1.1.1 Mixed ICUs								
Kollef 1997	3.33	1.2	179	3.56	0.96	178	12.1%	-0.23 [-0.46, -0.00]
Marelich 2000	4.22	1.2	166	4.82	1.36	169	11.3%	-0.60 [-0.87, -0.33]
Piotto 2008	4.27	1.39	18	3.81	1.44	18	3.7%	0.46 [-0.45, 1.38]
Rose 2008	4.793	0.752	51	4.828	0.863	51	10.7%	-0.04 [-0.35, 0.28]
Subtotal (95% CI)			**414**			**416**	**37.8%**	**-0.23 [-0.54, 0.09]**
Heterogeneity: $Tau^2 = 0.06$; $Chi^2 = 10.20$, df = 3 (P = 0.02); $I^2 = 71\%$								
Test for overall effect: Z = 1.42 (P = 0.16)								
1.1.2 Neuro ICUs								
Namen 2001	4.97	0.75	49	4.97	1.4	51	8.7%	0.00 [-0.44, 0.44]
Navalesi 2008	4.328	0.92	165	4.338	0.96	153	12.4%	-0.01 [-0.22, 0.20]
Subtotal (95% CI)			**214**			**204**	**21.1%**	**-0.01 [-0.20, 0.18]**
Heterogeneity: $Tau^2 = 0.00$; $Chi^2 = 0.00$, df = 1 (P = 0.97); $I^2 = 0\%$								
Test for overall effect: Z = 0.09 (P = 0.93)								

Mean Differnce IV, Random, 95% CI [log hours]

-1 -0.5 0 0.5 1

Favours protocol weaning Favours usual care

(Continued ...)

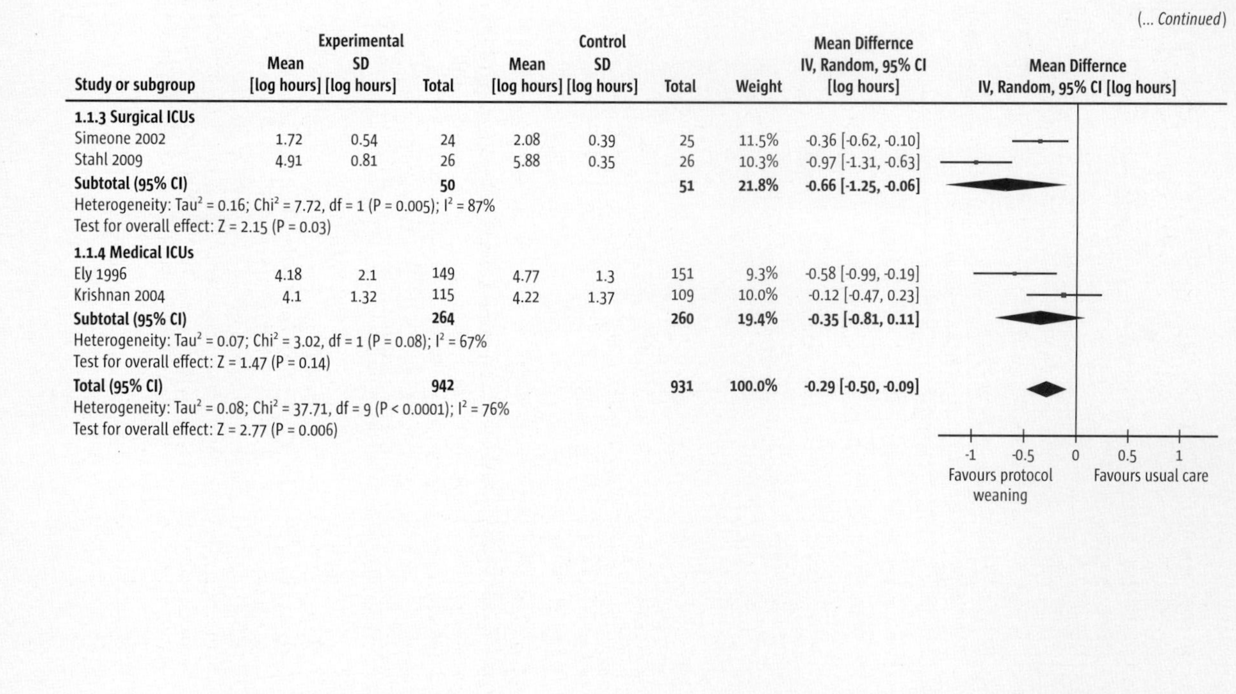

(... Continued)

Study or subgroup	Experimental Mean [log hours]	Experimental SD [log hours]	Experimental Total	Control Mean [log hours]	Control SD [log hours]	Control Total	Weight	Mean Differnce IV, Random, 95% CI [log hours]
1.1.3 Surgical ICUs								
Simeone 2002	1.72	0.54	24	2.08	0.39	25	11.5%	-0.36 [-0.62, -0.10]
Stahl 2009	4.91	0.81	26	5.88	0.35	26	10.3%	-0.97 [-1.31, -0.63]
Subtotal (95% CI)			**50**			**51**	**21.8%**	**-0.66 [-1.25, -0.06]**
Heterogeneity: $Tau^2 = 0.16$; $Chi^2 = 7.72$, df = 1 (P = 0.005); $I^2 = 87\%$								
Test for overall effect: Z = 2.15 (P = 0.03)								
1.1.4 Medical ICUs								
Ely 1996	4.18	2.1	149	4.77	1.3	151	9.3%	-0.58 [-0.99, -0.19]
Krishnan 2004	4.1	1.32	115	4.22	1.37	109	10.0%	-0.12 [-0.47, 0.23]
Subtotal (95% CI)			**264**			**260**	**19.4%**	**-0.35 [-0.81, 0.11]**
Heterogeneity: $Tau^2 = 0.07$; $Chi^2 = 3.02$, df = 1 (P = 0.08); $I^2 = 67\%$								
Test for overall effect: Z = 1.47 (P = 0.14)								
Total (95% CI)			**942**			**931**	**100.0%**	**-0.29 [-0.50, -0.09]**
Heterogeneity: $Tau^2 = 0.08$; $Chi^2 = 37.71$, df = 9 (P < 0.0001); $I^2 = 76\%$								
Test for overall effect: Z = 2.77 (P = 0.006)								

Secondary outcomes

Outcome	Results
Mortality	No statistically significant difference in hospital mortality (6 studies, $I^2 = 0\%$) or ICU mortality* (4 trials, n = 508, $I^2 = 57\%$)
Adverse events	No significant difference in: re-intubation* (8 trials, n = 1314); self-extubation (2 trials); or tracheostomy (6 trials). Only 1 out of 4 trials showed a significantly reduced likelihood of protracted MV in the protocolized group.
Quality of life	This was not reported by any of the trials
Weaning duration	Significantly reduced with protocolized weaning* 6 trials n = 854, (MD −39.41 hours, 95% CI −68.74 p −10.09). $I^2 = 97\%$
ICU LOS	Significantly reduced in the protocolized group by 18 hours 8 trials n = 1256 (MD −18.32, 95% CI −30.4 to −6.25, p = 0.008). $I^2 = 0\%$
Hospital LOS	No significant difference (4 trials)
Economic cost	No difference in ICU (2 trials) or hospital costs (3 trials)
*GRADE = low	

3

Sensitivity analysis

Excluding 2 studies with high risk of bias: This did not change the results of the primary analysis

Author's conclusion

Compared to usual weaning practice, protocolized weaning significantly reduces the total duration of mechanical ventilation, weaning duration and ICU length of stay, by 25%, 78% and 10% respectively (in geometric mean). This benefit must be interpreted with caution in view of the significant heterogeneity among studies which statistical analysis could not explain in terms of type of unit or method of protocol delivery.

Problems & limitations

- Heterogeneity in terms of frequency of assessment and weaning criteria; this ranged from 5 to 19 parameters which include oxygenation in all studies but not CVS, neurological or inflammatory indices
- Marked variation in weaning methods: 7 studies used SBT duration of which ranged from 30 minutes to 2 hours; with support ranging from PEEP 8 cmH_2O + PS 8 cmH_2O to CPAP 2–3 cmH_2O. 2 computerised systems used SIMV + PS, one used PS. 1 computerized weaning methods used SIMV
- Exploratory subgroup analysis to ascertain if weaning approach was the cause of the heterogeneity could not be undertaken due to the wide variety of protocols used

Advantages

- There was an acceptable number of patients in the pooled analysis for the primary outcome
- Important implications for research have arisen: the use of protocolized weaning may indeed improve clinically relevant outcomes and warrants further investigation. The pitfalls encountered with this review may help establish a framework for future research

3

Expert opinion

Richard Venn

How valid and robust are the data?
This review, despite its limitations, supports the concept that proactively addressing the weaning process reduces the duration of mechanical ventilation even if the detail of the benefit hasn't been elucidated.

Should clinical practice be influenced by this?
The review supports a change in clinical practice for individual ICUs to be consistent in their approach to weaning patients from mechanical ventilation. Consistency can be simply achieved by using protocols.

What is the next step?
The data are sufficiently reliable to inform & facilitate further research in this field. The research however should not focus on the precise prescription of the protocol since one solution may not fit all. Nevertheless heterogeneity of protocols needs to be minimised to encourage widespread acceptance of this intervention.

Citation

Blackwood B, Alderdice F, Burns K, Cardwell C, Lavery G, O'Halloran P. Protocolized versus non-protocolized weaning for reducing the duration of mechanical ventilation in critically ill patients. Cochrane database of systematic reviews 2010, Issue 5. Art NO.: CD006904. DOI: 10.1002/14651858.CD006904.pub2.

Blackwood B, Alderdice F, Burns K, Cardwell C, Lavery G, O'Halloran P. Use of weaning protocols for reducing duration of mechanical ventilation in critically ill adult patients: Cochrane systematic review and meta-analysis. BMJ 2011;342:c7237 doi:10.1136/bmj.c7237

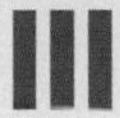

AMSTAR: methodological quality of the review

1.	Was "a priori" design provided?	Y
2.	Was study selection and data extraction adequate?	Y
3.	Was the literature search comprehensive?	Y
4.	Was 'Grey Literature' used?	Y
5.	Was a list of excluded studies provided?	Y
6.	Were the characteristics of included studies provided?	Y
7.	Was the scientific quality of studies assessed & documented?	Y
8.	Was the scientific quality of studies weighted appropriately in forming conclusions?	Y
9.	Were the methods used for data synthesis appropriate?	Y
10.	Was the potential for publication bias assessed?	Y
11.	Were any conflicts of interest stated?	Y

Overall quality of trials included	Varies from low to high
Overall quality of the review	High

NPPV for weaning

Condition: mechanical ventilation for acute respiratory failure
Intervention: noninvasive positive pressure ventilation (NPPV)
Clinical question: Does the use of NPPV for weaning critically ill patients from mechanical ventilation improve outcomes compared to invasive ventilation weaning?

NPPV augments the tidal volume, reduces breathing frequency and rests the respiratory muscles thereby providing partial respiratory support and improving gas exchange. NPPV has been shown to reduce mortality and intubation rates in patients with acute exacerbations of chronic obstructive pulmonary disease (COPD). While invasive ventilation may be essential in critically ill patients with respiratory failure, prolonged mechanical ventilation is associated with complications such as respiratory muscle weakness, upper airway pathology, sinusitis and ventilator associated pneumonia which significantly increases morbidity and demonstrates a trend towards increased mortality. NPPV may be used to wean patients and therefore minimise the duration of mechanical ventilation. Since no tracheal prosthesis is required for NPPV, the cough reflex, speech and potential for eating are preserved and sedation is usually not required. The main disadvantages relate to the lack of airway protection and desiccation of airway secretions.

Review characteristics

- **Eligibility criteria**: randomised and quasi-randomised trials comparing NPPV and IPPV for weaning
- **Exclusions**: trials of NPPV versus IPPV in the immediate postoperative period or following unplanned extubation
- **A priori**: sensitivity analysis excluding the effect of quasi-randomised studies on mortality and VAP outcomes. Subgroup analysis to assess the impact of aetiology of respiratory failure (COPD verses mixed population)
- **Population**: adults with acute or chronic respiratory failure of any aetiology for at least 24 hours in or outside ICU
- **Number of studies**: 12 (1 of which was quasi-randomised), 4 studies in COPD patients with pulmonary infection; in 2 studies ~ 75% of patients had COPD; in 2 further studies ~ 33% had COPD
- **Number of patients**: 530 (range 21–90)
- **Study dates**: 1998–2008

Definitions

- **Mixed population**: study population of less than 50% with COPD
- **Pulmonary infection control (PIC) criteria**: improved radiograph, temperature, WCC or neutrophil count, reduced volume and tenacity of respiratory secretions

Results

Primary outcome: all-cause mortality

Strong evidence that NPPV reduced mortality

RR	95% CI	*p*	I^2
0.55	0.38–0.79	0.001	0%

This was reported at different time intervals

Morality timing	30 day	60 day	90 day	Hospital (variable)
Studies	1	1	2	5

Secondary outcomes

Outcome	Trials/N	Result
Weaning Failure	4/141	Non-significant reduction in weaning failures (RR 0.72, 95% CI 0.37–1.42, $p = 0.34$, $I^2 = 9.2\%$)
VAP	11/509	Significant reduction with NPPV (RR 0.29, 95% CI 0.19–0.45, $p < 0.00001$, $I^2 = 0\%$)
ICU LOS	10/485	Significant reduction of 6 days in the NPPV group (WMD −6.27 days, 95% CI −8.77 to −3.78, $p < 0.00001$, $I^2 = 77.4\%$)
Hospital LOS	8/401	Significant reduction of 7 days in NPPV group (WMD −7.19 days, 95% CI −10.8 to −3.58, $p < 0.0001$, $I^2 = 76.8\%$)
Mean total duration of MV	7/385	Significant reduction in the NPPV group (WMD −5.64, 95% CI −9.5 to −1.77, $p = 0.004$, $I^2 = 85.6\%$)
Mean duration of weaning ventilation	6/224	No significant difference (WMD −0.94, 95% CI −3.24 to 1.36, $p = 0.42$, $I^2 = 91.8\%$)
Mean duration of endotracheal MV	9/391	Significant decrease in the NPPV group (WMD−7.81, 95% CI −11.31 to −4.31, $p < 0.0001$, $I^2 = 89.9\%$)
Re-intubation	6/328	Non-significant trend towards lower rate in the NPPV group (RR 0.73, 95% CI 0.40–1.34, $p = 0.31$, $I^2 = 32.4\%$)
Tracheostomy	3/141	Significant reduction in the NPPV group (RR 0.16, 95% CI 0.04–0.75, $p = 0.02$, $I^2 = 17.2\%$)
Arryhthmia	2/63	Non-significant increase in the NPPVC group (RR 1.05, 95% CI 0.17–6.67, $p = 0.96$, $I^2 = 0\%$)
Quality of life	0	Not reported

3

Fig. 7 Comparison 1 Noninvasive versus invasive weaning, Outcome 1 mortality [from Burns KEA, Adhikari NKJ, Keenan SP, Meade MO. Noninvasive positive pressure ventilation as a weaning strategy for intubated adults with respiratory failure. Cochrane Database of Systematic Reviews 2010, Issue 8. Art. No.: CD004127, © Cochrane Collaboration, reproduced with permission]

Review: Noninvasive positive pressure ventilation as a weaning strategy for intubated adults with respiratory failure
Comparison: 1 Noninvasive versus invasive weaning
Outcome: 1 Mortality

Study or subgroup	Noninvasive weaning n/N	Invasive weaning n/N	Risk Ratio M-H, Random, 95% CI	Weight	Risk Ratio M-H, Random, 95% CI
1 COPD					
Chen 2001	0/12	3/12		1.6%	0.14 [0.01, 2.50]
Nava 1998a	2/25	7/25		6.1%	0.29 [0.07, 1.24]
Prasad 2008	5/15	9/15		19.3%	0.56 [0.24, 1.27]
Rabie 2004	1/19	2/18		2.5%	0.47 [0.05, 4.78]
Wang 2004	1/14	2/14		2.5%	0.50 [0.05, 4.90]
Wang 2005	1/47	7/43		3.1%	0.13 [0.02, 1.02]
Zheng 2005	3/17	3/16		6.3%	0.94 [0.22, 4.00]
Zou 2006	3/38	11/38		9.2%	0.27 [0.08, 0.90]
Subtotal (95% CI)	**187**	**181**		**50.7%**	**0.42 [0.25, 0.69]**

Total events: 16 (Noninvasive weaning), 44 (Invasive weaning)
Heterogeneity: $Tau^2 = 0.0$; $Chi^2 = 4.48$, $df = 7$ ($P = 0.72$); $I^2 = 0.0\%$
Test for overall effect: $Z = 3.37$ ($P = 0.00075$)

0.001 0.01 0.1 1 10 100 1000
Favours noninvasive Favours invasive

(Continued ...)

(... *Continued*)

Study or subgroup	Noninvasive weaning n/N	Invasive weaning n/N	Risk Ratio M-H, Random, 95% CI	Weight	Risk Ratio M-H, Random, 95% CI
2 mixed					
Ferrer 2003	6/21	13/22		22.8%	0.48 [0.23, 1.03]
Girault 1999	0/17	2/16		1.5%	0.19 [0.01, 3.66]
Hill 2000	1/12	1/9		1.9%	0.75 [0.05, 10.44]
Trevisan 2008	9/28	10/37		23.1%	1.19 [0.56, 2.53]
Subtotal (95% CI)	**78**	**84**		**49.3%**	**0.72 [0.39, 1.32]**
Total events: 16 (Noninvasive weaning), 26 (Invasive weaning)					
Heterogeneity: $Tau^2 = 0.07$; $Chi^2 = 3.54$ df = 3 (P = 0.32); $I^2 = 15\%$					
Test for overall effect: Z = 1.06 (P = 0.29)					
Total (95% CI)	**265**	**265**		**100.0%**	**0.55 [0.38, 0.79]**
Total events: 32 (Noninvasive weaning), 70 (Invasive weaning)					
Heterogeneity: $Tau^2 = 0.0$; $Chi^2 = 10.46$, df = 11 (P = 0.49); $I^2 = 0.0\%$					
Test for overall effect: Z = 3.24 (P = 0.0012)					

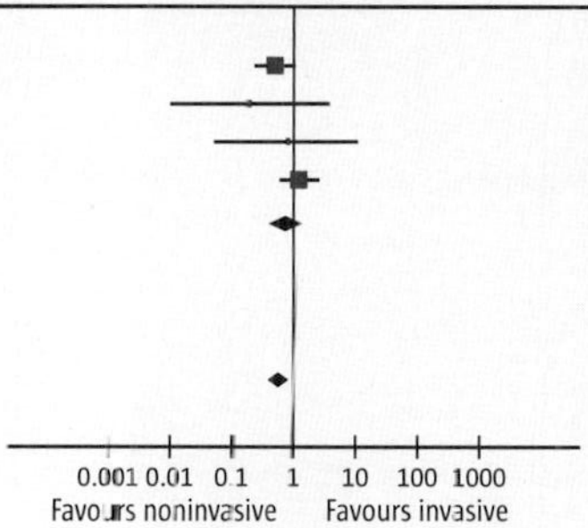

0.001 0.01 0.1 1 10 100 1000
Favours noninvasive
Favours invasive

3

Subgroup analysis

There was a significantly beneficial effect of NPPV weaning in COPD on mortality in the studies that enrolled at least 50% COPD patients (RR 0.4, 95% CI 0.28–0.65) compared to those enrolling less than 50% COPD patients (RR 1.15, 95% CI 0.56–2.37)

Author's conclusion

NPPV weaning significantly reduces mortality, ICU and hospital LOS, duration of invasive ventilation as well as total duration of mechanical ventilation and VAP incidence. However we acknowledge that direct access to the respiratory secretions may have enhanced VAP detection in the intubated group. Subgroup analysis suggested greater benefit in patients with COPD. Whether other aetiologies of respiratory failure are as amenable to NPPV remains to be determined. The optimal timing for the transition to NPPV weaning also remains to be determined. Varied weaning methods and the absence of adequately power RCTs limits the strengths of the conclusion.

Problems & limitations

- Small number of patients in the trials
- Differences between trials in terms of eligibility for weaning criteria, ventilation modes and weaning strategies for both the NPPV and IPPV groups e.g. some trials used ventilator settings, others physiologic parameters, and some used PIC criteria. Only 2 studies specified expectoration and improved GCS in their criteria; only 3 trials screened daily for spontaneous breathing trial (SBT) readiness
- Different definitions for weaning success or failure between studies
- Variable reporting of adverse events precluded pooling of data

Advantages

- Eligibility for inclusion was based on predefined weaning criteria for all the studies
- The sensitivity analysis maintained the statistically significant reduction in mortality and VAP in favour of NPPV weaning
- The funnel plot did not suggest any publication bias

Expert opinion

Jonathan Ball

How valid and robust are the data?
This review pooled data from 12 studies (530 patients) conducted over 10 years. All of the studies were small with significant heterogeneity between their methodologies. These data are not robust but are adequate to inform detailed hypothesis generation.

Should clinical practice be influenced by this?
No. However, consideration of weaning using noninvasive ventilation, especially in patients with COPD, is both reasonable and rationale.

What is the next step?
Weaning from ventilatory support remains a complex process, which is influenced by multiple and uncontrollable factors. A large scale randomised control trial comparing different ventilator modalities is an unrealistic proposal due to complexity of the process. In centres with expertise at delivering NIV, it should be considered as an option and used where appropriate. A prospective registry of cases in such centres is more likely to inform practice than a randomised control trial.

Citation

Burns KEA, Adhikari NKJ, Keenan SP, Meade MO. Noninvasive positive pressure ventilation as a weaning strategy for intubated adults with respiratory failure. Cochrane Database of Systematic Reviews 2010, Issue 8. Art. No.: CD004127. DOI: 10.1002/14651858.CD004127.pub2

AMSTAR: methodological quality of the review

1.	Was "a priori" design provided?	Y
2.	Was study selection and data extraction adequate?	Y
3.	Was the literature search comprehensive?	Y
4.	Was 'Grey Literature' used?	Y
5.	Was a list of excluded studies provided?	Y
6.	Were the characteristics of included studies provided?	Y
7.	Was the scientific quality of studies assessed & documented?	Y
8.	Was the scientific quality of studies weighted appropriately in forming conclusions?	Y
9.	Were the methods used for data synthesis appropriate?	Y
10.	Was the potential for publication bias assessed?	Y
11.	Were any conflicts of interest stated?	Y

Overall quality of trials included	Moderate to high
Overall quality of the review	High

Heated humidification versus HME

Condition: mechanical ventilation

Intervention: humidification

Clinical question: Are heated humidifiers (HH) or heat and moisture exchangers (HME) more effective in preventing mortality and other complications in mechanically ventilated patients?

Normally the upper airway humidifies inspired gas such that it is saturated at body temperature but artificial tracheal airways bypass this area. Inspiration of cold dry gases leads to a number of serious complications including: inflammation, necrosis and squamous metaplasia of the airways; airway collapse and deterioration in lung function occur; the tenacity of respiratory secretions increases and may lead to mucus plugging, a potentially life threatening situation. In neonatal and paediatric patients, water vapour and heat loss from the respiratory tract is an important component of fluid and heat balance.

3

HHs provide active humidification by heating water in a reservoir whereas HMEs passively conserve the patient's expired heat and moisture and then return them to the patient on inspiration. Both techniques have complications: HHs can lead to over humidification which can also damage the lung; increase the work of breathing and cause bacterial contamination. HMEs on the other hand are associated with an increased risk of tracheal tube occlusion; and may increase dead space leading to carbon dioxide retention and increased work of breathing. This effect is also more relevant in paediatrics as the HME volume forms a larger proportion of the normal tidal volume. The optimal level of humidity and how this is best achieved remains controversial.

Review characteristics

- **Eligibility criteria:** RCTs that compared HHs to HMEs. Cross-over studies were included if the order was randomised
- **Exclusions:** studies involving patient on NIV or patients self-ventilating via a tracheostomy or T-tube
- **A priori:** to perform subgroup analysis by age: i. neonates ii. infants and children and iii. adults; and by duration of mechanical ventilation: i. short-term ii. medium-term and iii. long-term
- **Population:** children and adults who are mechanically ventilated
- **Number of studies:** 33 studies in total. 30 adult studies, (25 parallel group design, 8 cross-over design). Only 3 studies reported data for infants or children
- **Number of patients:** total of 2,833 (2,710 in parallel design, 123 in cross-over studies)
- **Study dates:** 1996–2006

Definitions

- **HH and HME:** any model or type was included
- **Short-term MV:** up to 6 hours
- **Medium-term MV:** 6–48 hours
- **Long-term MV:** more than 48 hours

Results

Primary outcomes: all data from parallel studies

Outcome	Trials	N	RR	95% CI	GRADE
Artificial airway occlusion	15	2171	1.59	0.6–4.19	High
All-cause Mortality	12	1951	1.04	0.9–1.21	High
Pneumonia	12	2236	0.92	0.71–1.2	High

Secondary outcomes: data from parallel studies

Outcomes	Trials/N	Results
Atelectasis	3/303	No statistical difference
Pneumothorax	1/56	No statistical difference
PaO_2	1/30	Significantly higher in the HME group (MD 2.8 kPa, 95% CI 0.13 to −5.47, p = 0.04)
$PaCO_2$	1/30	No statistical difference
Tidal volume	1/85	No statistical difference
Minute ventilation	1/85	No statistical difference
Tracheal aspirations	3/290	No significant difference
Saline instillations	1/56	Significantly higher volume of saline used in the HME group
	but 2/204	Significantly lower number of saline instillations in the HME group
Body temperature	6/321	Actual temperature was significantly lower in the HME group MD −0.40, 95% CI −0.06 to −0.02, p = 0.04
Change in temperature	3/78	Mean change MD −0.58, 95% CI −0.79 to −0.37, p < 0.0001
ICU & Hospital LOS	NA	Data couldn't be included in meta-analysis. There was no consistent pattern in either group
Cost	6/1284	Data could not be added to meta-analysis. All studies reported lower costs for HMEs compared to HHs

3

Secondary outcomes: data from cross-over studies

Outcome	Trials/N	Results
SaO_2	1/11	No significant difference
PaO_2	4 /78	No significant difference
$PaCO_2$	5/88	Significantly higher in the HME group at all correlation estimates
Breathing rate	4/65	Significantly higher in the HME group at the low correlation No difference at the moderate or high correlation estimates
Tidal volume	5/76	No difference at low or moderate correlation estimates but Significantly higher with HME at higher correlation estimates
Work of breathing (J)	2/21	Higher in both studies but data were too skewed to be added to meta-analysis
Minute ventilation	5/76	Significantly higher in HME group at all correlation estimates
Body temperature	2/21	No significant difference

Subgroup analysis

No difference in artificial airway occlusion or all-cause mortality when paediatric (1 study, n = 56) and adult studies were analysed separately
Significant increase in artificial airway occlusion when 5 medium-term studies (n = 362) were combined. There was no difference when long-term or medium plus long-term studies were combined, however it should be noted that in some studies, patients were removed from the study if they were prone to artificial airway blockage.
There was no difference in all-cause mortality or pneumonia with length of ventilation
Types or HMEs: hygroscopic versus hydrophobic No difference in artificial airway occlusion or all-cause mortality Significantly lower prevalence of pneumonia with hydrophobic HMEs (3 trials, n = 569) No difference when a hygroscopic HME was used (8 trials, n = 1663)

Author's conclusion

There was some evidence that the prevalence of pneumonia may be lowered by using heat and moisture exchangers that capture less moisture. A heat and moisture exchanger may however also increase blockage of the artificial airway. Overall there was no increase in artificial airway occlusion; however there was an increase with the use of HMEs in the subgroup which was ventilated between 6–48 hours. This may be explained by the fact in some studies patients were changed from HME to HH for a variety of reasons such as thick secretions, to minimize dead space or because of

hypothermia. Overall there was no difference in mortality or prevalence of pneumonia. However a hydrophobic HME may reduce pneumonia compared to HH. HMEs may increase the CO_2 and decrease body temperature. Results do need to be interpreted with caution because several studies excluded patients that were not considered suitable for HMEs. More studies are need in neonates and paediatric populations who are more susceptible to the potential complications of HMEs.

Problems & limitations

- The use of cross-over studies
- Significant statistical heterogeneity although this was really an issue with the crossover trials and not so much the parallel trials
- Four out of eight studies comparing HHs with hygroscopic HMEs used HHs with a heated wire while one of those comparing hydrophobic HMEs did

Advantages

- Other reviews also reported no difference in the prevalence of artificial airway occlusion overall
- HMEs are considerably cheaper

Expert opinion

Jonathan Ball

How valid and robust are the data?

These data are very heterogeneous resulting in no clear signal with regard to inferiority or superiority for either heated humidification (HH) or heat and moisture exchange (HME) devices. This heterogeneity originates from the variability of study designs, the specific devices used (variable design and performance characteristics of different HMEs), their mode of use (settings/change frequency etc) and uncontrolled for variables (practice variation over time – included studies range from 1984–2006, geographical variation in clinical practice etc.). In short, there is no clear signal amongst the noise. One cannot conclude that there is no signal, merely that no consistent signal can be observed from the reasonable volume of generated over a prolonged period.

Should clinical practice be influenced by this?

Yes. In adult sized patients HME devices should be the standard of care – due to non-inferiority and cheaper cost. Escalation to HH devices should have a clearly documented rational with demonstrable objective benefit to the individual patient based upon the identified indication. In neonates, infants and children there is insufficient evidence to guide decision making.

What is the next step?

Airway humidification forms an essential part of the complex package of care required to optimise invasive mechanical ventilation, as well as minimise secondary complications and iatrogenic harm. Future research must protocolize all the elements of this package in order to generate meaningful outcome data. Reports from registries of single centre experience with protocolized care packages (including adherence rates), which include clear indications for, and objective measures of the efficacy of, HH, should be used to generate hypotheses worthy of future randomised studies and provide reliable estimates of effect size to ensure such studies are sufficiently powered.

3

Citation

Kelly M, Gillies D, Todd DA, Lockwood C. Heated humidification versus heat and moisture exchangers for ventilated adults and children. Cochrane Database of Systematic Reviews 2010, Issue 4. Art.No.: CD004711. DOI: 10.1002/14651858.CD004711.pub2

AMSTAR: methodological quality of the review

1.	Was "a priori" design provided?	Y
2.	Was study selection and data extraction adequate?	Y
3.	Was the literature search comprehensive?	Y
4.	Was 'Grey Literature' used?	Y
5.	Was a list of excluded studies provided?	Y
6.	Were the characteristics of included studies provided?	Y
7.	Was the scientific quality of studies assessed & documented?	Y
8.	Was the scientific quality of studies weighted appropriately in forming conclusions?	Y
9.	Were the methods used for data synthesis appropriate?	Y
10.	Was the potential for publication bias assessed?	Y
11.	Were any conflicts of interest stated?	Y

Overall quality of trials included	Variable
Overall quality of the review	High

Pleural effusions drainage

Condition: pleural effusions
Intervention: thoracentesis and drainage
Clinical question: What are the clinical and physiological risks and benefits of drainage?

Pleural effusions are common in critically ill patients with a reported incidence up to 60%. Animal studies suggest that they reduce respiratory system compliance and increase intrapulmonary shunting. Effusions cause hypoxaemia by collapsing adjacent lung when chest wall compliance is reduced or the effusion is large because smaller effusion are accommodated by the compliant chest wall and diaphragm. In spontaneously breathing patients, thoracentesis has only been associated with minor improvements in lung mechanics and oxygenation but significantly relieves dyspnoea. The presence of pleural effusions has been associated with a longer duration of mechanical ventilation and ICU LOS but the impact of drainage on clinically relevant outcomes remains unclear. 3

Review characteristics

- **Eligibility criteria:** controlled trial or observational studies
- **Exclusions:** case reports and studies of patients who had absolute indications for drainage e.g. empyema
- **Population:** mechanically ventilated adults (and non-ventilated if outcomes were recorded separately)
- **Number of studies:** 19 cohort studies (15 prospective and 4 retrospective)
- **Number of patients:** 1,690 in total. 1,124 of these were mechanically ventilated and only these outcomes were included
- **Study dates:** 1990–2009

Definitions

- **Thoracentesis:** 12 studies used a one-time needle/catheter thoracentesis procedure
- **Drainage:** 6 studies used drainage catheter or thoracostomy

Results

Outcome	Studies/n	Result
Clinical	3/189	Drainage of pleural effusions changed the diagnosis and/or management in 31% to 75% of patients
	2/157	No difference was found in duration of MV or ICU LOS but one of these compared less (< 500 ml) versus more pleural fluid removal (> 500 ml)
Oxygenation	5/118	Meta-analysis demonstrated 18% improvement in the PaO_2:FiO_2 1 study suggested that a ratio < 180 mmHg was the sole independent predictor of improvement In 1 study improvement correlated with the volume of effusion drained
Lung Mechanics		Thoracentesis
	2/28	Reported reduction in respiratory rate but no change in compliance
	1/22	Reported improvement in dynamic compliance
Complications	7/660	No pneumothoraxes
	8/305	Pneumothorax incidence ranged from 1.3% to 15% in procedures performed by staff of varying seniority (from student to staff intensivist)
	2/228	Haemothorax rate of 1.1–4.5% Use of US guidance did not reduce risk of pneumothorax

Author's conclusion

There is no evidence for or against drainage of pleural effusions in mechanically ventilated patients to improve important clinical outcomes such as duration of mechanical ventilation, ICU length of stay or mortality. Drainage does improve oxygenation; is associated with a low risk of peri-procedural complications and may even alter diagnosis and management. The minimal important drainage volume; the importance of lung recruitment following drainage; and whether the improvement in oxygenation depends upon the severity of underlying hypoxaemia or amount of fluid removed remains to be determined.

Problems & limitations

- Absence of controlled studies
- Heterogeneity between studies in terms of severity of illness, effusion volume, and timing of post procedure observations
- Skill of operators with regards to thoracentesis, chest drain insertion and ultrasound use

Fig. 8 Forest plot of meta-analysis of studies reporting change in oxygenation after pleural drainage. $PaO_2:FiO_2$ ratios before and after thoracentesis analysed by (A) relative mean difference (ratio of means) and (B) absolute mean difference [from Ewan C Goligher, Jerome A Leis, Robert A Fowler, Ruxandra Pinto, Neill KJ Adhikari, Niall D Ferguson, Goligher et al. Utility and safety of draining pleural effusions in mechanically ventilated patients: a systematic review and meta-analysis. Critical Care 2011, 15:R46]

Study Name	N	Pre-Mean (SE)	Post-Mean (SE)	Ratio of means (95% CI)	Weight (%)
Talmor 1998	19	151.0 (15.3)	244.5 (29.1)	1.52 (1.28, 2.05)	14.7
De Waele 2003	24	190.0 (17.1)	216.0 (15.1)	1.14 (0.95, 1.35)	20.5
Ahmed 2004	22	245.0 (22.0)	270.0 (21.5)	1.10 (0.92, 1.32)	19.7
Roch 2005	44	209.6 (10.8)	242.4 (15.0)	1.16 (1.02, 1.31)	26.7
Doelken 2006	9	96.0 (9.9)	102.0 (7.3)	1.06 (0.87, 1.29)	18.5
Overall	**118**				**100.0**

Overall effect: ratio of means 1.18; 95% CI (1.05, 1.33); p-value = 0.0052

Heterogenity: I^2 = 53.7%

A)

Study Name	N	Pre-Mean (SE)	Post-Mean (SE)	Mean difference (95% CI)	Weight (%)
Talmor 1998	19	151.0 (15.3)	244.5 (29.1)	93.5 (40.8, 146.2)	13.0
De Waele 2003	24	190.0 (17.1)	216.0 (15.1)	26.0 (-8.8, 60.8)	20.1
Ahmed 2004	22	245.0 (22.0)	270.0 (21.5)	25.0 (-21.7, 71.7)	15.0
Roch 2005	44	209.6 (10.8)	242.4 (15.0)	32.7 (4.1, 61.3)	23.3
Doelken 2006	9	96.0 (9.9)	102.0 (7.3)	6.0 (-13.0, 25.0)	28.5
Overall	**118**				**100.0**

Overall effect: mean difference 30.5; 95% CI (6.4, 54.6); p-value = 0.013

Heterogenity: I^2 = 61.5%

B)

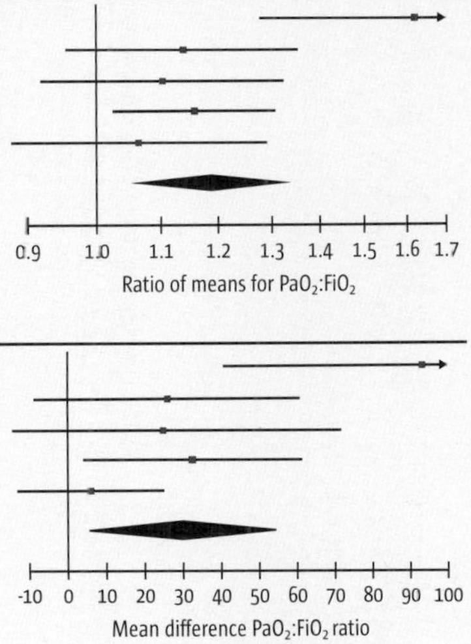

Fig. 9 Forest plot of meta-analysis of studies reporting the rate of pneumothorax after pleural drainage [from Ewan C Goligher, Jerome A Leis, Robert A Fowler, Ruxandra Pinto, Neill KJ Adhikari, Niall D Ferguson, Goligher et al. Utility and safety of draining pleural effusions in mechanically ventilated patients: a systematic review and meta-analysis. Critical Care 2011, 15:R46]

Study Name	Events (n)	Total (N)	Weight (%)
Godwin 1990	2	32	9.6
Yu 1992	1	14	6.8
McCartney 1993	3	31	11.0
Gervais 1997	6	90	13.3
Lichtenstein 1999	0	45	4.5
De Waele 2003	5	33	12.5
Singh 2003	0	12	4.4
Ahmed 2004	0	31	4.4
Mayo 2004	3	232	11.3
Roch 2005	0	44	4.5
Vignon 2005	0	17	4.4
Balik 2006	0	92	4.5
Tu 2006	0	184	4.5
Liang 2009	0	108	4.5
Overall	**20**	**965**	**100**

Overall effect: 3.4%; 95% CI (1.7%, 6.5%)
Heterogenity: I^2 = 52.5%

0 5 10 15 20 25 30
Percentage (%)

Advantages

- 1 study (n = 19) that showed the greatest benefit in oxygenation had pre-selected patients that had hypoxaemia refractory to high PEEP. This may indicate group of patients with low compliance that are more likely to benefit from the resultant lung re-inflation

Expert opinion

Jonathan Ball

How valid and robust are the data?
The data presented in this review are surprisingly limited given the high incidence of this pathology. The studies reported, fail to determine whether and in whom, thoracocentesis improves clinically meaningful outcomes. In addition the optimal method, aspiration verses drain left in situ, remains to be determined.

Should clinical practice be influenced by this?
No.

What is the next step?
A first step would be to define 2 groups of patients, those with high ventilatory demands and/ or poor gas exchange and pleural effusions, and those who have delayed weaning from mechanical ventilation and pleural effusions. The underlying cause, size and biochemical nature of these effusions should to be determined. In the first group, the addition of thoracocentesis (drain left in situ), to a comprehensive, protocolized, package of care with the outcome of

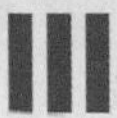

time to successful weaning from mechanical ventilation and the incidence of complications, especially empyema, should be investigated. In the second group, studies comparing protocolized weaning, including active management of fluid balance and oedema, with or without the addition of thoracocentesis (drain left in situ) should be undertaken, with time to successful weaning being the primary outcome. The difficulty with such studies is developing the comprehensive protocols that legislate for all the other interventions that affect the weaning process. It could be argued that this is unrealistic given that treatment of the underlying pathology, sedation practice, mode of ventilation, weaning programme, fluid balance, nutrition, physical rehabilitation, determination and treatment of cardiac and neuromuscular pathologies, timing of tracheotomy etc. is not possible in a large enough group of patients to sufficiently power a randomised control trial. More information might be gleaned from further reports of small cohorts of patients from single centres with protocolized care (and monitoring of adherence), especially where thoracocentesis has clear indications such us, failure to respond to diuretics, optimising ventilatory settings to enhance pleural drainage, consideration of oncotic therapy and the possible effects of co-incident anti-inflammatory therapy. Additional insights might also emerge from large single centres, which develop registries of patients who require prolonged mechanical ventilation. Retrospective analysis might be valuable in determining which interventions appear to have the greatest effect on clinically important outcomes.

Citation

Goligher EC, Leis JA, Fowler RA, Pinto R, Adhikari NKJ, Ferguson ND, Goligher et al. Utility and safety of draining pleural effusions in mechanically ventilated patients: a systematic review and meta-analysis. Critical Care 2011, 15:R46

AMSTAR: methodological quality of the review

1.	Was "a priori" design provided?	Y
2.	Was study selection and data extraction adequate?	Y
3.	Was the literature search comprehensive?	Y
4.	Was 'Grey Literature' used?	Y
5.	Was a list of excluded studies provided?	N
6.	Were the characteristics of included studies provided?	Y
7.	Was the scientific quality of studies assessed & documented?	NA
8.	Was the scientific quality of studies weighted appropriately in forming conclusions?	Y
9.	Were the methods used for data synthesis appropriate?	Y
10.	Was the potential for publication bias assessed?	Y
11.	Were any conflicts of interest stated?	Y

Overall quality of trials included	No RCTs
Overall quality of the review	High

4

Cardiovascular dynamics

Atrial fibrillation 100
Therapeutic hypothermia 104
Vasopressin for vasodilatory shock 109
Pre-emptive haemodynamic intervention 114

Also see:
Section 7: Health technology
Oesophageal doppler monitoring

Atrial fibrillation

Condition: atrial fibrillation (AF)

Intervention: pharmacological treatments

Clinical question: Which are the most efficacious drugs to use in the control of new-onset AF in ICU patients?

AF is the most common dysrhythmia amongst adult critically ill patients; prevalence is between 10–20% in general surgical and medical intensive care patients and much higher following cardiac surgery. New-onset AF is associated with at least a 2-fold increased risk of mortality, however this relationship might suggest that AF is a marker of illness severity rather than an independent risk factor for death.

Review characteristics

- **Eligibility criteria:** peer-reviewed RCTs comparing inert or active control for new-onset AF
- **Exclusions:** cardiac surgery patients, patients treated for AF before ICU admission
- **Number of studies:** 4
- **Number of patients:** 143 [89 (76%) had AF, the rest had other atrial arrhythmias]
- **Population:** adult patients admitted to ICU
- **Study dates:** 1993–1998

Definitions

- **New-onset atrial tachyarrhythmia:** AF, atrial flutter or other SVT
- **Cardioversion:** conversion to normal sinus rhythm (NSR) at 1 hour, 12 hours or 24 hours

Results

Primary outcome: cardioversion to normal sinus rhythm

Drug comparison	N	NSR AT 1–2 h	NSR AT 12 h	NSR AT 24 h
Amiodarone vs. procainamide	24	– –	70% 71%	50% –
Amiodarone (+ digoxin) vs. magnesium (+ digoxin)	34	– –	50% 77%	– –
Esmolol vs. diltiazem	55	68% 33% ($p < 0.05$)	85% 62% ($p = 0.116$)	– –
Flecanide vs. verapamil	30	80% 33% ($p < 0.001$)	– –	– –

Unable to pool estimates due to heterogeneity

NSR = Normal Sinus Rhythm

4

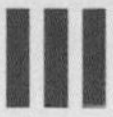

Fig. 1 Conversion rates (and 95% confidence intervals) for all drugs evaluated. Conversion rates reported as per cent with 95% confidence intervals for reported conversion rates at 12 hours for each drug except flecainide and verapamil, which are presented as 1-hour conversion rates [Treatment of new-onset atrial fibrillation in noncardiac intensive care unit patients: A systematic review of randomized controlled trials. Salmaan Kanji, PharmD; Robert Stewart, MD; Dean A. Fergusson, Lauralyn McIntyre, Alexis F. Turgeon, Paul C. Hébert. Crit Care Med 2008 Vol. 36, No. 5]

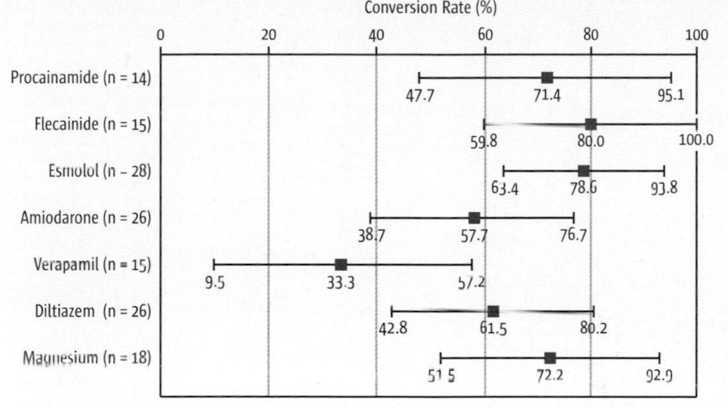

Adverse events

Drug	Frequency	Event
Amiodarone	2	Hypotension
	2	Death: cause not given
Flecainide	3	Significantly prolonged QRS: with VEs in 1 & hypotension in 2 patients
Verapamil	3	Hypotension
Esmolol	10	Hypotension (drug had to be discontinued in 2 patients)
Diltiazem	12	Hypotension (drug had to be discontinued in 1 patient)

Author's conclusion

Heterogeneity and trial design preclude recommendation of any particular drug. In a comparable review evaluating pharmacological cardioversion rates after cardiac surgery the conclusion was similar in that heterogeneity in both trial methodology and results prohibited specific recommendation. DC cardioversion may be a viable alternative, although its success rate of 70–95% is only described in 1 observational study in non-critically ill patients. The substrate for AF in this population may not be eliminated until the disease process is treated, therefore targeting rate rather than rhythm may be of greater value.

Problems & limitations

- 1 trial of flecainide versus verapamil only evaluated rhythm up to 1 hour after intervention
- No trial collected data beyond 24 hours
- Maintenance of rhythm control was not evaluated in any of the studies
- No studies were carried out against placebo
- Patient numbers were very small
- 3 out of 4 studies excluded haemodynamically unstable patients, presumably due to the emergent nature of intervention in this situation

Advantages

- All trials evaluated the same outcomes albeit at different times: cardioversion and safety

Expert opinion

Fernando Clau-Terré and Maurizio Cecconi

How valid and robust are the data?
The review contains 4 randomized trials that go beyond the methodological power level admitted, and these studies were conducted from 1993 to 1998. The number of patients is small and the sample of patients, heterogeneous, is poorly identified in relation to gravity risk scale, its evolution and follow up. The term supraventricular arrhythmia covers different types of arrhythmias as flutter or atrial fibrillation, in the same way the definition used for successful cardioversion into sinus rhythm is different in each one of the articles.

Should clinical practice be influenced by this?
The review has an absence of scientific evidence regarding the most effective drugs, cardioversion doses and type of patient. It is difficult from the data to understand the real efficacy of drugs used and to recommend a change in practice.

What's the next step?
Properly designed studies are needed with larger samples and longer monitoring to have a stronger evidence of morbidity and mortality of atrial fibrillation (AF) in critically ill patients and which drugs may be more useful in their treatment.

Citation

Salmaan K, Pharm D, Robert Stewart MD, Fergusson DA, McIntyre L, Turgeon AF, Hébert PC. Treatment of new-onset atrial fibrillation in noncardiac intensive care unit patients: A systematic review of randomized controlled trials. Crit Care Med 2008 Vol. 36, No. 5 DOI: 10.1097/CCM.0b013e3181709e43

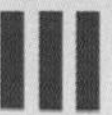

AMSTAR: methodological quality of the review

1.	Was “a priori” design provided?	Y
2.	Was study selection and data extraction adequate?	Y
3.	Was the literature search comprehensive?	Y
4.	Was ‘Grey Literature’ used?	P
5.	Was a list of excluded studies provided?	N
6.	Were the characteristics of included studies provided?	Y
7.	Was the scientific quality of studies assessed & documented?	Y
8.	Was the scientific quality of studies weighted appropriately in forming conclusions?	Y
9.	Were the methods used for data synthesis appropriate?	Y
10.	Was the potential for publication bias assessed?	Y
11.	Were any conflicts of interest stated?	N

Overall quality of trials included	Low
Overall quality of the review	Moderate-high

Therapeutic hypothermia

Condition: cardiac arrest

Intervention: therapeutic hypothermia

Clinical question: Does therapeutic hypothermia improve neurological outcome following cardiac arrest?

Out of hospital cardiac arrest is common; up to 40% are successfully resuscitated (ROSC) and reach hospital but only between 7–30% of those patients achieving a good neurological outcome. Cerebral reperfusion after resuscitation can trigger harmful chemical cascades resulting in multifocal brain damage, "post resuscitation syndrome". The protective effect of hypothermia has been recognised for decades and has been used pre-emptively in surgical procedures requiring circulatory arrest states however its application in patients following arrest is relatively novel.

4

Review characteristics

- **Eligibility criteria**: RCTs and "quasi-randomised" RCTs
- **Exclusions**: patients aged less than 18 years
- **Number of studies**: 5 studies (4 papers and 1 abstract)
- **Number of patients**: 481
- **Population**: adults who suffered cardiac arrest either in or out of hospital
- **Study dates**: 2001–2005

Definitions

- **Therapeutic hypothermia**: body temperature reduced to below 35°C within 6 hours of arrival in hospital, achieved by any means
- **Primary outcome**:
  1. Good cerebral performance: normal but +/– minor deficits
  2. Moderate cerebral disability: sufficient for activities of daily living (ADL) but with obvious deficit
  3. Severe cerebral disability: dependent on others for ADLs
  4. Coma/vegetative state
  5. Brain death certified

Results

Primary outcome: good neurological outcome

Cooling method	Trials	Patients	RR	95% CI	I^2
Comparable/conventional	3	383	1.54	1.22–1.95	32%
Haemofiltration	1	42	0.71	0.31–1.54	NA
Not stated	1	54	4.5	1.17–17.30	NA

Fig. 2 Comparison 1 Neurological. Outcome: cooling versus no cooling, outcome 1 good neurological outcome [from Arrich J, Holzer M, Herkner H, Müllner M. Hypothermia for neuroprotection in adults after cardiopulmonary resuscitation. Cochrane Database of Systematic Reviews 2009, Issue 4. Art. No.: CD004128. DOI: 10.1002/14651858.CD004128.pub2, © Cochrane Collaboration, reproduced with permission]

Review: Hypothermia for neuroprotection in adults after cardiopulmonary resuscitation
Comparison: 1 Neurological Outcome cooling vs. no cooling
Outcome: 1 Good neurological outcome

Study or subgroup	Experimental n/N	Control n/N	Risk Ratio M-H, Fixed, 95% CI	Weight	Risk Ratio M-H, Fixed, 95% CI
1 Conventional cooling without extracorporeal methods (IPD, best ever reached CPC of 1 or 2 during hospital stay)					
Bernard 2002	21/43	9/34		12.9%	1.84[0.97, 3.49]
HACA 2002	75/136	54/137		69.1%	1.40 [1.08, 1.81]
Hachimi-Idrissi 2001	8/16	2/17		2.5%	4.25 [1.06, 17.08]
Subtotal (95% CI)	**195**	**188**		**84.5%**	**1.55 [1.22, 1.96]**
Total events: 104 (Experimental), 65 (Control)					
Heterogeneity: $Chi^2 = 2.92$, df = 2 (P = 0.23); $I^2 = 32\%$					
Test for overall effect: Z = 3.64 (P = 0.00025)					
2 Cooling with haemofiltration (no IPD, CPC of 1 or 2 at six months)					
Laurent 2005	7/22	9/20		12.1%	0.71 [0.32, 1.54]
Subtotal (95% CI)	**22**	**20**		**12.1%**	**0.71 [0.32, 1.54]**
Total events: 7 (Experimental), 9 (Control)					
Heterogeneity: not applicable					
Test for overall effect: Z = 0.87 (P = 0.38)					

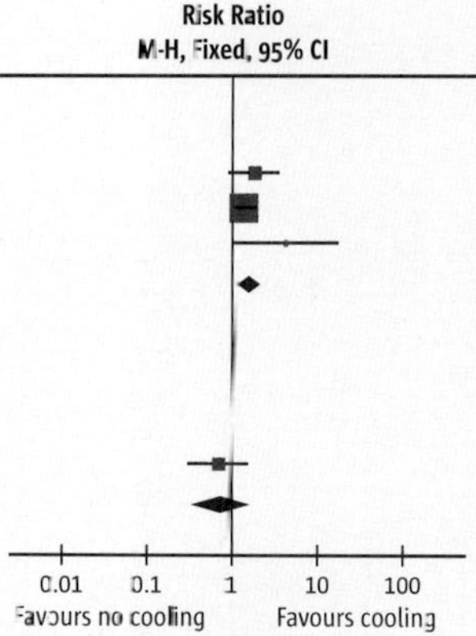

0.01 0.1 1 10 100
Favours no cooling Favours cooling

(Continued ...)

4

4

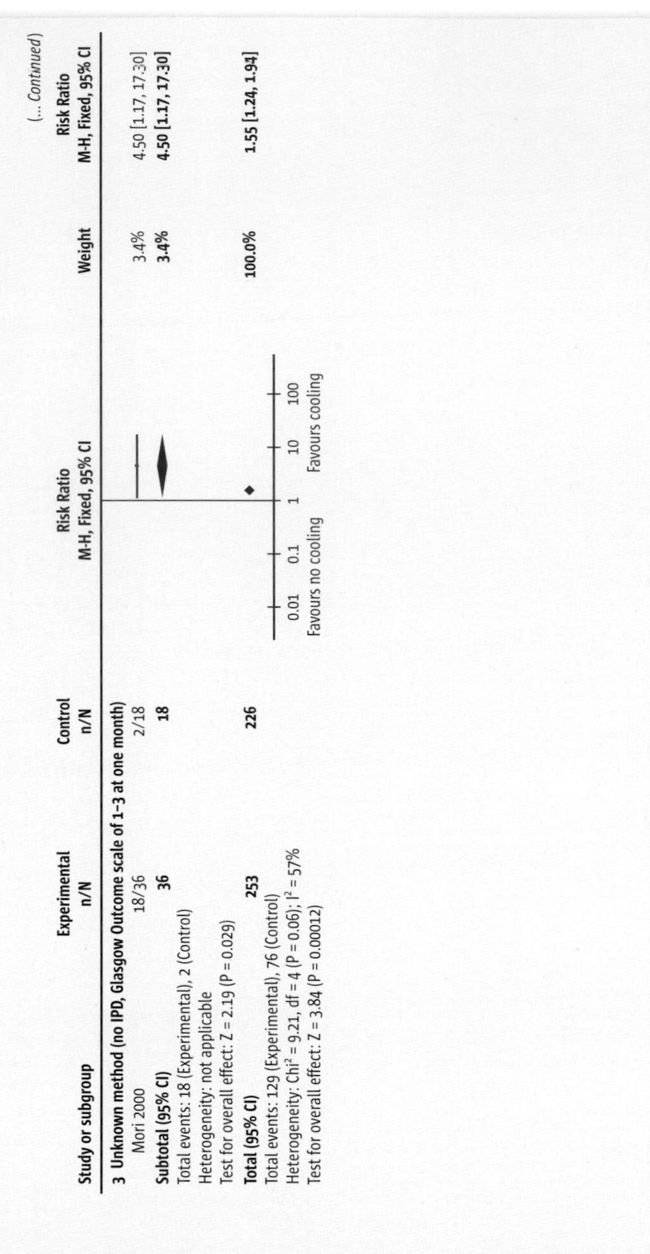

(... *Continued*)

Study or subgroup	Experimental n/N	Control n/N	Risk Ratio M-H, Fixed, 95% CI	Weight	Risk Ratio M-H, Fixed, 95% CI
3 Unknown method (no IPD, Glasgow Outcome scale of 1–3 at one month)					
Mori 2000	18/36	2/18		3.4%	4.50 [1.17, 17.30]
Subtotal (95% CI)	**36**	**18**		**3.4%**	**4.50 [1.17, 17.30]**
Total events: 18 (Experimental), 2 (Control)					
Heterogeneity: not applicable					
Test for overall effect: Z = 2.19 (P = 0.029)					
Total (95% CI)	**253**	**226**		**100.0%**	**1.55 [1.24, 1.94]**
Total events: 129 (Experimental), 76 (Control)					
Heterogeneity: $Chi^2 = 9.21$, df = 4 (P = 0.06); $I^2 = 57\%$					
Test for overall effect: Z = 3.84 (P = 0.00012)					

Secondary outcomes

No data were available on: survival at 6 months and 1 year; quality of life at 6 months and long term dependency; or cost effectiveness.

Adverse events

There were no significant differences between the groups.

Author's conclusion

Therapeutic hypothermia with conventional cooling methods seems to improve neurological outcome and survival of patients following cardiac arrest. The currently available evidence suggests that patients with out-of-hospital cardiac arrest and for patients with VT/VF rhythm as the first recorded cardiac rhythm benefit from therapeutic hypothermia. For in hospital and non-cardiac cause of arrest there were insufficient data to draw any conclusion.

Problems & limitations

- There were only a small number of randomised controlled trials
- In some subgroups the number of patients was too small to make any reliable inferences
- There was some heterogeneity with cooling methods but those studies were analysed separately
- Control groups varied with regards to temperature control, in 2 studies, mean temperatures were above 37°C. Inadequate temperature control in some control groups may have affected overall outcome as it is well recognised that even small temperature rises can increase the risk of an unfavourable neurological outcome

Advantages

- Overall quality of trials was good
- This review was academically initiated
- The data represent individual patient analyses

Expert opinion

Ian Poelaert

How valid and robust are the data?

From selected studies with availability of individual patient data, results after either out-of-hospital or in-hospital cardiac arrest were enrolled. For each study, specific criteria of inclusion were withheld after which quality was assessed; only randomized studies with primary focus on cerebral performance as first outcome variable were enrolled. Hence, this review contains a very limited number (5) of publications, based on the above mentioned strict inclusion criteria.

Should clinical practice be influenced by this review/result?

In principle, controlled hypothermia as a first measure in patients suffering from cardiac arrest, should already be implemented, if medicine and supportive measures have been implemented "lege artis". For those, not yet persuaded based on previous publications, this review may change their minds, providing an overview and summary of performed studies.

What should be the next step?

Setup of a larger follow up creating a larger database, including assessment of cerebral performance, should be the next step to obtain a continuous quality assessment. Large participation should allow inclusion of many new centres, enlarging the usage of this technique considerably.

Citation

Arrich J, HolzerM, HerknerH, MüllnerM. Hypothermia for neuroprotection in adults after cardiopulmonary resuscitation. Cochrane Database of Systematic Reviews 2009, Issue 4. Art. No.: CD004128. DOI: 10.1002/14651858.CD004128.pub2

AMSTAR: methodological quality of the review

1.	Was "a priori" design provided?	Y
2.	Was study selection and data extraction adequate?	Y
3.	Was the literature search comprehensive?	Y
4.	Was 'Grey Literature' used?	Y
5.	Was a list of excluded studies provided?	Y
6.	Were the characteristics of included studies provided?	Y
7.	Was the scientific quality of studies assessed & documented?	Y
8.	Was the scientific quality of studies weighted appropriately in forming conclusions?	Y
9.	Were the methods used for data synthesis appropriate?	Y
10.	Was the potential for publication bias assessed?	Y
11.	Were any conflicts of interest stated?	Y

Overall quality of trials included	Good in 3/5 studies
Overall quality of the review	High

Vasopressin for vasodilatory shock

Condition: vasodilatory shock
Interventions: vasopressin and terlipressin
Clinical question: Does the use of vasopressin or its analogue terlipressin for vasodilatory shock reduce morbidity or mortality?

Mortality from septic shock remains high at 40–60% and is usually associated with refractory hypotension. Initial management consists of fluid resuscitation and vasopressors such as norepinephrine however a significant number of patients remain unresponsive with subsequent deterioration in organ function and death. As an endogenous stress hormone, vasopressin has little if any effect in normal subjects; however patients with vasodilatory shock have inappropriately low vasopressin levels. In the latter, a low dose infusion of vasopressin can restore vascular tone in patients and although it can improve blood pressure, its effect on mortality remains controversial. Furthermore the impact of side effects such as arrhythmias; skin, myocardial, and gut ischaemia remains to be elucidated.

4

Review characteristics

- **Eligibility criteria:** RCTs and quasi-randomised controlled trials with or without blinding that compared vasopressin with standard therapy or placebo in patients with vasodilatory shock
- **Population:** children and adults with septic and non septic vasodilatory shock
- **Number of studies:** 10 RCTs. 2 multicentre trials, 1 at 2 centres and 7 single centre trials
  6 trials used vasopressin and 4 used terlipressin
  8 trials of adults, 2 trials included children
- **Number of patients:** 1,134. Range 10–778 (VASST, Russell et al., 2008)
  Adults, n = 1,007; children < 17 years old, n = 127
- **Study dates:** 1999–2009

Definitions

- **Intervention:** intravenous vasopressin or terlipressin
- **Replacement therapy:** vasopressin given at a fixed dose of 0.04 UI/hour
- **Vasopressor therapy:** vasopressin titrated to achieve a particular haemodynamic goal e.g. MAP
- **Standard therapy:** fluid replacement and/or vasopressors; mechanical ventilation; RRT
- **Short-term mortality:** varied (28-day, 30-day, ICU or hospital mortality)
- **Control:** 2 trials of vasopressin versus placebo; 4 trials of vasopressin versus norepinephrine; 2 trials of terlipressin to norepinephrine; 1 trial of terlipressin versus vasopressin + norepinephrine; 1 trial of terlipressin versus dopamine, dobutamine and epinephrine

Populations

- **8 trials:** patients with septic shock
- **2 trials:** mixed population – patients with septic and non-septic shock (n = 117)

Some patients were treated with corticosteroids or recombinant activated protein C (rhAPC) however these were distributed equally between intervention and control groups.

Results

Primary Outcome: short-term all-cause mortality

Study type	Trials/n	Intervention Gp mortality	Control Gp mortality	RR	95% CI	*p*	I^2
Vasopressin/terlipressin in adults	6/973	40.2%	42.9%	0.91	0.8–1.0	0.21	0%
Vasopressin/terlipressin in septic shock	5/910	38.5%	41.4%	0.9	0.8–1.0	0.20	0%
Vasopressin for vasodilatory shock	4/879	37.5%	41.8%	0.91	0.78–1.06	0.20	0%
Terlipressin for vasodilatory shock	3/109	59.4%	62.2%	0.91	0.68–1.24	0.58	0%
Paediatric trials	2/127	46.1%	40.3%	1.2	0.56–2.54	0.64	58%

Meta-regression analysis

There was no association between vasopressin dose ($p = 0.65$) or age ($p = 0.93$) and short-term mortality.

Secondary outcomes

Outcome	Results
Epinephrine dose	Meta-regression analysis showed a significant association between vasopressin and epinephrine dose
Serious adverse events	In 4 trials (n = 463) there was no significant difference in complications (Intervention group 10.6% and control group 11.8%)
Urine output	In 5 trials (n = 171) within 24 hours from vasopressin/terlipressin infusion the WMD between intervention and control group was 0.49 ml/kg/h difference (95% CI −0.18 to 1.16, p = 0.15, I^2 = 72%)

Author's conclusion

Overall there was no survival benefit from vasopressin/terlipressin therapy. Although there was no statistical heterogeneity between trials, there were important clinical differences between the dose and duration of therapy. Vasopressin therapy did significantly reduce norepinephrine requirement and may improve urine output. There was no increase in the incidence of adverse events with either vasopressin or terlipressin.

Fig. 3 Mortality in adults (CI indicates confidence interval) [from Polito A, Parisini E, Ricci Z, Picardo S, Annane D on behalf of the ESICM systematic Review Unit. Vasopressin for the treatment of vasodilatory shock: an ESICM systematic review and meta-analysis. (Not yet published)]

Study or subgroup	Experimental		Control		Weight	Risk Ratio M-H, Random 95% CI
	Events	Total	Events	Total		
Albanese 2005	5	10	4	10	2.1%	1.25 [0.47, 3.33]
Dunser 2003	17	24	17	24	15.0%	1.00 [0.70, 1.44]
Lauzier 2006	3	13	3	10	1.0%	0.77 [0.20, 3.03]
Morelli 2008	26	39	14	20	15.0%	0.95 [0.66, 1.37]
Morelli 2009	15	30	10	15	7.7%	0.75 [0.45, 1.24]
Russell 2008	140	396	150	382	59.2%	0.90 [0.75, 1.08]
Total (95% CI)		**512**		**461**	**100.0%**	**0.91 [0.79, 1.05]**
Total events:	206		198			

Heterogeneity: $Tau^2 = 0.00$; $Chi^2 = 1.36$, $df = 5$ ($P = 0.93$); $I^2 = 0\%$

Test for overall effect: $Z = 1.25$ ($P = 0.21$)

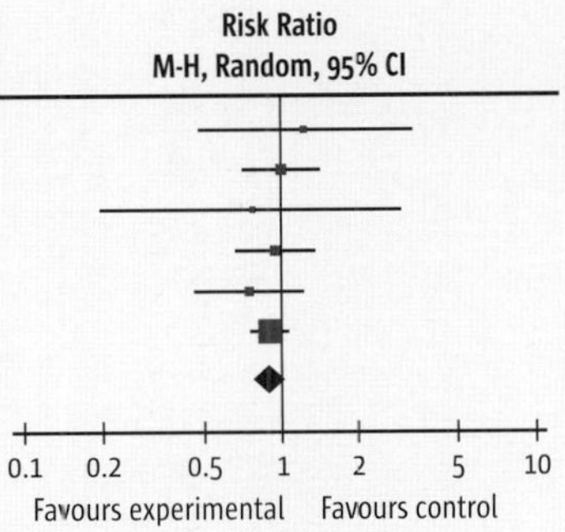

Risk Ratio M-H, Random, 95% CI

0.1 0.2 0.5 1 2 5 10

Favours experimental Favours control

Problems & limitations

- Vasopressor duration varied from 4 hours (1 trial) to > 24 hours (5 trials) or was titrated to haemodynamics and side effects (2 trials)
- Vasopressin and terlipressin have markedly different pharmacokinetic properties
- There was a marked difference between trials for mortality time points
- 1 study used 24 hours mortality but this was not included in the pooled analysis
- Small numbers of patients in all but the VASST trial

Advantages

- Subgroup analysis excluding various studies to explore the impact of the between trial differences consistently yielded similar results

Expert opinion

Anthony Gordon

How valid and robust are the data?
This systematic review and meta-analysis includes studies of both vasopressin and terlipressin in comparison to other catecholamine vasopressors or placebo, often unblinded. Amongst the studies different dosing regimens have been used for varying durations and the patients studied include both septic and non-septic shock. Although more than 1,100 patients have been included, ~70% come from one study. These factors severely limit the validity and robustness of the data.

Should clinical practice be influenced by this?
Despite the limitations outlined above the data for this review support the 2008 guidelines of the Surviving Sepsis Campaign; "vasopressin ... may be added to norepinephrine subsequently with anticipation of an effect equivalent to that of norepinephrine alone."

What is the next step?
The data from this review suggest that vasopressin is an effective vasopressor and appears as safe as alternative catecholamine vasopressors. Further work is required to determine if vasopressin (or terlipressin) administered according to different dosing regimens, used earlier in less severely ill patients, possibly in combination with other treatments offers any benefit on outcome.

4

Citation

Polito A, Parisini E, Ricci Z, Picardo S, Annane D on behalf of the ESICM systematic Review Unit. Vasopressin for the treatment of vasodilatory shock: an ESICM systematic review and meta-analysis. [Not yet published]

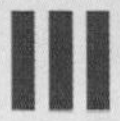

AMSTAR: methodological quality of the review

1.	Was "a priori" design provided?	Y
2.	Was study selection and data extraction adequate?	Y
3.	Was the literature search comprehensive?	Y
4.	Was 'Grey Literature' used?	Y
5.	Was a list of excluded studies provided?	Y
6.	Were the characteristics of included studies provided?	Y
7.	Was the scientific quality of studies assessed & documented?	Y
8.	Was the scientific quality of studies weighted appropriately in forming conclusions?	Y
9.	Were the methods used for data synthesis appropriate?	Y
10.	Was the potential for publication bias assessed?	Y
11.	Were any conflicts of interest stated?	Y

Overall quality of trials included	5 high quality on Jadad score
Overall quality of the review	High

Pre-emptive haemodynamic intervention

Condition: major surgery
Intervention: haemodynamic optimisation
Clinical question: Can a pre-emptive strategy of haemodynamic monitoring and manipulation improve outcomes in moderate to high risk surgical patients?

Major surgery, particularly emergency surgery is associated with significant morbidity and mortality. The risks are further amplified in patients with limited cardiorespiratory reserve. Many studies have shown benefit from flow-based haemodynamic monitoring and optimisation however this has not been adapted as standard care. This may be due to the small numbers of patients in the existing predominantly single centre studies.

Review characteristics

4

- **Eligibility criteria:** RCTs examining a pre-emptive, monitored haemodynamic approach that reported hospital mortality as an outcome on an intention-to-treat basis
- **Population:** moderate to high risk surgical patients
- **A priori:** subgroup and sensitivity analyses based on a) the type of monitoring used, b) fluid versus fluids plus inotropes, c) therapeutic goals and d) normal versus supranormal resuscitation target
- **Number of studies:** 29 RCTs
- **Number of patients:** 4,805
- **Study dates:** 1985–2008

Definitions

- **Haemodynamic intervention:** the proactive use of haemodynamic monitoring, and therapies such as intravenous fluid and inotropes to manipulate haemodynamics in the perioperative period
- **Perioperative period:** 24 hours preoperatively, intraoperatively or up to 24 hours postoperatively
- **Moderate to high risk patient:** criteria initially published by Shoemaker et al. and later modified by Pearse et al. (see "Additional information")
- **Supranormal:** oxygen delivery index more than or equal to 600 ml/min/m^2
- **Optimization goals:** studies varied in their specific optimisation goals but most studies used either cardiac index, oxygen delivery or FTc (oesophageal Doppler – flow time corrected)
- **Control group:** 17 studies used "standard care" which may have varied significantly between studies. The remaining studies had specific targets

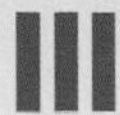

Results

Primary outcome

Mortality

Pooled OR from all 29 studies showed a significant reduction in mortality in the haemodynamic intervention group (OR 0.48, 95% CI 0.33–0.78, p = 0.0002)

3 studies had no mortality in either group

There was a reduction in control group mortality over time with mortality halving every decade from 29.5% in the 1980s to 7% in the last decade.

Subgroup analysis

Mortality was reduced in the studies using:

Pulmonary artery catheter (OR 0.35, 95% CI 0.19–0.65, p = 0.001)

Fluids and inotropes (OR 0.47, 95% CI 0.29–0.76, p = 0.002) as compared to fluids alone

Cardiac index or oxygen delivery (OR 0.38, 95% CI 0.21–0.68)

Supranormal resuscitation targets (OR 0.29, 95% CI 0.18–0.47)

Secondary outcome

Morbidity

23 studies reported complications

There was a significant reduction in complications in the haemodynamic intervention group (OR 0.43, 95% CI 0.34–0.53)

This result was consistent across all 4 subgroups

Complication rates remain constant over time, approximately one third of patients are affected

Author's conclusion

Pre-emptive targeted haemodynamic therapy reduces mortality and morbidity after major surgery. The beneficial effects on morbidity were observed even in the lower risk groups. Better overall care, improvements in technology and availability of less invasive monitoring techniques may explain the reduction in control group mortality over time. This review demonstrated a significant benefit with the use of the pulmonary artery catheter in contrast to studies that caused much controversy over its use.

Fig. 4 Effects of pre-emptive haemodynamic intervention in protocol group versus control on mortality rate, grouped by quality of the study as assessed by a Jadad score of more than or less than 3. M-H = Mantel-Haenszel [from Hamilton MA, Cecconi M, Rhodes A. A systematic review and meta-analysis on the use of pre-emptive haemodynamic intervention to improve post-operative outcomes in moderate and high risk surgical patients. Anesthesia and analgesia DOI:10.1213/Ana.0b013e3181eeaae5]

Study or subgroup	Protocol		Control		Weight	Odds Ratio M-H, Random, 95% CI
	Events	Total	Events	Total		
1.7.1 Jadad Score ≥ 3						
Chytra 2007 (26)	13	80	18	82	9.4%	0.69 [0.31, 1.52]
Gan 2002 (23)	0	50	0	50		Not estimable
Lobo 2000 (22)	3	19	9	18	4.6%	0.19 [0.04, 0.88]
Lobo 2006 (21)	2	25	7	25	4.0%	0.22 [0.04, 1.21]
Mckendry 2004 (18)	4	89	2	90	3.9%	2.07 [0.37, 11.60]
Noblett 2006 (16)	0	51	1	52	1.4%	0.33 [0.01, 8.37]
Pearse 2005 (15)	7	62	9	60	7.3%	0.72 [0.25, 2.08]
Polonen 2000 (14)	2	196	6	197	4.3%	0.33 [0.07, 1.65]
Sandham 2003 (13)	78	997	77	997	13.7%	1.01 [0.73, 1.41]
Valentine 1998 (8)	3	60	1	60	2.5%	3.11 [0.31, 30.73]
Venn 2002 (7)	3	30	2	29	3.5%	1.50 [0.23, 9.70]
Wakeling 2005 (6)	0	67	1	67	1.4%	0.33 [0.01, 8.21]
Wilson 1999 (5)	3	92	8	46	5.3%	0.16 [0.04, 0.64]
Subtotal (95% CI)		**1818**		**1773**	**61.2%**	**0.62 [0.39, 1.01]**
Total events	118		141			

Heterogeneity: $Tau^2 = 0.21$; $Chi^2 = 17.70$, df = 11 (P = 0.09); $I^2 = 38\%$

Test for overall effect: Z = 1.94 (P = 0.05)

Odds Ratio M-H, Random, 95% CI

0.01 0.1 1 10 100

Favours experimental Favours control

(*Continued ...*)

(... *Continued*)

Study or subgroup	Protocol Events	Protocol Total	Control Events	Control Total	Weight	Odds Ratio M-H, Random, 95% CI
1.7.2 Jadad Score < 3						
Bender 1997 (32)	1	51	1	53	1.8%	1.04 [0.06, 17.08]
Berlauk 1991 (31)	1	68	2	21	2.2%	0.14 [0.01, 1.65]
Bishop 1995 (30)	9	50	24	65	8.6%	0.38 [0.16, 0.90]
Bonazzi 2002 (29)	0	50	0	50		Not estimable
Boyd 1993 (28)	3	53	12	54	5.6%	0.21 [0.06, 0.79]
Buettner 2008 (27)	0	40	1	40	1.4%	0.33 [0.01, 8.22]
Conway 2002 (25)	0	29	1	28	1.4%	0.31 [0.01, 7.95]
Kapoor 2008 (19)	0	15	0	15		Not estimable
Lopes 2007 (20)	2	17	5	18	3.6%	0.29 [0.05, 1.80]
Mythen 1995 (17)	0	30	1	30	1.4%	0.32 [0.01, 8.24]
Schultz 1985 (12)	1	35	10	35	2.8%	0.07 [0.01, 0.61]
Shoemaker 1988 (11)	1	28	18	60	2.9%	0.09 [0.01, 0.69]
Sinclair 1997 (10)	1	20	2	20	2.2%	0.47 [0.04, 5.69]
Ueno 1998 (9)	0	16	2	18	1.5%	0.20 [0.01, 4.49]
Ziegler 1997 (4)	3	32	2	40	3.5%	1.97 [0.31, 12.54]
Subtotal (95% CI)		**534**		**545**	**38.8%**	**0.31 [0.18, 0.52]**
Total events	22		81			
Heterogeneity: $Tau^2 = 0.00$; $Chi^2 = 8.97$, df = 12 (P = 0.71); $I^2 = 0\%$						
Test for overall effect: Z = 4.46 (P < 0.00001)						
Total (95% CI)		**2312**		**2318**	**100.0%**	**0.46 [0.31, 0.69]**
Total events	140		222			
Heterogeneity: $Tau^2 = 0.27$; $Chi^2 = 37.57$, df = 24 (P = 0.04); $I^2 = 36\%$						
Test for overall effect: Z = 3.80 (P = 0.0001)						

Odds Ratio M-H, Random, 95% CI: 0.01 0.1 1 10 100

Favours experimental | Favours control

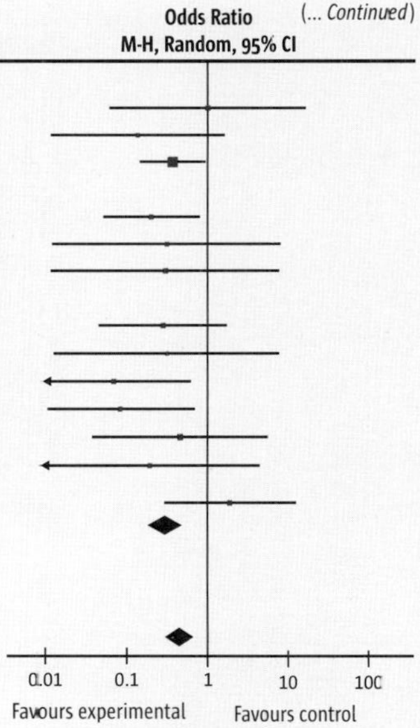

4

Problems & limitations

- The pooled analysis of the higher quality studies does not show any mortality benefit whereas that of the lower quality studies does
- The reporting of postoperative complications was variable as was the definition of these complications. Only 2 studies used standardized methods of outcome reporting e.g. the postoperative morbidity survey

Advantages

- There was a significant reduction in morbidity with haemodynamic intervention regardless of trial quality
- Results agree with previous reviews

Citation

Hamilton MA, Cecconi M, Rhodes A. A systematic review and meta-analysis on the use of pre-emptive haemodynamic intervention to improve post-operative outcomes in moderate and high risk surgical patients. Anesthesia and analgesia DOI:10.1213/Ana.0b013e3181eeaae5

4

Additional information

The original criteria for high risk surgery/patients can be found in the following reference:

Shoemaker WC, Appel PL, Kram HB, Waxman K, Lee TS. Prospective trial of supranormal values of survivors as therapeutic goals in high risk surgical patients. Chest 1988; 94: 1176–86

The modified criteria:

1. Severe cardiac or respiratory illness resulting in severe functional limitation
2. Extensive surgery planned for carcinoma involving bowel anastomosis
3. Acute massive blood loss (> 2.5 litres)
4. Aged over 70 years with moderate functional limitation of one or more organ systems
5. Septicaemia (positive blood cultures or septic focus)
6. Respiratory failure (PaO_2 < 8 kPa on FiO_2 > 0.4 i.e. PaO_2: FiO_2 ratio < 20 kPa or ventilation > 48 hours)
7. Acute abdominal catastrophe (e.g. pancreatitis, perforated viscous, gastro-intestinal bleed)
8. Acute renal failure (urea > 20 mmol/l, creatinine > 260 μmol/l)
9. Surgery for abdominal aortic aneurysm

Citation: Pearse R, Dawson D, Fawcett J, Rhodes A, Grounds RM, Bennett ED. Early goal-directed therapy after major surgery reduces complications and duration of hospital stay. A randomised, controlled trial [ISRCTN38797445]. Crit Care 2005; 9: R687–93, http://www.biomedcentral.com/content/supplementary/cc3887-S1.doc

On-going study: Pre-emptive haemodynamic optimization of high risk patients undergoing elective major surgical procedures. NCT00725972. This study is currently recruiting and aims to enrol 200 patients. The estimated completion date was May 2011

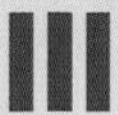

AMSTAR: methodological quality of the review

1.	Was "a priori" design provided?	Y
2.	Was study selection and data extraction adequate?	Y
3.	Was the literature search comprehensive?	Y
4.	Was 'Grey Literature' used? Restricted to English language	P
5.	Was a list of excluded studies provided? 68 excluded studies	NA
6.	Were the characteristics of included studies provided?	Y
7.	Was the scientific quality of studies assessed & documented?	Y
8.	Was the scientific quality of studies weighted appropriately in forming conclusions?	Y
9.	Were the methods used for data synthesis appropriate?	Y
10.	Was the potential for publication bias assessed?	N
11.	Were any conflicts of interest stated?	Y

4

Overall quality of trials included	14 high quality based on Jadad score
Overall quality of the review	High

5
Ethics

Organ donation ____ 122

Organ donation

Condition: organ donation/brain stem death

Task: obtaining consent

Clinical question: Is there anything we can do to influence the relatives of brain stem dead patients to offer or decline organ donation?

The number of patients on organ transplant lists has increased by 70% in the UK over a 10-year period, whereas the supply of organs for transplantation has remained static, and as a result, one patient dies every day awaiting transplantation. In the UK, the Human Tissue Act 2004 priorities the wishes of the potential donor over the relatives' wishes but it would be practically impossible to proceed without the family's consent. Thus obtaining consent remains the most significant barrier to organ retrieval in suitable donors. This review addresses the question as to which factors can be modified to increase the consent rate.

Review characteristics

5

- **Eligibility Criteria**: RCTs, observational studies and audits
- **Excluded**: studies that examined non-modifiable factors e.g. religion, racew
- **Study characteristics**: request for organ donation – successful versus unsuccessful
  - Observational studies
  - Audits with "before and after" factors
  - Prospective, retrospective, structured interview, postal survey or staff questionnaire
- **Number of studies**: 20
- **Number of patients**: 8,966
- **Population**: adult and paediatric
- **Study dates**: 1994–2006

Results

6 modifiable factors were identified

1. Information discussed during the request
2. Perceived quality of care of the donor
3. Understanding of brainstem death
4. Timing of the request
5. Setting in which the request is made
6. Approach and expertise of the person making the request

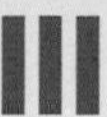

Modifiable Factor	Papers/n	Impact on decision	Specific factors
Information	5 papers/ 1434 patients	+	Families which felt they were given enough information
		+	Cost of donation, funeral arrangements, choice of donated organs
		–	Telling families to enquire about donation
Quality of Care	3 papers/ 869 patients	–	Negative perception of care
Understanding BSD	5 papers/ 1208 patients	+	Understanding the concept of brainstem death increase consent
		+	Accepting that recovery is not possible after brain death
		+	Using nuclear medicine brain flow imaging
Timing	9 papers/ 4001 patients	+	Separating notification of and acceptance of BSD from request for organ donation
		+	Giving families enough time to make a decision
Setting	2 out of 3 papers/ 871 patients	+	Private setting to make the request
Expertise	14 studies/ 7638 patients	+	Procurement of an in-house organ donation coordinator was the most significant factor
		+	Combined approached by hospital staff and coordinator
		+	Procurement of race specific coordinator especially for minority groups

5

Authors' conclusion

Many of the findings of the review were not surprising as these are considered to be good practice when "breaking bad news".

Only factors studied at the hospital level were identified; however there may be more modifiable factors that can be addressed at a population level

Most of the studies were conducted in the US where organ donation rates are higher than in the UK; therefore these strategies may have an even greater impact in the UK.

Problems & limitations

- No RCTs. Some studies would be considered too small to draw convincing evidence
- Some of the studies didn't specify if the donor and non-donor families were representative of the whole population
- Interviews and questionnaires are subject to recall bias

Advantages

- Two studies had more than 1,000 patients, overall combined numbers were impressive

Expert opinion

Jozef Kesecioglu

The authors performed a systematic review to study the modifiable determinants of consent to organ donation requests. Nearly 250 potentially relevant papers were screened from a total of almost 900 identified abstracts. Nonetheless, the actual knowledge base on the topic proved to be quite limited, which resulted in the inclusion of not more than 20 observational studies and surveys into this review. No interventional studies were identified.

The authors found that the provision of adequate information during the donation request, the perceived quality of medical care of the potential donor, ensuring a clear understanding of the concept of brain stem death, separating the notification of death and the request for donation, making the request in a private setting, and using trained and experienced individuals to make the request were the main factors associated with success.

How valid and robust are these findings?

The studies included in this review originated almost entirely from the U.S. (where donation rates may be higher than in some European settings) and exclusively relate to heart beating donation procedures (where there is time to reflect on the donation request). Therefore, the findings of this review may not be generalizable to all settings; in particular they may not be applicable to non-heart beating procedures.

It is also important to stress that the studies were purely observational and that factors correlated with consent to organ donation thus might not be causative. Furthermore, many of the studies were retrospective chart reviews and relied on hospital or organ procurement staff to collect the data. This introduces the possibility of observation bias, since accounts about the communication with relatives may be recorded more extensively, or with a more positive connotation, when a request for organ donation was granted compared to when it was denied. Finally, a number of studies were based on telephone interviews with donor and non-donor families several months after the events, which introduces the possibility of recall bias.

Should clinical practice be influenced by this?

The two factors that had the largest effect on consent rates were the individual making the request and the timing of this conversation. Consent rates were higher when an organ procurement coordinator and hospital staff made the request together. Although it is clearly not cost-effective to place a dedicated donor transplant coordinator in every hospital, this might be feasible in hospitals with a large number of potential organ donors.

What is the next step?

There is a clear need for interventional studies to assess the factors of organ donation requests that can be modified in order to maximise consent rates. The randomised controlled ACRE (assessment of collaborative requesting) trial is one such study, which is currently under way in the UK.

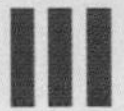

Citation

Simpkin AL, Robertson LC, Barber VS and Young JD. Modifiable factors influencinq relative's decision to offer organ donation: systematic review. BMJ 2009; 339: b991

Additional information

This review was part of the background work for the ACRE study of "collaborative requesting" (ACRE Trial Collaborators. Effect of "collaborative requesting" on consent rate for organ donation: randomised controlled trial [ACRE trial].BMJ. 2009 Oct 8;339).

AMSTAR: methodological quality of the review

1.	Was "a priori" design provided?	Y
2.	Was study selection and data extrartion adequate?	Y
3.	Was the literature search comprehensive?	Y
4.	Was 'Grey Literature' used?	P
5.	Was a list of excluded studies provided?	NA
6.	Where the characteristics of included studies provided?	Y
7.	Was the scientific quality nf studies assessed & documented?	NA
8.	Was the scientific quality of studies weiqhted appropriately in forming conclusions?	Y
9.	Were the methods used for data synthesis appropriate?	Y
10.	Was the potential for publication bias assessed?	U
11.	Were any conflicts of interest stated?	Y

Overall quality of trials included	No RCTs
Overall quality of the review	High

6

General

Stress ulcer prophylaxis 128
Critical illness polyneuropathy and polymyopathy 134
Thromboprophylaxis 139
Music therapy 143

Stress ulcer prophylaxis

Condition: stress ulceration
Intervention: H_2 blockers
Clinical question: What are the benefits and risks of stress ulcer prophylaxis (SUP)?

The role of SUP in preventing GI bleeding in high risk critically ill patients was established in the 1980s when it was common to keep ICU patients 'nil-per-os', and has been reinforced more recently by the introduction of 'care bundles' in the UK, where SUP is considered a core 'quality' measure for mechanically ventilated patients. 90% of patients admitted to ICU receive SUP either in the form of histamine-2 receptor blockers (H_2RB) or proton pump inhibitors (PPI), however, this is not without risk. Acid suppression (maintaining pH > 3.5) is associated with increased colonisation of the upper GI tract with pathogenic organisms resulting in increased risk of hospital (or ventilator) acquired pneumonia (HAP). Gastric acid forms important defence against Clostridium Difficile therefore suppression can cause C. Difficile infection. Evidence from recent observational studies suggests that because of early enteral feeding stress ulceration is very uncommon (1%), and therefore SUP may place the patient at unnecessary risk.

Review characteristics

6

- **Eligibility criteria:** RCTs that compared histamine-2 receptor blocker with a placebo (as PPIs have only been assessed in 1 trial)
- **Subgroups:** enteral nutrition (EN) versus no enteral nutrition (includes parenteral nutrition)
- **Number of studies:** 17 RCTs
- **Number of patients:** 1,836 (range 28–223)
- **Population:** adults from MICU, SICU, GICU or NICU
- **Study dates:** 1980–2004 (6 from 1980's; 10 from 1990's; 1 from 2004)

Definitions

- **EN:** enteral nutrition. Adequate being > 50% of nutritional requirement
- **Clinical gastrointestinal bleed (GIB):** not defined
- **H_2RB:** dose and route not defined

Results

Primary outcome: clinically evident GI bleeding (16 studies) or on endoscopy (2 studies) for SUP

Group	Trials/n	OR	95% CI	p	I^2	Result
All	17/1836	0.47	0.29–0.76	0.002	44%	SS
Enteral feed	3/262	1.26	0.43–3.7	–	–	NSS

Fig. 1 Effect of stress ulcer prophylaxis (SUP) on the risk of gastrointestinal (GI) bleeding. Studies are grouped by the use or nonuse of enteral nutrition. Weight is the relative contribution of each study to the overall treatment effect (odds ratio [OR] and 95% confidence interval [CI]) on a log scale assuming a random effects model. H2RB, histamine-2 receptor blocker [from Paul E. Marik, Tajender Vasu, Amyn Hirani, Monvasi Pachinburavan. Stress ulcer prophylaxis in the new millennium: A systematic review and meta-analysis. Crit Care Med 2010 Vol. 38(11): 2222–2228]

Study or subgroup	H2RB Events	H2RB Total	Control Events	Control Total	Weight	Odds Ratio M-H, Random, 95% CI	Year
1.3.1 No Enteral Nutrition							
Halloran 1980	2	26	8	24	5.6%	0.17 [0.03, 0.89]	1980
Zinner 1981	14	100	20	100	11.8%	0.65 [0.31, 1.38]	1981
Feura 1985	1	21	7	18	3.7%	0.08 [0.01, 0.72]	1985
Cheadle 1985	2	98	3	97	5.0%	0.65 [0.11, 4.00]	1985
Groll 1986	6	114	11	107	9.4%	0.48 [0.17, 1.36]	1986
Reusser 1990	0	19	0	21		Not estimable	1990
Karlstadt 1990	1	54	7	33	3.9%	0.07 [0.01, 0.60]	1990
Ruiz-Santana 1991	2	19	1	30	3.1%	3.41 [0.29, 40.50]	1991
Metz 1993	3	85	15	81	7.7%	0.16 [0.04, 0.57]	1993
Martin 1993	9	65	22	66	10.7%	0.32 [0.13, 0.77]	1993
Chan 1995	9	52	21	49	10.4%	0.28 [0.11, 0.70]	1995
Burgess 1995	0	16	5	18	2.3%	0.07 [0.00, 1.47]	1995
Hanisch 1998	3	57	2	57	4.9%	1.53 [0.25, 9.51]	1998
Kantorova 2004	2	71	1	75	3.2%	2.14 [0.19, 24.19]	2004
Subtotal (95% CI)		**798**		**776**	**31.7%**	**0.37 [0.23, 0.61]**	
Total events	54		123				

Heterogeneity: $Tau^2 = 0.26$; $Chi^2 = 18.60$, df = 12 ($P = 0.10$); $I^2 = 35\%$

Test for overall effect: $Z = 3.90$ ($P < 0.0001$)

Odds Ratio M-H, Random, 95% CI: 0.01 0.1 1 10 100 — Favours H2RB / Favours control

(Continued ...)

6

(… *Continued*)

Study or subgroup	H2RB Events	H2RB Total	Control Events	Control Total	Weight	Odds Ratio M-H, Random, 95% CI	Year
1.3.2 Enteral Nutrition							
van den Berg 1985	5	14	1	14	3.5%	7.22 [0.72, 72.70]	1985
Apte 1992	5	16	6	18	6.7%	0.91 [0.22, 3.84]	1992
Ben-menachen 1994	5	100	6	100	8.1%	0.82 [0.24, 2.79]	1994
Subtotal (95% CI)		**130**		**132**	**18.3%**	**1.26 [0.43, 3.70]**	
Total events	15		13				
Heterogeneity: $Tau^2 = 0.28$; $Chi^2 = 2.86$, df = 2 (P = 0.24); $I^2 = 30\%$							
Test for overall effect: Z = 0.43 (P = 0.67)							
Total (95% CI)		**928**		**908**	**100.0%**	**0.47 [0.29, 0.76]**	
Total events	69		136				
Heterogeneity: $Tau^2 = 0.38$; $Chi^2 = 26.62$, df = 15 (P = 0.03); $I^2 = 44\%$							
Test for overall effect: Z = 3.07 (P = 0.002)							

Odds Ratio
M-H, Random, 95% CI

0.01 0.1 1 10 100

Favours H2RB Favours control

Secondary outcomes: HAP and hospital mortality in patients who received SUP

Outcomes	Trials/n	OR	95% CI	P	I^2	Result
HAP overall	17/1836	1.53	0.89–2.61	0.12	41%	NSS
HAP: EN	2/234	2.81	1.20–6.56	0.02	0%	SS
Mortality	17/1836	1.03	0.78–1.37	0.82	-	NSS
Mortality: EN	2/234	1.89	1.04–3.44	0.04	0%	SS

There was no difference between treatment effect and the year the study was reported (by meta regression analysis).

Author's conclusion

This meta-analysis shows that SUP does not reduce the risk of GI bleeding in patients who are enterally fed, and that H2RB in these patients may increase the risk of HAP and death. EN improves mucosal blood flow and immunity and may even blunt stress related vagal stimulation of the stomach. Studies that have compared other types of acid suppression (PPIs or sucralfate) have not found any difference in the incidence of GI bleeding, HAP or mortality. However some studies suggest that EN is more effective at acid suppression especially if administered continuously compared to antacids and cimetidine. Both H_2RB and EN are effective at acid suppression resulting in a higher gastric pH which may explain the increased risk of HAP compared to either intervention alone.

6

Problems & limitations

- Eligibility into the enteral group only required 50% of patients in the study to have adequate enteral nutrition. This may have underestimated the combined effect of H2RB and EN on HAP and mortality
- Only 3 studies had enterally fed patients thus numbers were small

Advantages

- Only RCTs were included and most studies were of high quality as determined by Jadad score
- Results are supported by results from recent observational studies

Citation

Marik PE, Vasu T, Hirani A, Pachinburavan M. Stress ulcer prophylaxis in the new millennium: A systematic review and meta-analysis. Crit Care Med 2010 Vol. 38(11): 2222–2228. DOI: 10.1097/CCM.0b013e3181f17adf

Additional information

In the UK and USA, stress ulcer prophylaxis forms an integral part of the ventilator care bundle, which was designed to reduce the incidence of VAP and other complications associated with mechanical ventilation.

In the UK the Patient safety First Campaign describes four interventions (www.patientsafetyfirst.nhs.uk):

1. Patient positioning – head elevation to 30–45 degrees
2. Ventilator weaning – daily sedative interruption and assessment of readiness to extubate
3. Peptic ulcer disease prophylaxis
4. Venous thromboembolism prophylaxis

In the USA the Institute for Healthcare Improvement (IHI) ventilator bundle includes the above four components and an additional element (www.ihi.org):

5. Daily oral care with chlorhexidine

This IHI ventilator bundle document on peptic ulcer disease (PUD) prophylaxis states:

> *"While it is unclear if there is any association with decreasing rates of ventilator acquired pneumonia, our experience is that when applied as a package of interventions for ventilator care, the rate of pneumonia decreases precipitously. The intervention remains excellent practice in the general care of ventilated patients."*

6

However this document also acknowledges that the recommendations for PUD prophylaxis are based on a meta-analysis of studies conducted before 1990's that did not find an increased incidence of hospital acquired pneumonia with gastric pH elevation and that there was a reduced rate of pneumonia with sucralfate compared to H_2 blockers. However recent Surviving Sepsis campaign review of the evidence concluded that H_2 blockers were more efficacious than sucralfate.

The European Care Bundle developed for the prevention of ventilator associated pneumonia does not include peptic ulcer disease prophylaxis.

This document proposes the following components:

1. No ventilator circuit tube changes unless specifically indicated
2. Strict hand hygiene practice with the use of alcohol-based hand rub
3. Appropriately educated and trained staff
4. Sedation vacation and weaning protocol
5. Oral care with the use of chlorhexidine

The development of this bundle "used a formalized methodology to assess the supporting data, based on multi-criteria decision analysis."

Rello J, Lode H, Cornaglia G, Masterton R. A European care bundle for prevention of ventilator-associated pneumonia. Intensive Care Med 2010; 36:773–780.

AMSTAR: methodological quality of the review

1.	Was "a priori" design provided?	Y
2.	Was study selection and data extraction adequate?	Y
3.	Was the literature search comprehensive?	Y
4.	Was 'Grey Literature' used?	Y
5.	Was a list of excluded studies provided? Reasons for exclusion were provided	N
6.	Were the characteristics of included studies provided?	Y
7	Was the scientific quality of studies assessed & documented?	Y
8.	Was the scientific quality of studies weighted appropriately in forming conclusions?	Y
9.	Were the methods used for data synthesis appropriate?	Y
10.	Was the potential for publication bias assessed?	Y
11.	Were any conflicts of interest stated?	N

Overall quality of trials included	High
Overall quality of the review	High

6

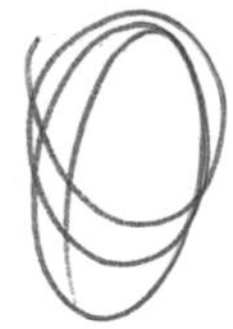

Critical illness polyneuropathy and polymyopathy

Condition: critical illness polyneuropathy (CIPN) and critical illness myopathy (CIM)
Interventions: pharmacological and non-pharmacological
Clinical question: Is there any intervention that can reduce the incidence of CIPN or CIM?

CIPN and CIM occur in critically ill patients and result in weakness of the limbs and respiratory muscles, less commonly the facial or ocular muscles are involved. Their clinical features are almost identical therefore it can be difficult to distinguish the two conditions, however as they often co-exist the term critical illness polyneuromyopathy (CIPNM) has recently been coined. CIPN is a primary axonal motor and sensory polyneuropathy therefore distal loss of sensation also occurs. Diagnosis can be established by the use of EMG, NCS or muscle biopsy for CIM. The reported incidence is between 49–84% in patients who have been on ICU for at least 7 days. The most consistently recognised risk factors are sepsis, SIRS and MOF; whereas the role of corticosteroids has been controversial and they may even be protective. CIPNM is associated with difficulties weaning from mechanical ventilation due to phrenic nerve and diaphragm involvement, increased ICU LOS and mortality.

Review characteristics

6

- **Eligibility criteria**: RCTs comparing any treatment to prevent CIPN or CIM compared to placebo, no treatment or a different treatment
- **Number of studies**: 9 trials were analysed but only 3 reported the primary outcome
- **Number of patients**: 3 trials n = 1005 (other 6 trials n = 8325)
- **Population**: aged over 18 years, admitted to either medical, surgical or mixed ICU
- **Study dates**: 1996–2007

Definitions

- **Intervention**: any that has been linked to a decreased risk of CIPNM – nutritional, hormonal, antioxidant, immunoglobulin, physiotherapy and rehabilitation, and electrical were all considered
- **CIP/CIM**: (author's definition) weakness of the limbs or respiratory muscles, or EMG documented peripheral neuropathy or myopathy for which other causes have been excluded. In the included trials this was examined at least on day 7
- **Intensive insulin therapy (IIT)**: maintain blood glucose levels within 80–110 mg/dl (4.4–6.1 mmol/l)
- **Conventional insulin therapy**: avoid hyperglycaemia (glucose > 215 mg/dl) or 11.9 mmol/l
- **Corticosteroids dose**: 2 mg/kg/day then gradually tapered over 3 weeks

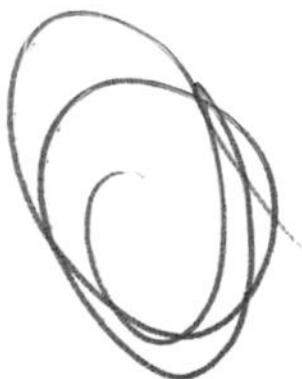

Results

Primary outcome: Incidence of CIPN/CIM

Intervention	Trials	N	Intervention Gp	Control Gp	p
Intensive insulin therapy (IIT) Surgical ICU	1	405	49%	25%	0.0001
Intensive insulin therapy medical ICU	1	420	50%	39%	0.02
Corticosteroids in ARDS	1	180	25%	23%	0.67

Pooled data

Intervention	Trials	Patients	RR	95% CI	I^2
Intensive insulin therapy	2	825	0.65	0.55–0.77	> 50%

Secondary outcomes

Outcome	Trials	N	Result
Duration of MV	2	825	Significantly reduced in the intensive insulin therapy group
ICU LOS	2	825	Significantly reduced in the intensive insulin therapy group
In-hospital mortality (and at 30 and 180 days)	2	522	Statistically significant increase in those treated with growth hormone
Mechanical ventilation	1	40	No significant difference with inspiratory muscle training
Mortality at 30 days	2	825	No significant difference with IIT
Mortality at 60 days	1	180	No significant difference with steroids treatment
Mortality at 180 days	2	825	Significantly reduced with IIT

Adverse events

In the insulin trials, there was a significantly higher incidence of hypoglycaemia but this was not associated with increased death within 24 hours after the last hypoglycaemic event.

Corticosteroids were not associated with higher incidence of CIPN/CIM, higher blood glucose levels or new serious infections. They appeared to have a protective effect from new episodes of shock and pneumonia.

Fig. 2 Comparison 1 Intensive insulin therapy (IIT) versus conventional insulin therapy (CIT), Outcome 1 Occurence of CIP/CIM [from Hermans G, De Jonghe B, Bruyninckx F, Van den Berghe G. Interventions for preventing critical illness polyneuropathy and critical illness myopathy. Cochrane Database of Systematic Reviews 2009, Issue 1. Art. No.: CD006832, © Cochrane Collaboration, reproduced with permission]

Review: Interventions for preventing critical illness polyneuropathy and critical illness myopathy
Comparison: 1 Intensive insulin therapy (IIT) versus conventional insulin therapy (CIT)
Outcome: 1 Occurence of CIP/CIM

Study or subgroup	IIT n/N	CIT n/N	Risk Ratio M-H, Fixed, 95% CI	Weight	Risk Ratio M-H, Fixed, 95% CI
1 In total population randomised					
Hermans 2007	81/595	107/605		49.6%	0.77 [0.59, 1.00]
Van den Berghe 2005	46/765	109/783		50.4%	0.43 [0.31, 0.60]
Subtotal (95% CI)	**1360**	**1388**		**100.0%**	**0.60 [0.49, 0.74]**
Total events: 127 (IIT), 216 (CIT)					
Heterogeneity: $Chi^2 = 7.20$, $df = 1$ ($P = 0.01$); $I^2 = 86\%$					
Test for overall effect: $Z = 4.88$ ($P < 0.00001$)					
2 In screened patients					
Hermans 2007	81/208	107/212		52.1%	0.77 [0.62, 0.96]
Van den Berghe 2005	46/181	109/224		47.9%	0.52 [0.39, 0.69]
Subtotal (95% CI)	**389**	**436**		**100.0%**	**0.65 [0.55, 0.77]**
Total events: 127 (IIT), 216 (CIT)					
Heterogeneity: $Chi^2 = 4.68$, $df = 1$ ($P = 0.03$); $I^2 = 79\%$					
Test for overall effect: $Z = 4.86$ ($P < 0.00001$)					

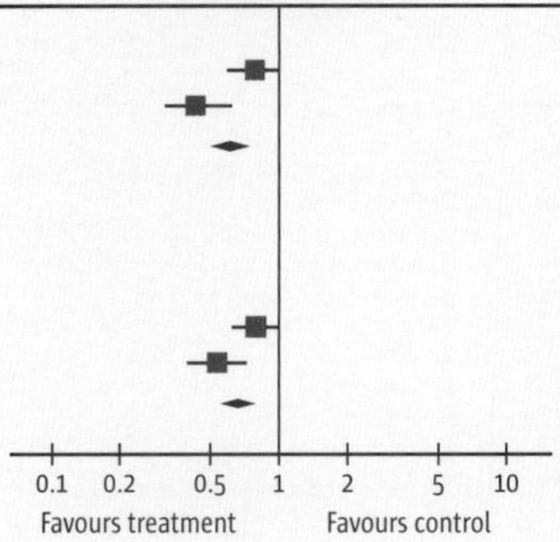

0.1 0.2 0.5 1 2 5 10
Favours treatment Favours control

Author's conclusion

The results showed a significant reduction in CIPN/CIM amongst patients who had been on ICU for at least one week and received intensive insulin therapy. Patients who were discharged or deceased before this time were not screened for CIPN/CIM therefore imputation of data was necessary which is not ideal. Duration of mechanical ventilation and 180-day mortality was also reduced by IIT. The most common adverse effect was hypoglycaemia but retrospective analysis did not show any long lasting detrimental effects.

Problems & limitations

- The 2 trials comparing intensive versus conventional insulin therapy were sub-analyses of larger RCTs
- Diagnostic limitations mean that some cases of CIM may have been missed
- There were only 3 trials evaluating the incidence of CIPN/CIM, one of the main reasons for this is the absence of clear diagnostic criteria making it hard to distinguish from normal weakness
- Very few trials reported either primary or secondary outcomes

Advantages

- Most trials were of adequate quality
- Data on electrophysiology were present in the 3 trials that reported the primary outcome

Expert opinion

Pedro Navarrete-Navarro

How valid and robust are the data?
This review found 2 RCTs, from the same group, conducted over the last 10 years period, examining the effect of intensive insulin therapy aiming at maintaining normoglycaemia versus conventional insulin therapy on overall mortality and morbidity in ICU patients. A sub-analysis of both trials to examine the effects of both treatment regimens on the incidence and need for prolonged mechanical ventilation, showed that strict glycaemic control reduced the electrophysiological incidence of CIPN/CIM, duration of mechanical ventilation, duration of ICU stay and 180-day mortality but not 30-day mortality. Intensive insulin therapy significantly increased hypoglycaemic events and recurrent hypoglycaemia. Death within 24 hours of the hypoglycaemic event was not different between groups.

A third trial examined the effects of corticosteroids versus placebo in 180 patients with prolonged acute respiratory distress syndrome, no significant effect of corticosteroids on CIPN/CIM was found, nor effect on 180-day mortality, or nor new serious infections and glycaemia at day seven were found.

Should clinical practise be influenced by this?
Many different pathophysiological mechanism are presumed to be involved in the development of CIPN/CIM. Until now, actual beneficial effects have been demonstrated only for strict glycaemic control, reducing the electrophysiological incidence of CIPN/CIM.

What's the next step?
I believe that glycaemic control has to be a standard practice for ICUs patients. We need properly designed, large RCTs, for other risk factors involved in CIPN/CIM development.

Citation

Hermans G, De Jonghe B, Bruyninckx F, Van den Berghe G. Interventions for preventing critical illness polyneuropathy and critical illness myopathy. Cochrane Database of Systematic Reviews 2009, Issue 1. Art. No.: CD006832. DOI: 10.1002/14651858.CD006832.pub2.

Additional information

The reader should be aware that this review did not include the NICE-SUGAR study. A multicentre randomised controlled trial that enrolled 6,104 ICU patients and compared intensive versus conventional. Intensive insulin therapy was associated with increased severe hypoglycaemic episode and increased mortality.

Citation: The NICE-SUGAR Study Investigators. Intensive versus Conventional Glucose Control in Critically Ill Patients. N Engl J Med 2009; 360:1283–1297. ClinicalTrials.gov number, NCT00220987

AMSTAR: methodological quality of the review

1.	Was "a priori" design provided?	Y
2.	Was study selection and data extraction adequate?	Y
3.	Was the literature search comprehensive?	Y
4.	Was 'Grey Literature' used?	Y
5.	Was a list of excluded studies provided?	Y
6.	Were the characteristics of included studies provided?	Y
7.	Was the scientific quality of studies assessed & documented?	Y
8.	Was the scientific quality of studies weighted appropriately in forming conclusions?	Y
9.	Were the methods used for data synthesis appropriate?	Y
10.	Was the potential for publication bias assessed?	Y
11.	Were any conflicts of interest stated?	Y

Overall quality of trials included	5 high quality
Overall quality of the review	High

Thromboprophylaxis

Condition: venous thromboembolism (VTE)

Intervention: thromboprophylaxis

Clinical question: Does the use of low molecular weight heparin (LMWH) in critically ill medical and surgical patients reduce the incidence of VTE and is it safe?

Venous thromboembolism is a common and potentially life threatening complication of critical illness, with the estimated incidence of DVT being between 9–40% over the course of ICU stay. The most commonly used mode of prophylaxis is LMWH largely because it is easier to administer than unfractionated heparin (UFH) and no monitoring of levels is required. However the efficacy of LMWH has not been studied in this population.

If Anti-Xa activity should be measured: the therapeutic target is 0.25–0.29 IU/ml in the first 3 days, then 0.33–0.37 IU/ml on days 4–10 for optimal prophylaxis whilst minimising the risk of bleeding.

Review characteristics

- **Eligibility criteria:** prospective cohort studies or RCTs
- **Number of studies:** 8 prospective cohort studies (1 multicentre), 1 RCT
- **Number of patients:** 629 patients
- **Population:** medical, surgical, trauma or mixed ICUs
- **Study dates:** 2000–2008

6

Definition

- **4 types of LMWH used, Inconsistent dosing:** approximately half the patients may have received the higher prophylaxis dose
- **Renal impairment:** standard definitions: severe (creatinine clearance < 30 ml/min), moderate (CC 30–50 ml/min)
- **Control groups:** only defined in 4/9 studies
- **DVT:** Venography in the 1 RCT & USS in 2 other studies
- **Bleeding:** variable definitions

Results

Laboratory outcomes

a. Anti-Xa Levels in patients without renal insufficiency
b. Anti-Xa Levels in patients with renal insufficiency
c. Thombocytopenia

	General summary (but be aware of inconsistency between studies)
a	Levels were sub-therapeutic with lower doses Oedema or twice daily dosing made no difference to levels The number of patients with therapeutic levels decreased with time Higher levels with inotropes/lower levels with vasopressors (but n = 15) ICU patients had lower clearance than medical patients
b	No evidence of accumulation even in severe renal impairment for up to 17 days
c	Only 1 study reported on thrombocytopenia: no difference

Clinical Outcomes

VTE	Not all studies reported all outcomes
	45/326 (13.8%) patients had VTE Range 5.1–15.5% with LMWH c.f. 28.2% with placebo (1 RCT), $p < 0.045$ Most DVTs were associated with femoral venous catheters
Bleeding	Total incidence of bleeding: 55/378 (55%) 7.2%–23.1% with LMWH c.f. 15.9% with placebo No clear correlation between LMWH use and bleeding
Mortality	No difference in mortality (1 RCT, n = 223)

6

Author's conclusion

The number of patients in the review is small, most were from cohort studies and without a comparison group. The efficacy and safety of LMWH thromboprohylaxis remain unknown; mortality and morbidity remain unknown and no comparison has been made with alternatives.

The pharmacokinetics of LMWH are predictable in other patient groups but have not been studied in critically ill patients who have multiple compounding factors.

VTE was still observed despite prophylaxis (14%).

No recommendations can be made based on these data.

Problems & limitations

- Most studies concentrated on laboratory rather than clinical end-points
- Large heterogeneity of the studies
- Lack of statistical analysis within studies and within the review

Advantages

- The participants represented a typical general ICU population

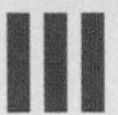

Expert opinion

Miguel Tavares and Maurizio Cecconi

How valid and robust are the data?
This review has found only 1 randomized trial and 8 observational studies. The total number of patients is relatively small (629) and quite heterogeneous (4 medical, 4 mixed medical-surgical patients and 1 in trauma). Outcome data (clinical and laboratory) are also reported in very different ways. The overall data available therefore are limited.

Should clinical practise be influenced by this?
This review does not provide sufficient evidence to prove that LMWH should be used in ICU or preferred to unfractionated heparin. Based on the available laboratory data LMWH does not seem to accumulate at current regimes in medical-surgical intensive care patients. From the available data though, it is not possible to determine if the dose currently used is effective to prevent VTE.

What's the next step?
A large RCT is needed to address if LMWH is effective and safe as a VTE prophylaxis measure in medical-surgical ICU patients.

Citation

Ribic C, Lim W, Cook D and Crowther M. Low-molecular-weight-heparin thromboprophylaxis in medic-surgical critically ill patients: a systematic review. Journal of Critical Care 2009; 24(2): 197–205

Additional information

Also see: Dalteparin versus unfractionated heparin in critically ill patients.

This was a multicentre RCT that enrolled 3,764 patients that was published after this review. This trial compared subcutaneous dalteparin to subcutaneous heparin. There was no difference in the incidence of deep vein thrombosis, bleeding or in-hospital mortality, however there was less heparin-induced thrombocytopenia and there were significantly less patients with pulmonary emboli in the dalteparin group.

Dalteparin versus Unfractionated Heparin in Critically Ill Patients. The PROTECT Investigators for the Canadian Critical Care Trials Group and the Australian and New Zealand Intensive Care Society Clinical Trials Group. 10.1056/nejmoa1014475, March 2011, nejm.org (NCT00182143.)

AMSTAR: methodological quality of the review

1.	Was "a priori" design provided?	Y
2.	Was study selection and data extraction adequate?	Y
3.	Was the literature search comprehensive?	Y
4.	Was 'Grey Literature' used?	P
5.	Was a list of excluded studies provided?	N
6.	Were the characteristics of included studies provided?	Y
7.	Was the scientific quality of studies assessed & documented?	Y
8.	Was the scientific quality of studies weighted appropriately in forming conclusions?	Y
9.	Were the methods used for data synthesis appropriate?	Y
10.	Was the potential for publication bias assessed?	Y
11.	Were any conflicts of interest stated?	Y

Overall quality of trials included	Low
Overall quality of the review	High

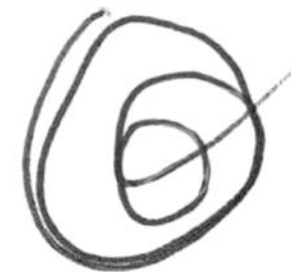

Music therapy

Condition: mechanical ventilation

Intervention: music

Clinical question: Can music intervention reduce anxiety and physiological responses in mechanically ventilated patients?

Mechanically ventilated patients often experience breathing difficulties, severe distress, anxiety and fear. The discomfort caused by the artificial airway and frequent suctioning is compounded by the inability to talk, unfamiliar surroundings and uncertainty about their condition. Distress causes constriction of arteries and bronchioles, and weaning difficulties. Analgesia and sedation are used to minimise these unpleasant experiences however heavy sedation can also be harmful and is undesirable during the weaning process. Immobility as a result of sedation leads to increased risk of venous thrombosis, pressure damage to skin and nerves, and may prolong the duration of mechanical ventilation and its associated complications.

Four non-pharmacological interventions have been investigated i. hypnosis and relaxation ii. patient education and information sharing iii. supportive touch and iv. music therapy, and results have been promising. The anxiolytic effects of music therapy have been studied in a number of medical and surgical fields and have been shown to reduce pain and anxiety as well as enhance feelings of control and well-being (Chlan 1995, Wong 2001) in mechanically ventilated patients. It cannot be assumed that sedative music will have a positive impact on all patients. Many factors affect the individual's response including: age, gender, culture, cognitive function, severity of anxiety and discomfort as well as training in music and music preference. Personal associations with music are important to consider as music can evoke various types of imagery which will influence the individual's response.

6

There is a clear distinction between music intervention delivered by healthcare professionals (music medicine) and that implemented by trained music therapists (music therapy). The latter is tailored to individual needs, employs a systematic approach and has been shown to be significantly more effective than music medicine (Dileo & Bradt, 2005).

Review characteristics

- **Eligibility criteria:** RCTs and quasi-randomised controlled trials that compared music intervention with standard care to standard care alone or with other therapies or placebo
- **Population:** mechanically ventilated patients in ICUs, long-term acute care hospitals or 'step-down' units
- **Number of studies:** 8 trials. 4 in the USA, 2 in China and 2 in Europe
- **Number of patients:** 213 (range 10–64)
- **Study dates:** 1995–2007

Definitions

- **Placebo:** headphones with no music stimuli or some form of auditory stimulus e.g. white noise (hiss), pink noise (ocean sounds), or nature sounds

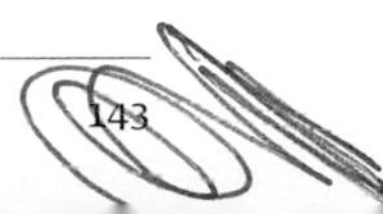

- **State anxiety:** "a temporary unpleasant emotional arousal in the face of threatening demands or danger". This is different to trait anxiety which is stable individual differences in reactions

Results

Population characteristics

Ventilatory support
Reported by 4 studies: most patients were on SIMV or PS modes
Type of airway
3 studies reported this: most patients had oral ETTs or tracheostomy. Few had nasal ETTs
ICU LOS before study enrolment
5 studies: average LOS ranged from 2.5 days to 14 days
Diagnosis
Mostly pulmonary in 7 studies. Overall mixed population of post-surgical, trauma, cardiac, oncology and septic patients
Type of music intervention
7 studies: music medicine where patients simply listened to pre-recorded music 1 study used music therapy where patients selected live music played by the music therapist. Initial music tempo matched the patient's respiratory rate and was then gradually decreased to tempo/RR compatible with extubation Duration of music sessions was 20–30 minutes mostly (60 minutes in one study) Music styles were: jazz, easy listening, country & western and classical Only 1 study provided composition specific information and another study (music medicine) provided information on music tempo.
Music Choice
1 study used researcher selected music 7 studies used patient selected music but from a limited selection of music styles 2 studies reported that on average 5 patients disliked the music or refused to participate because they didn't like the music options

6

Primary outcome: state anxiety

Measured using the Spielberg state and trait anxiety inventory (STAI)

The pooled estimate form 3 studies (n = 135) indicates that music listening may be beneficial (SMD -1.06, 95% CI 2.09 to -0.04, p = 0.04). GRADE = very low

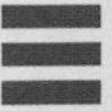

Fig. 3 Comparison 1 Music versus standard care, Outcome 1 State Anxiety [Bradt J, Dileo C, Grocke D. Music interventions for mechanically ventilated patients. Cochrane Database of Systematic Reviews 2010, Issue 12. Art. No.: CD006902, © Cochrane Collaboration, reproduced with permission]

Review: Music interventions for mechanically ventilated patients
Comparison: 1 Music versus standard care
Outcome: 1 State Anxiety

Study or subgroup	Experimental N	Experimental Mean (SD)	Control N	Control Mean (SD)	Weight	Std. Mean Difference IV, Random, 95% CI
Chlan 1997	24	-7.17 (3.85)	27	-1.55 (4.08)	35.2%	-1.39 [-2.01, -0.77]
Lee 2005	32	-1.6 (3.31)	32	-1 (2.31)	36.9%	-0.17 [-0.66, 0.32]
Wong 2001	10	-14 (5.62)	10	-3.84 (4.97)	27.9%	-1.83 [-2.92, -0.75]
Total (95% CI)	**66**		**69**		**100.0%**	**-1.06 [-2.09, -0.04]**

Heterogeneity: $Tau^2 = 0.68$; $Chi^2 = 13.43$, df = 2 (P = 0.001); $I^2 = 85\%$
Test for overall effect: Z = 2.03 (P = 0.043)

6

Secondary outcomes

Outcome	Trials	N	Result	GRADE
Sedation	1	10	Narrative report that patients in the music group didn't require additional sedation but the control group did	–
Heart rate	5	167	Significantly lower in the music group (MD −4.75, 95% CI −6.98 to −2.51, $p = 0.001$)	Very low
Respiratory rate	6	187	Significantly lower in the music group (MD −3.18, 95% CI −4.41 to −1.95, $p < 0.001$)	Low
Blood Pressure	3	98	Both SBP & DBP were slightly lower but not statistically significant	Low
SaO_2	2	40	No significant difference but some patients already had 100% saturation	Very low
Hormones levels	2	20	1 study found significant decreases in some stress hormones. The other did not however some patients in the music group required suction during the study	–

6

Author's conclusion

The results suggest that music may have a beneficial effect on anxiety in mechanically ventilated patients however the evidence is not strong.

The magnitude of the anxiety-reducing effect differed across the studies but the trials agreed on the direction of the point estimates. The results furthermore indicate that listening to music reduces heart rate and respiratory rate consistently across studies . Music interventions did not improve oxygen saturation levels but the usefulness of oxygen saturation as an indicator of a relaxation response in mechanically ventilated patients is questionable as this outcome is greatly influenced by ventilator settings.

No studies were found that examined outcomes such as: patient satisfaction, quality of life, post discharge outcomes, mortality or cost effectiveness.

Problems & limitations

- Small number of studies and patients
- Most studies did not use a trained music therapist
- Variable reporting: insufficient data reporting in some studies and only 2 studies reported ethnicity
- Inability to include all the studies in the pooled analysis due to confounding factors

Advantages

- The effect on heart rate and respiratory rate was consistent in all studies
- Results were not changed by sensitivity analysis

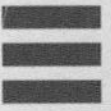

Fig. 4 Comparison 1 Music versus standard care, Outcome 2 Heart Rate [Bradt J, Dileo C, Grocke D. Music interventions for mechanically ventilated patients. Cochrane Database of Systematic Reviews 2010, Issue 12. Art. No.: CD006902, © Cochrane Collaboration, reproduced with permission]

Review: Music interventions for mechanically ventilated patients
Comparison: 1 Music versus standard care
Outcome: 2 Heart Rate

Study or subgroup	Experimental N	Experimental Mean (SD)	Control N	Control Mean (SD)	Mean Difference IV, Fixed, 95% CI	Weight	Mean Difference IV, Fixed, 95% CI
Chlan 1995	11	-8.9 (5.56)	9	-1.6 (3.63)		30.4%	-7.30 [-11.35, -3.25]
Chlan 1997	26	85.9 (15.6)	23	91.5 (18.9)		5.2%	-5.60 [-15.38, 4.18]
Jaber 2007	7	84.7 (15)	7	89.1 (14.9)		2.0%	-4.40 [-20.06, 11.26]
Lee 2005	32	-3.8 (7)	32	-0-3 (4.4)		60.8%	-3.50 [-6.36, -0.64]
Phillips 2007	10	0.2 (24.69)	10	1.3 (15.77)		1.5%	-1.10 [-19.26, 17.06]
Total (95% CI)	**86**		**81**			**100.0%**	**-4.75 [-6.98, -2.51]**

Heterogeneity: $Chi^2 = 2.44$, $df = 4$ ($P = 0.66$); $I^2 = 0.0\%$
Test for overall effect: $Z = 4.16$ ($P = 0.000031$)

-10 -5 0 5 10
Favours experimental Favours control

6

Fig. 5 Comparison 1 Music versus standard care, Outcome 3 Respiratory Rate [Bradt J, Dileo C, Grocke D. Music interventions for mechanically ventilated patients. Cochrane Database of Systematic Reviews 2010, Issue 12. Art. No.: CD006902, © Cochrane Collaboration, reproduced with permission]

Review: Music interventions for mechanically ventilated patients
Comparison: 1 Music versus standard care
Outcome: 3 Respiratory Rate

Study or subgroup	Experimental N	Experimental Mean (SD)	Control N	Control Mean (SD)	Mean Difference IV, Fixed, 95% CI	Weight	Mean Difference IV, Fixed, 95% CI
Chlan 1995	11	-5 (3.8)	9	-0.2 (2.45)		19.9%	-4.80 [-7.56, -2.04]
Chlan 1997	23	16.4 (5.5)	26	18.7 (6.1)		14.4%	-2.30 [-5.55, 0.95]
Jaber 2007	7	23.73 (3.22)	7	25.9 (2.7)		15.7%	-2.17 [-5.28, 0.94]
Lee 2005	32	-3.6 (4.9)	32	-0.1 (3.4)		35.5%	-3.50 [-5.57, -1.43]
Phillips 2007	10	-0.2 (7.6)	10	2.7 (7.9)		3.3%	-2.90 [-9.69, 3.89]
Wong 2001	10	17.35 (4.16)	10	19.25 (4.23)		11.2%	-1.90 [-5.58, 1.78]
Total (95% CI)	**93**		**94**			**100.0%**	**-3.18 [-4.41, -1.95]**

Heterogeneity: $Chi^2 = 2.58$, df = 5 (P = 0.76); $I^2 = 0.0\%$
Test for overall effect: Z = 5.06 (P < 0.00001)

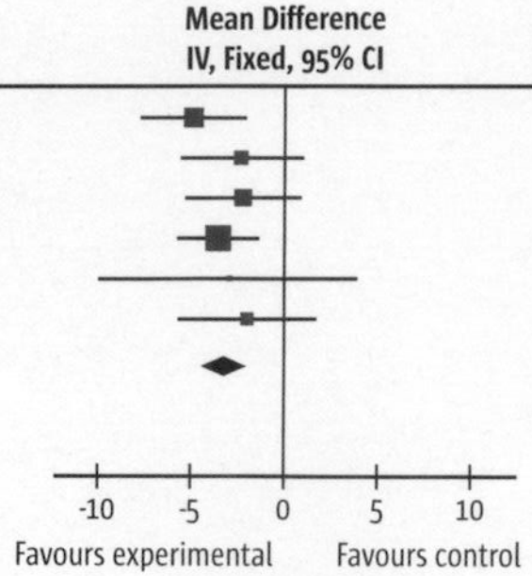

-10 -5 0 5 10
Favours experimental Favours control

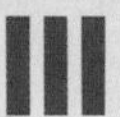

Citation

Bradt J, Dileo C, Grocke D. Music interventions for mechanically ventilated patients. Cochrane Database of Systematic Reviews 2010, Issue 12. Art. No.: CD006902. DOI: 10.1002/14651858.CD006902.pub2.

AMSTAR: methodological quality of the review

1.	Was "a priori" design provided?	Y
2.	Was study selection and data extraction adequate?	Y
3.	Was the literature search comprehensive?	Y
4.	Was 'Grey Literature' used?	Y
5.	Was a list of excluded studies provided?	Y
6.	Were the characteristics of included studies provided?	Y
7.	Was the scientific quality of studies assessed & documented?	Y
8.	Was the scientific quality of studies weighted appropriately in forming conclusions?	Y
9.	Were the methods used for data synthesis appropriate?	Y
10.	Was the potential for publication bias assessed?	Y
11.	Were any conflicts of interest stated?	Y

Overall quality of trials included	1 high quality, 5 low quality
Overall quality of the review	High

7

Health technology

Chest radiography ______ 152
Oesophageal doppler monitoring ______ 157
Computerised decision support systems ______ 165

Chest radiography

Technology: chest radiography (CXR)
Clinical questions: Does abandoning daily chest radiography adversely affect ICU patients? Is there a subgroup of ICU patients that may benefit from daily CXRs?

The American College of Radiology recommends daily chest radiography for patients with acute cardiopulmonary problems and those who are mechanically ventilated to allow early detection of abnormalities that may otherwise not be found. This is based on observational studies from the 1980's and 1990's that report a high incidence of unexpected findings. This approach not only increases healthcare costs and the work burden, but also puts patients at risk of complications associated with repositioning, and both patients and staff have increased radiation exposure.

Review characteristics

- **Eligibility criteria:** RCTs and observational studies that compared the impact of daily routine versus clinically indicated chest radiography that reported at least one of the primary outcomes: (mortality, LOS or duration of MV, or adverse events) and had at least 30% ventilated patients
- **Exclusions:** studies that did not score at least 5 out of 22 on quality criteria as determined by CONSORT or STROBE criteria
- **Number of studies:** 8 (2 RCTs n = 259, 6 observational n = 6,819)
- **Number of patients:** 7,078 (59% medical, 61% mechanically ventilated)
- **Population:** adults aged 18 or above in medical or surgical ICUs
- **Study dates:** 1997–2008

Definitions

- **Adverse events:** inadvertent extubations and reintubations; complications requiring intervention (malpositioned tubes and catheters, mediastinal bleeding, pneumothoraces and pleural effusions); and readmissions to ICU

Results

Outcome	Results
Mortality	No significant difference in hospital or ICU mortality (I^2 = 0%)
LOS	No difference in ICU or hospital LOS with pooled analysis
Adverse events	Incidence was similar between the 2 groups

These results remained unchanged when RCTs and observational studies were examined separately.

Fig. 1 Forest plot for effect of daily routine chest radiography on ICU LOS. CXR = chest radiography, RCT = randomized controlled trial, SD = standard deviation [from Yuji Oba, Tareq Zaza. Abandoning Daily Routine Chest Radiography in the Intensive Care Unit: Meta-Analysis. Radiology: Volume 255: Number 2. May 2010, © Radiological Society of North America]

Review: CXR in ICU
Comparison: 02 On-Demand vs Routine 01
Outcome: 03 ICU LOS

Study or sub-category	On-demand N	On-demand Mean (SD)	Routine N	Routine Mean (SD)	Weight %	WMD (random) 95% CI
01 RCT						
Clech 2008	81	23.40 (15.50)	84	22.30 (15.6[illegible])	0.44	1.10 [-3.69, 5.89]
Krivopal 2003	51	9.55 (7.19)	43	11.93 (9.91)	0.79	-2.38 [-5.94, 1.18]
Subtotal (95% CI)	**132**		**127**		**1.23**	-1.14 [-4.00, 1.71]
Test for heterogeneity: $Chi^2 = 1.31$, df = 1 (P = 0.25); $I^2 = 23.4\%$						
Test for overall effect: Z = 0.60 (P = 0.55)						
02 Observational						
Brivet 2006	957	3.00 (6.30)	572	2.00 (2.22)	19.86	1.00 [0.56, 1.44]
Hendrikse 2007	250	1.00 (0.74)	486	1.00 (0.74)	30.47	0.00 [-0.11, 0.11]
Krinsley 2003	1267	3.57 (5.27)	1297	3.55 (5.14)	21.08	0.02 [-0.38, 0.42]
Kroner 2008	743	2.00 (2.22)	747	2.00 (2.22)	27.37	0.00 [-0.23, 0.23]
Subtotal (95% CI)	**3217**		**3102**		**98.77**	**0.21 [-0.12, 0.53]**
Test for heterogeneity: $Chi^2 = 18.98$, df = 3 (P = 0.0003); $I^2 = 84.2\%$						
Test for overall effect: Z = 1.25 (P = 0.21)						
Total (95% CI)	**3349**		**3229**		**100.00**	**0.19 [-0.13, 0.51]**
Test for heterogeneity: $Chi^2 = 20.95$, df = 5 (P = 0.0008) $I^2 = 76.1\%$						
Test for overall effect: Z = 1.16 (P = 0.25)						

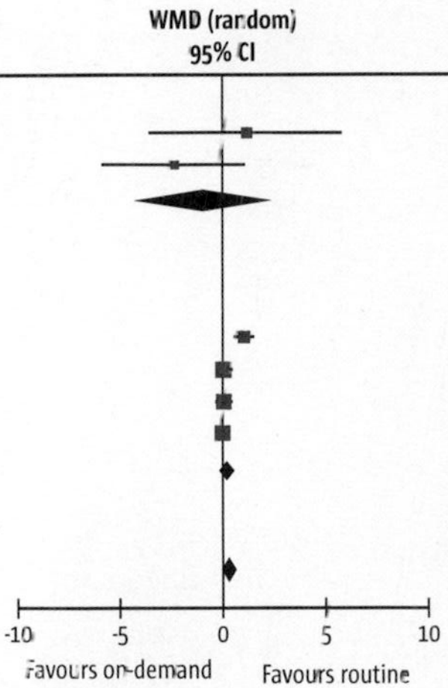

WMD (random) 95% CI: -10 -5 0 5 10
Favours on-demand Favours routine

7

Subgroup analysis: did not identify any patients groups where daily routine CXR may be beneficial

Number of CXRs: mean number of CXRs ranged from 2.4–10.5 in the daily routine groups and 0.4–4.4 in the on-demand group. This difference was statistically significant.

Author's conclusion

This study suggests that daily routine chest radiography can be eliminated without increasing adverse outcomes in patients. Further studies are required to ascertain whether or not there is any group of patients that may benefit from routine screening such as patients with PACs. More recent studies report a much lower incidence of radiographic abnormalities that require clinical intervention. Differences in opinion may arise as a result of various definitions of efficacy (unexpected findings versus findings that lead to treatment change).

Problems & limitations

- Mostly observational studies are included due to the paucity of RCTs in this area.
- Baseline characteristics of patients were not the same in 3 of the observational studies, adjustments for severity of illness were made in 1 study
- The observed mortality was between 3–33% therefore daily CXR may be beneficial in subgroup with higher severity of illness and mortality

Advantages

- Large number of patients
- Sensitivity analysis did not change the results
- Results concur with a recent French survey that found that 75% of ICU specialists did not feel that daily routine CXR was necessary in an intubated patient

Expert opinion

Pierre Squara

The objective of this study was to examine whether abandoning daily routine chest radiography in Intensive Care Medicine would adversely affect outcomes and identify a subgroup in which daily routine chest radiography might be beneficial.

Height studies were extracted from 128 including a total of 7,078 patients in which 3,429 underwent daily routine chest radiography and 3,649 underwent only clinically indicated chest radiography.

The meta-analysis found no difference between the two groups in mortality, duration of mechanical ventilation, length of stay and the occurrence of adverse effects. Univariate and multivariate analyses failed to identify any subgroup in which routine chest radiograph was beneficial.

How valid and robust are the data?
I am not a statistician; this is only the opinion of a clinician. Among the traditional limitations of meta-analyses listed by Berk & Freedman (2003), I was especially concerned in this study by the heterogeneity of the pool.

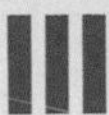

Heterogeneity of the studies
- Random/observational (2/6)
- Quality of the quality of data (from 5/22 to 15/22, 22 is the max score)

Heterogeneity of patients
- Medical ICU/surgical (from 0 to 100%, overall 60%)
- Mechanically ventilated (from 36 to 100%, overall 60%)
- Predicted mortality (based on APACHE II) from 16 to 60%

Heterogeneity of the range of daily number of chest radiographs
- From 2.5–10.5 (daily routine group) to 0.4–4 (on-demand group)

In addition, I do not admit their conclusion. "... our systematic analysis demonstrates that the elimination of daily routine chest radiography did not adversely affect hard outcomes, ..." They were just unable to prove the benefit of one strategy versus another. The absence of evidence is not evidence of absence. In this study the statistical power of the results was not discussed. This is especially critical for a meta-analysis in which changing the models used may completely change the results (See for example Ropp et al., Fertility and Sterility 2008; 90:71–76).

Should clinical practice be influenced by this?
The daily routine use of the chest radiograph needs a reappraisal but the controversy observed in the literature and discussed in this study will not be solved by this study for the reasons listed above.

As observed in several complementary tests, the impact of daily routine use on outcome is probably varying according to different situations. So, for me the objective is not to determine if routine chest X ray is globally beneficial or not but to determine in which patients it is beneficial.

What's the next step?
If you share this objective, I would recommend:
- Determining a limited number of clearly identified situations in which the daily routine use is likely to be beneficial
- Designing a multicentre randomized study to test the hypothesis
- Then discussing the generalizability of the observed findings

I was asked to additionally review another paper not included in this meta-analysis because it was published in 2009 after the reviewers closed their search in December 2008.

Comparison of routine and on-demand prescription of chest radiographs in mechanically ventilated adults: a multicentre, cluster-randomised, two-period crossover study. Gilles Hejblum et al., Lancet 2009; 374: 1687–93

Interestingly, this new study is in accordance with three of my recommendations.
- The study is limited to patient with mechanical ventilation > 2 days.
- It is a multicentre randomized study.
- The primary outcome is clear.

However, I do not believe that this study has closed the debate.

The main finding is robust. I admit that we can generalize that the on-demand strategy reduces roughly by 30% the number of chest radiographs as compared to the routine daily strategy. This is expected, and the methodology used to show this evidence is adequate.

This main result is paralleled by an equivalent number of interventions in the two groups, suggesting that the routine chest radiographs in excess as compared to the on-demand radiographs are ineffective. Again, absence of evidence is not evidence of absence. This finding is provocative enough to ask for a type 2 error analysis.

Last, no difference in mortality, length of stay, and duration of mechanical ventilation was observed between the two groups. However, the study was not designed for that purpose. Statistical power was neither studied nor discussed.

Then, we can state that on-demand strategy decreases the number of radiographs and the cost but we cannot conclude that it has no side effects. One or several patient may have died from unsuspected event in the on demand group, therefore no intervention was done and the study does not have enough power to show it.

Citation

Oba Y, Zaza T. Abandoning Daily Routine Chest Radiography in the Intensive Care Unit: Meta-Analysis. Radiology: Volume 255: Number 2 May 2010

AMSTAR: methodological quality of the review

1.	Was "a priori" design provided?	Y
2.	Was study selection and data extraction adequate?	Y
3.	Was the literature search comprehensive?	Y
4.	Was 'Grey Literature' used?	Y
5.	Was a list of excluded studies provided?	N
6.	Were the characteristics of included studies provided?	Y
7.	Was the scientific quality of studies assessed & documented?	Y
8.	Was the scientific quality of studies weighted appropriately in forming conclusions?	Y
9.	Were the methods used for data synthesis appropriate?	Y
10.	Was the potential for publication bias assessed?	Y
11.	Were any conflicts of interest stated?	N

Overall quality of trials included	Generally low
Overall quality of the review	High

7

Oesophageal doppler monitoring

Technology: oesophageal doppler monitoring (ODM)
Clinical question: Is the use of ODM effective clinically and financially compared to conventional clinical assessment and other techniques for measuring cardiac function?

Optimizing the haemodynamic state of high-risk and critically ill patients is considered paramount in improving outcomes. Several devices, both invasive and non-invasive, can be used for haemodynamic monitoring, although the traditional and more invasive pulmonary artery catheter has fallen out of favour as more recent studies have failed to show any benefit from its use. The ODM is placed into the patient's oesophagus and uses doppler ultrasound to measure blood velocity in the descending aorta. Cardiac output is calculated using a nomogram that estimates the aortic cross-sectional area based on the patient's age, height and weight. ODM has generally been used in unconscious patients however newer probes that may be tolerated by awake patients have been manufactured but these remain to be evaluated.

Review characteristics

- **Eligibility criteria:** RCTs and systematic reviews
- This review was based the US Agency for Healthcare Research and Quality (AHRQ) review (8 studies) and supplemented by additional studies (2 studies). The discussions and conclusions below may refer to the AHRQ report separately or overall results with the additional studies
- **Exclusions:** studies where ODM was used as a measure of outcome rather than as a monitoring tool
- **Population:** adult patients undergoing certain types of major surgery (colorectal; elective general, urology, gynaecology and cardiac surgery; hip fracture repair) or critically ill patients
- **Number of studies:** 10 RCTs (8 RCTs of surgical patients, 2 RCTs of ICU patients)
- **Number of patients:** 959 (surgical n = 623, ICU n = 336)
- **Study dates:** 1997–2007

Definitions

- **Major surgery:** surgical procedures which are associated with substantial blood loss or fluid shifts requiring replacement
- **Critically ill patients:** two distinct groups in each of the studies. 1 study was in a post cardiac surgery unit and the other was in a unit focused on major trauma
- **EORTC QLQ-C30:** European Organisation for Research and Treatment of Cancer 30 item QOL questionnaire used for patients with cancer
- **QLQ-CR38:** a 38-item colorectal cancer specific QOL questionnaire designed for use with the EORTC QLQ-C30

Results

5 outcomes were considered: mortality, major complications, total complications, hospital LOS and quality of life for the for 4 different comparisons below.

1. ODM + CVP + CA versus CVP + CA intra-operatively

5 studies (n = 453) used this comparison and reported the following:

There were fewer deaths in the ODM group (Peto OR 0.13, 95% CI 0.02–0.96)

Mortality however was very low in the control group and there was a low overall number of events

LOS was shorter in the ODM group (pooled estimate not provided, 95% CI −2.21 to −0.57)

3 studies reported the following:

Major complications were significantly less in the ODM group
(OR 0.12, 95% CI 0.04–0.31)

There were less total complications in the ODM group (OR 0.43, 95% CI 0.26–0.71)

2. ODM + CVP + CA versus CVP + CA in critically ill patients

2 studies (n = 366) in different groups: cardiac and major trauma patients

There was no difference in mortality (OR 0.84, 95% CI 0.41–1.70)

There were less complications in the ODM group (OR 0.49, 95% CI 0.30–0.81)

Median LOS was significantly shorter in the ODM group

3. ODM + CA versus CA intra-operatively

3 studies (n = 139) used this comparison

There was no difference in mortality (OR 0.81, 95% CI 0.23–2.77)

LOS was shorter in all 3 studies in the ODM group

7

4. ODM + CA versus CVP + CA intra-operatively

1 study (n = 61) showed no statistical difference in mortality, total complications or LOS. Major complications were not reported separately

CA = Conventional clinical assessment

Quality of Life

None of the studies reported quality of life data.

1 study (Wakeling 2005) reported that the EORTC QLQ-C30 and QLQ-CR38 at 4–6 weeks after surgery showed no difference between the groups (ODM + CVP + CA versus CVP + CA intra-operatively)

Cost

None of the studies reported cost

Individual probes cost £ 60–£ 120 (plus shared costs of the monitor and maintenance)

Cost effectiveness

The overall differences in costs and effectiveness is unclear

The cost of ODM may be offset by reductions in LOS

Economic modelling shows that ODM is likely to be cost-effective but this is based heavily on analysis assumptions

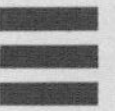

Fig. 2 Meta-analysis of studies reporting mortality (Aberdeen TAR group) [from Mowatt G, Houston G, Hernández R, de Verteuil R, Fraser C, Cuthbertson B, Vale L. Systematic review of the clinical effectiveness and cost-effectiveness of oesophageal Doppler monitoring in critically ill and high-risk surgical patients. Health Technol Assess 2009;13(7)]

Review: Oesophageal Doppler monitoring
Comparison: ODM + CVP + conventional assessment vs CVP + conventional assessment
Outcome: Mortality

Study or subcategory	ODM n/N	Control n/N	Peto OR 95% CI	Weight %	Peto OR 95% CI	Order
Gan, 2002	0/50	0/50			Not estimable	0
Conway, 2002	0/29	1/28		24.99	0.13 (0.00–6.59)	0
Mythen, 1995	0/30	1/30		25.00	0.14 (0.00–6.82)	0
Noblett, 2006	0/51	1/52		25.00	0.14 (0.00–6.95)	0
Wakeling, 2005	0/64	1/64		25.00	0.14 (0.00–6.82)	0
Total (95% CI)	**224**	**224**		**100.0**	**0.13 (0.02–0.96)**	

Total events: 0 (ODM), 4 (Control)
Test for heterogeneity: $\chi^2 = 0.00$, df = 3 (p = 1.00); $I^2 = 0\%$
Test for overall effect: z = 2.00 (p = 0.05)

Fig. 3 Meta-analysis of studies reporting major complications (Aberdeen TAR group) [from Mowatt G, Houston G, Hernández R, de Verteuil R, Fraser C, Cuthbertson B, Vale L. Systematic review of the clinical effectiveness and cost-effectiveness of oesophageal Doppler monitoring in critically ill and high-risk surgical patients. Health Technol Assess 2009;13(7)]

Review: Oesophageal Doppler monitoring
Comparison: ODM + CVP + conventional assessment vs CVP + conventional assessment
Outcome: Major complications

Study or subcategory	ODM n/N	Control n/N	Peto OR 95% CI	Weight %	Peto OR 95% CI	Order
Conway, 2002	0/29	5/28		29.31	0.11 (0.02–0.69)	0
Mythen, 1995	0/30	6/30		34.67	0.11 (0.02–0.60)	0
Noblett, 2006	0/51	6/52		36.02	0.12 (0.02–0.64)	0
Total (95% CI)	**110**	**110**		**100.0**	**0.12 (0.04–0.31)**	

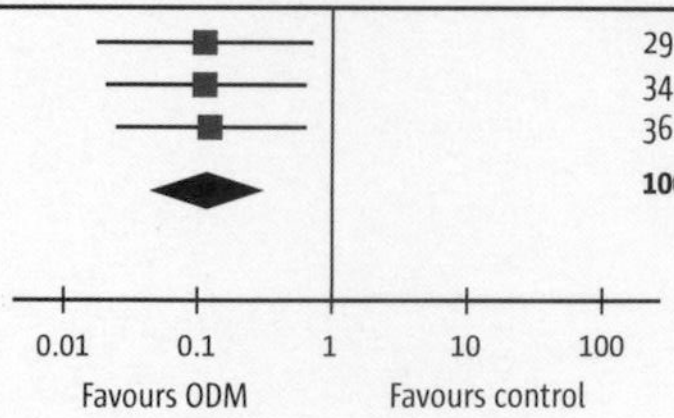

Total events: 0 (ODM), 17 (Control)
Test for heterogeneity: $\chi^2 = 0.01$, df = 2 ($p = 0.99$); $I^2 = 0\%$
Test for overall effect: $z = 4.28$ ($p < 0.0001$)

0.01 0.1 1 10 100
Favours ODM Favours control

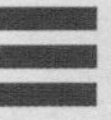

Fig. 4 Meta-analysis of length of hospital stay (Aberdeen TAR group) [from Mowatt G, Houston G, Hernandez R, de Verteuil R, Fraser C, Cuthbertson B, Vale L. Systematic review of the clinical effectiveness and cost-effectiveness of oesophageal Doppler monitoring in critically ill and high-risk surgical patients. Health Technol Assess 2009;13(7)]

Review: Oesophageal Doppler monitoring
Comparison: ODM + CVP + conventional assessment vs CVP + conventional assessment
Outcome: Length of hospital stay

Study or subcategory	n	ODM Mean (SD)	n	Control Mean (SD)	WMD (fixed) 95% CI	Weight %	WMD (fixed) 95% CI	Order
Conway, 2002	29	18.70 (20.20)	23	12.70 (6.00)		2.29	6.00 (-1.68 to 13.68)	0
Gan, 2002	50	5.00 (3.00)	50	7.00 (3.00)		97.71	-2.00 (-3.18 to -0.82)	0
Total (95% CI)	**79**		**78**			**100.0**	**-1.82 (-2.98 to -0.65)**	

Test for heterogeneity: $\chi^2 = 4.07$, df = 1 ($p = 0.04$), $I^2 = 75.4\%$
Test for overall effect: $z = 3.06$ ($p = 0.002$)

7

Discussion points

Cardiac and non-cardiac studies are non-comparable groups and are not usually analysed together however cardiac patients were included in this review and results were generally consistent to those from other studies. It is also unclear whether data from the critically ill population should be combined with surgical patients.

1 study of critically ill poly-trauma patients (Chytra 2007) noted that the ODM probe was difficult to keep in place and that the 12 hour protocol was time consuming.

The original AHRQ report concluded that the number of deaths was too low to permit pooling and none of the individual studies showed a significant difference between the ODM and non-ODM groups. The authors of this review used different statistical methods (Peto method) which showed significantly fewer deaths in the ODM group (comparison 1: ODM + CVP + CA versus CVP + CA).

The AHRQ report also considered 23 studies (RCTs, case series and case reports) that reported complications associated with ODM use. 4 studies reported minor complications, but none of these were the RCTs. The AHRQ concluded that ODM probes were relatively low risk.

In terms of cost-effectiveness, limited data are available; thus more research is required to enable more complete economic modelling.

Author's conclusion

The use of ODM-guided fluid optimization combined with CVP monitoring and conventional clinical assessment during major surgery leads to a reduction in complications, hospital stay and possibly mortality and based on this may be cost-effective. There is some evidence suggesting fewer complications and shorter hospital stay for certain critically ill subgroups but this is not enough to recommend widespread use in this population.

Problems & limitations

- Small studies: 5 of the studies had less than 100 patients
- There were significant differences in the ODM protocol between groups e.g. 4 hours for the post-operative cardiac patients and 12 hours for the trauma patients
- Mortality results need to be interpreted with caution because of the low number of events
- The evidence for reduced LOS in the ODM for comparison 3 (ODM + CA versus CA) is weak

Advantages

- This review only considered RCTs therefore is less prone to bias
- Based on AHRQ conclusions the strength of the evidence for the reduction in major complications, total complications and LOS in the ODM for comparison 1 (ODM + CVP + CA versus CVP + CA) is strong
- Other reviews in certain surgical groups have also shown that fluid optimization (some with invasive monitoring) may reduce hospital LOS

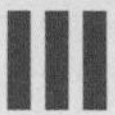

Expert opinion

Claudia Spies and Aarne Feldheiser

How valid and robust are the data?
This review found eight RCTs conducted with oesophageal Doppler monitoring (ODM) in the last 15 years with a low level of heterogeneity and with a relatively high number of patients. The review classifies the studies according to the algorithm if the oesophageal Doppler was used in combination with other monitoring opportunities like central venous pressure. The overall effect of the use of ODM has to be stated as valid and robust.

Should clinical practice be influenced by this?
The review highlights the impact of ODM on postoperative morbidity and hospital length of stay indicating that the method is clinically effective. Especially in any kind of major abdominal surgery or high-risk traumatic procedure ODM should be considered to improve clinical care.

What is the next step?
The further evaluation of the cost-effectiveness of ODM in combination with the definition of surgical procedures and groups of patients which benefit most of ODM needs to be clarified in more detail in the future.

Citation

Mowatt G, Houston G, Hernández R, de Verteuil R, Fraser C, Cuthbertson B, Vale L. Systematic review of the clinical effectiveness and cost-effectiveness of oesophageal Doppler monitoring in critically ill and high-risk surgical patients. Health Technol Assess 2009;13(7). DOI: 10.3310/hta13070

Additional information

Potentially relevant study identified and largest of on going studies

Stroke Volume Optimisation in Patients with hip fracture (FRACTALE). NCT00444262

Intervention: haemodynamic optimization with ODM using voluven and other solutes

This was due to run from April 2007 to April 2010 and aimed to enrol 800 patients.

AMSTAR: methodological quality of the review

1.	Was "a priori" design provided?	Y
2.	Was study selection and data extraction adequate?	Y
3.	Was the literature search comprehensive?	Y
4.	Was 'Grey Literature' used? Limited to English language	P
5.	Was a list of excluded studies provided?	Y
6.	Were the characteristics of included studies provided?	Y
7.	Was the scientific quality of studies assessed & documented?	Y
8.	Was the scientific quality of studies weighted appropriately in forming conclusions?	Y
9.	Were the methods used for data synthesis appropriate?	Y
10.	Was the potential for publication bias assessed?	Y
11.	Were any conflicts of interest stated?	Y

Overall quality of trials included	8 high quality, 2 moderate
Overall quality of the review	High

Computerised decision support systems

Technology: computerized decision-support systems (CDSS)

Clinical question: What are the characteristics of effective CDSS and what are their effects on tight glycaemic control (TGC)?

A CDSS is a computer program that is designed to help healthcare workers in making clinical decisions. These systems are characterized by the level of support provided, consultation style and communication style used. Support level ranges from simply displaying the protocol to suggesting a specific therapy; consultation may be active providing regular feedback or only on-demand. Communication style can be critical, pointing out deviations from protocol and non-critical, providing advice whether or not the protocol has been followed.

Tight glycaemic control is the ideal test application as it must applied in a highly controlled environment where additional efforts are required such as timing of blood glucose level (BGL) measurements to avoid harmful complications such as hypoglycaemia.

Review characteristics

- **Eligibility criteria:** controlled trials and observational studies that evaluated a given TGC protocol with a CDSS
- **Number of studies:** 17 studies (3 RCTs, 7 controlled trial before/after, 7 observational studies)
- **Number of patients:** 6,200
- **Population:** medical, surgical or trauma ICU patients + patients from a progressive care unit.
- **Study dates:** 2005 2008

7

Definitions

- **Quality indicator:** "a measurable quantity of the TGC process that may alone or in combination with other quantities, indicate some aspect of its quality". 24 different indicators of glycaemic control were extracted
- **Hypoglycaemic event:** 6 different thresholds between 40–70 mg/dl (2.2–3.9 mmol/l)
- **Target glucose range:** lower limit ranged from 80–100 mg/dl (4.4–5.5 mmol/l) to upper limit 110–150 mg/dl (6.1–8.3 mmol/l)

Main findings

Several recommendations are consequently made by the authors to improve the practical usefulness of future studies aimed at validating the use of CDSS:

1. The TGC protocol should be integrated into clinical workflows
2. Preliminary researches are necessary to determine the CDSS most appropriate implementation site, target user, and time of advice

3. It is essential to determine a common glycaemic vocabulary. What are exactly the consensual indicators of hyperglycaemia, hypoglycaemia and glycaemic control?
4. In case of passive CDSS, the usage of the system frequency must be clearly described
5. In case of active CDSS, the usage, usability and acceptability of the messages must be detailed
6. TGC impact on care is dependent on the quality of data. It must be known if data are entered manually, with or without systematic verification

Author's conclusion

In most studies, an improvement in at least one indicator of TGC was observed in terms of quality indicators. It is however impossible to define the successful factors nevertheless this review did result in key recommendations for future research.

Problems & limitations

- In 5 studies, a modified version of the TGC was used after CDSS implementation and 11 studies evaluated a new TCG protocol at the same time as CDSS implementation, both scenarios can cause considerable staff confusion
- Due to the variability in case-mix, insulin therapy, associated therapies, and end points used, a meta-analysis was not performed as the results would have been unreliable
- Reminders for BGL were only active in 9 studies

Advantages

- In all the studies, the CDSS were operated in the same mode ('critiquing mode')
- 16 studies used the passive mode for pump speed adjustments necessitating clinician involvement
- CDSS may improve glycaemic control; with regards to hypoglycaemic events, 6 studies reported no change, 7 observation studies reported hypoglycaemic events to be in the acceptable range and 2 studies even reported a reduction

Expert opinion

Pierre Squara

The key recommendations as above where summarised

How valid and robust are the data?
There is no doubt that the heterogeneity of the available studies does not allow valid conclusions regarding the CDSS usefulness for TCG. The suggested subsequent recommendations may be considered as "expert opinion" for improving the reproducibility and generalizability of future studies.

Should clinical practice be influenced by this?
Not yet, but this paper illustrates how it is important to harmonize the definitions, the indicators and the protocols. It can be the task of a scientific society to help in this objective.

What's the next step?
Determining consensually the indicators of a hypoglycaemic episode, a hyperglycaemic episode, a glycemic control? Trying to determine one TGC quantitative quality criteria, which can be used to compare the effectiveness of the different modalities of TGC? Then restart studies using this quality criteria to show: i) which type of CDSS (active or passive) works best, ii) where should it be located, and iii) which type of data verification must be used?

Citation

Eslami S, Abu-Hanna A, de Jonge E, de Keizer NF. Tight Glycaemic control and computerised decision support. Intensive Care Med (2009) 35:1505–1517 DOI 10.1007/s00134-009-1542-0

AMSTAR: methodological quality of the review

1.	Was "a priori" design provided?	Y
2.	Was study selection and data extraction adequate?	Y
3.	Was the literature search comprehensive?	Y
4.	Was 'Grey Literature' used?	P
5.	Was a list of excluded studies provided?	N
6.	Were the characteristics of included studies provided?	Y
7.	Was the scientific quality of studies assessed & documented?	Y
8.	Was the scientific quality of studies weighted appropriately in forming conclusions?	Y
9.	Were the methods used for data synthesis appropriate?	Y
10.	Was the potential for publication bias assessed?	U
11.	Were any conflicts of interest stated?	N

Overall quality of trials included	U
Overall quality of the review	High

8

Infection

Peripheral venous catheters 170
Procalcitonin 174
Continuous beta-lactam antibiotics 179
Ventilator-associated pneumonia 183
Selective decontamination of the digestive tract 187
Antibiotic prophylaxis for pancreatic necrosis 191

Also see:

Section 3: Acute respiratory failure – Non-ARDS
Corticosteroids for pneumonia
Section 12: Paediatric intensive care
Bacterial meningitis
Section 13: Sepsis

Peripheral venous catheters

Condition: peripheral venous catheter infections

Clinical questions: Should peripheral venous catheters be replaced when clinically indicated instead of routinely after 3-4 days as recommended?
What are the costs associated with routine replacement?

Studies report a wide range in the incidence of phlebitis (2.3–60%) and bacteraemia rate of 0.8%. Routine peripheral cannula replacement is thought to reduce these complications, when this review was conducted, Centres for Disease Control (CDC) guidelines recommended replacement every 72–96 hours in adults. However, this was based on one observational study conducted in 1992. Furthermore, thrombophlebitis may result from mechanical factors such as cannula fabric, size, drug irritation or insertion technique rather than infection, therefore recent improvements in cannula design and composition should be considered. Some studies suggest that the risk of phlebitis is associated with the number of times a cannula is used rather than age per se and that the risk is highest in the first days post insertion.

[CDC recommendation for children: only replace cannula if clinically indicated]

Review characteristics

- **Eligibility criteria:** RCTs comparing routine versus clinically indicated removal of catheters in patients who require intermittent or continuous intravenous (iv) therapy for at least 3 days. Only studies where data was available per patient not per catheter (1 patient may have a catheter for 6 days or 2 catheters for 3 days each)
- **Exclusions:** crossover trials, participants receiving parenteral fluids
- **Number of studies:** 6 RCTs (4 published, 2 unpublished)
- **Number of patients:** 3,455 (range 47–1885)
- **Population:** patients with peripheral iv therapy either in the community or in hospital
- **Study dates:** 2004–2010

Definitions

- **Device-related bacteraemia:** bacteraemia while catheter is *in situ* or within 48 hours of removal if no other source is identified
- **Study Group:** when catheter was changed when clinically indicated
- **Thrombophlebitis:** any definition used by trial authors
- **Cost:** materials and labour associated with catheter insertion

Fig. 1 Forest plot of comparison: 1 Clinically indicated versus routine change outcome: 1.2 Phlebitis all studies [from Webster J, Osborne S, Rickard C, Hall J. Clinically-indicated replacement versus routine replacement of peripheral venous catheters. Cochrane Database of Systematic Reviews 2010, Issue 3. Art. No.: CD007798, © Cochrane Collaboration, reproduced with permission]

Study or subgroup	Clinically indicated Events	Clinically indicated Total	Routine replacement Events	Routine replacement Total	Weight %	Odds Ratio M-H, Fixed, 95% CI
1.2.1. Continuous infusion						
Barker 2004	11	26	1	21	0.6	14.67 [1.70, 126.39]
Rickard 2008	18	185	12	177	10.2	1.48 [0.69, 3.17]
Rickard 2009	73	944	71	941	60.5	1.03 [0.73, 1.44]
Webster 2007	1	103	2	103	1.8	0.50 [0.04, 5.55]
Webster 2008	15	379	12	376	10.6	1.34 [0.62, 2.87]
Subtotal (95% CI)		**1637**		**1618**	**83.7**	**1.21 [0.91, 1.59]**
Total events	119		98			
Heterogeneity: $Chi^2 = 6.90$, df = 4 (P = 0.14); $I^2 = 42\%$						
Test for overall effect: Z = 1.32 (P = 0.19)						
1.2.2. Intermittent infusion						
Van Donk 2009	37	105	26	95	16.3	1.44 [0.79, 2.64]
Subtotal (95% CI)		**105**		**95**	**16.3**	**1.44 [0.79, 2.64]**
Total events	37		26			
Heterogeneity: Not applicable						
Test for overall effect: Z = 1.19 (P = 0.23)						
Total (95% CI)		**1742**		**1713**	**100.0**	**1.24 [0.97, 1.60]**
Total events	156		124			
Heterogeneity: $Chi^2 = 7.30$, df = 5 (P = 0.20); $I^2 = 31\%$						
Test for overall effect: Z = 1.70 (P = 0.09)						
Test for subgroup differences: Not applicable						

0.05 0.2 1 5 20

Favours cl-indicated Favours 3-day

8

Results

Primary outcomes	Trials	N	Results
Bacteraemia	5	3408	Trend to lower incidence in study group but NSS
Phlebitis	6	3455	Increased in study group but NSS
Cost	2	961	Significantly reduced in study group

Secondary outcomes	Trials	N	Results
Local infection	3	1323	2 events in study group but NSS
Blockage	4	1523	Higher in the study group (P = 0.03)
Infiltration into tissue	3	1323	Higher in the study group but NSS

Author's conclusion

The review suggests that patients are not adversely affected if peripheral catheters are changed when clinically indicated, instead of routinely. The trend towards increases in phlebitis in the study group was less apparent if data were analysed per 1,000 device days or if only trials that used the accepted definition of phlebitis were included.

Problems & limitations

- In 3 trials, a third of the patients had protocol violations, mainly in the control group when catheters were not replaced within the specified time
- Incomplete reporting in 1 trial (47 patients)
- Lack of blinding in all the trials
- Varying definitions of phlebitis

Advantages

- Trials were recent eliminating major concerns with catheter technology
- Overall number of patients was large and trial quality was good

Expert opinion

George Dimopoulos

How valid and robust are the data?

This review found 6 RCTs (4 published, 2 unpublished) conducted over 6 years and including 3,455 patients (range 47–1,885). In 3 trials, a third of the patients had protocol violations mainly in the control group when catheters were not replaced within the specified time while incomplete reports have been observed in 1 trial (47 patients). In all of the trials a lack of blinding was noted while the definitions of phlebitis varied. Trials were recent eliminating major concerns with catheter technology while overall number of patients was large and trial quality was good.

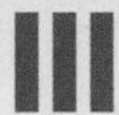

Should clinical practise be influenced by this?

The authors suggest that the clinically-indicated instead of routine replacement of peripheral catheters did not adversely affect the patients and a trend towards increases in phlebitis in the study group was less apparent if data was analysed per 1,000 device days or if only trials that used the accepted definition of phlebitis were included.

What's the next step?

I believe that this SR-MA strongly indicates the need for less interventions in the critically ill patients in order to avoid/minimize the infective complications.

Citation

Webster J, Osborne S, Rickard C, Hall J. Clinically-indicated replacement versus routine replacement of peripheral venous catheters. Cochrane Database of Systematic Reviews 2010, Issue 3. Art. No.: CD007798. DOI: 10.1002/14651858.CD007798.pub2.

Additional information

One of the unpublished trials in the review has recently been completed:

There were over 3,300 participants over three hospitals. Rates of bacteraemia and phlebitis were not affected by study allocation in this large study of over 5,000 cannulas.

New Guidelines: see critical care Medscape:

CDC Updates IV Catheter Infection Prevention Guidelines (http://www.medscape.org/viewarticle/740412?src=cmemp)

12 recommendations have been made, however, time-based rather than clinically-based change of peripheral cannula is only required if asepsis on insertion could not be assured

AMSTAR: methodological quality of the review

1.	Was "a priori" design provided?	Y
2.	Was study selection and data extraction adequate?	Y
3.	Was the literature search comprehensive?	Y
4.	Was 'Grey Literature' used?	Y
5.	Was a list of excluded studies provided?	Y
6.	Where the characteristics of included studies provided?	Y
7.	Was the scientific quality of studies assessed & documented?	Y
8.	Was the scientific quality of studies weighted appropriately in forming conclusions?	Y
9.	Were the methods used for data synthesis appropriate?	Y
10.	Was the potential for publication bias assessed?	Y
11.	Were any conflicts of interest stated?	Y

Overall quality of trials included	High
Overall quality of the review	High

8

Procalcitonin

Condition: infection/sepsis

Clinical question: Can procalcitonin be used effectively and safely as a biomarker for sepsis to guide antibiotic use and duration?

Emerging antimicrobial resistance has attracted a great deal of concern in the health care setting particularly with the advent of virulent multi-drug resistant (MDR) organisms. It is well recognized that the majority of patients on critical care will exhibit signs of infection and will receive antibiotics (ABx); however, systemic inflammation without sepsis is also common in ICU and often hard to distinguish from sepsis in the absence of positive microbiological cultures. The only effective means of combating the emerging antimicrobial resistance is to restrict antibiotic use and duration to that which is absolutely required to treat infections.

Procalcitonin is one of the many biomarkers studied for sepsis and appears to be the most promising. However procalcitonin displays wide inter-individual variability, therefore, interpretation may require serial measurements.

Review characteristics

- **Eligibility criteria**: only RCTs in critically ill adults, children and neonates
- **A priori**: not to include data from paediatric/neonatal ICUs in the pooled outcomes
- **Number of studies**: 7 RCTs (6 adult ICU, 1 neonatal ICU). 5 single centre, 2 multicentre. All published after 2007
- **Number of patients**: 1,010 adults + 121 neonates
- **Population**: 3 trials from surgical ICUs. Of 1,010 patients: 40% community acquired infection mostly pneumonia, 60% hospital acquired infection. Most surgical patients had abdominal surgery or multiple trauma, commonest infection was peritonitis

8

Results

Primary outcomes

- **Duration of antibiotic treatment for the first episode of infection**: 2 days shorter in PCT group
- **The antibiotic free days at 28 days after study enrolment**: 3 days more ABx-free days in the PCT group
- **Total antibiotic therapy with daily ABx use excluding antifungals, up to day 28**: 4 days less in the PCT group

Outcome	1. ABx Duration	1. ABx Duration	2. ABx Free days	Total ABx	Neonates
Trials/pts	5 trials/938	3 trials*/ 801	3 trials*/801	3 trials*/801	1 trial/101
FEM:WMD	2.14 days less	3.10 days less	2.94 days	4.19 days less	22 hours less
95% CI	-2.48 to -1.80	-3.88 to -2.32	1.92–3.96	-4.98 to -3.39	NA
p	< 0.01	< 0.001	< 0.00001	< 0.001	< 0.012
I^2	68%	NA	0%	71.5%	NA

* 3 highest quality trials

Secondary outcomes

Outcomes	Results
28-day all-cause mortality	No difference
Hospital mortality	No difference
ICU LOS	Shorter in the PCT group by 0.49 days but NSS
Hospital LOS	No difference
Days free from MV	No difference
Relapse/persistent infection/ superinfection	No difference
Cost (in 1 study only)	Significantly reduced in PCT group (17.8%, p < 0.01)
Adverse events	No difference
Other findings	Algorithm overruling occurred in 3 studies in the patients randomised to PCT group

Note: Not all studies had data for all secondary outcomes

Author's conclusion

PCT-guided algorithms for managing critically ill septic patients resulted in less antibiotic exposure with similar mortality rates, LOS and adverse events.

The use of these PCT guided algorithms appears to be safe.

The primary findings of the meta-analysis were concordant in all 3 outcome measures and confirmed by the sensitivity analysis.

Caution advised as the full clinical impact of reduction in antibiotic exposure remains unknown.

8

Fig. 2 Total duration of antibiotic treatment: forest plot showing the comparison of procalcitonin-guided algorithms vs. routine practice. The size of each square represents the proportion of information provided by each study. The vertical line depicts the point of "no difference" between the two groups, and the horizontal lines correspond to the 95% confidence intervals (CIs). Diamonds represent the weighted mean difference (WMD) for all studies. [from Petros Kopterides; Ilias I. Siempos; Iraklis Tsangaris; Argirios Tsantes; Apostolos Armaganidis. Procalcitonin-guided algorithms of antibiotic therapy in the intensive care unit: A systematic review and meta-analysis of randomized controlled trials. Crit Care Med 2010; 38:2229–2241]

Review: Procalcitonin-guided algorithms of antibiotic stewardship in the intensive care unit: systematic review and meta-analysis
Comparison: 01 Procalcitonin-guided algorithms versus routine practice
Outcome: 02 Total duration of antibiotic treatment

Study or sub-category	N	PCT-guided algorithm Mean (SD)	N	Routine practice Mean (SD)	WMD (fixed) 95% CI	Weight %	WMD (fixed) 95% CI
Bouadma	307	10.30 (7.70)	314	13.30 (7.60)		43.91	-3.00 [-4.20, -1.80]
Stolz	51	10.00 (2.50)	50	15.00 (3.25)		49.60	-5.00 [-6.13, -3.87]
Nobre	39	8.00 (5.75)	40	14.00 (8.25)		6.49	-6.00 [-9.13, -2.87]
Total (95% CI)	**397**		**404**			**100.00**	**-4.19 [-4.98, -3.39]**

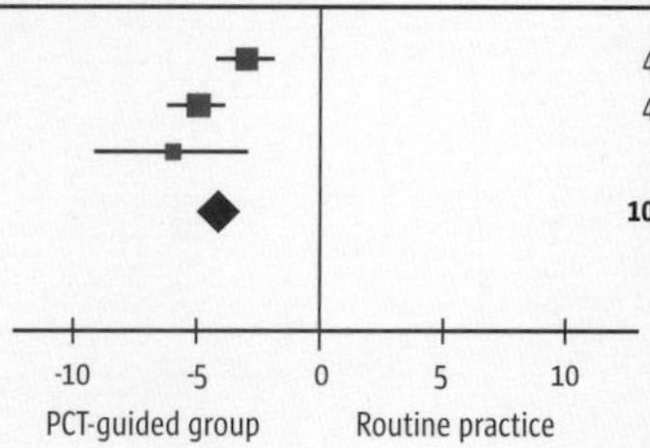

Test for heterogeneity: $Chi^2 = 7.01$, df = 2 (P = 0.03); $I^2 = 71.5\%$
Test for overall effect: Z = 10.29 (P < 0.00001)

-10 -5 0 5 10
PCT-guided group Routine practice

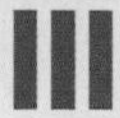

Problems & limitations

- Lack of blinding
- Small numbers of patients as not all studies reported all outcomes
- Heterogeneity between studies even in the PCT assays and algorithms
- "Routine practice" was not protocol-based or standardised
- Patient groups excluded include: difficult to treat organisms/infections and the severely immune-compromised

Advantages

- There was concordance between studies on the outcomes which were measured

Expert opinion

Jordi Rello

How valid and robust are the data?

These data have to be analysed with caution. In real ICU practice, the majority of patients required inotropes or have multi-resistant organisms, and they were excluded.

It is unclear how bacteraemia may influence outcomes. Blinding is not clear in the control arm. Caution to generalize data of pneumonia to peritonitis is needed. Each infectious site requires an individual analysis.

Should clinical practice be influenced by this?

No. A trial using 8 days of therapy for VAP, as used in standard practice should be reported.

What's the next step?

Assess duration of therapy for control patients. Standard of care in Europe, according to EUVAP study, the largest study in Europe is 8 days of antibiotic therapy for VAP-HAP.

To identify variables associated with short antibiotic therapy.

To assess performance in patients with septic shock or multi-resistant organisms.

Citation

Kopterides P, Siempos II, Tsangaris I, Tsantes A, Armaganidis A. Procalcitonin-guided algorithms of antibiotic therapy in the intensive care unit: A systematic review and meta-analysis of randomized controlled trials. Crit Care Med 2010; 38:2229–2241

AMSTAR: methodological quality of the review

1.	Was "a priori" design provided?	Y
2.	Was study selection and data extraction adequate?	Y
3.	Was the literature search comprehensive?	Y
4.	Was 'Grey Literature' used?	Y
5.	Was a list of excluded studies provided?	N
6.	Where the characteristics of included studies provided?	Y
7.	Was the scientific quality of studies assessed & documented?	Y
8.	Was the scientific quality of studies weighted appropriately in forming conclusions?	Y
9.	Were the methods used for data synthesis appropriate?	Y
10.	Was the potential for publication bias assessed?	Y
11.	Were any conflicts of interest stated?	Y

Overall quality of trials included	3 high quality, 4 low quality
Overall quality of the review	High

Continuous beta-lactam antibiotics

Condition: acute infections

Clinical question: Does the use of continuous or 'extended infusion' of β-lactam antibiotics confer any benefit to patients or reduce mortality?

Bacterial-killing properties of antimicrobials can be concentration-dependent or time-dependent. In the former, efficacy is optimised by increasing the ratio of the maximum antibiotic concentration to the minimum inhibitory concentration (C_{max}:MIC). With time-dependent antibiotics such as beta-lactams, antibacterial activity is optimized by maximizing the time for which their concentration is above the MIC. *In vitro* studies have established that different classes of beta-lactams have differing T > MIC targets e.g. carbapenems 40%; penicillins 50–60%; cephalosporins 60–70%. It is therefore important to determine what the ultimate dosing strategy is for this widely used group of antibiotics to improve efficacy and minimize side effects.

Review characteristics

- **Eligibility criteria:** RCTs and observational studies comparing β-lactam extended dose or infusion to bolus administration
- **Exclusions:** inadequate randomisation, cross-over studies, and those that lacked data on either clinical cure or mortality
- **Number of studies:** 14 RCTs, 2 observational studies (not included in the pooled analysis)
- **Number of patients:** total 846 patients
- **Population:** any hospitalised with an infection
- **Study dates:** 1 study from 1979, 1 from 1983 and the rest are from 2000–2007

Definitions

- **Infection:** any infection in hospitalised patients
- **Extended administration of antibiotic:** dose given over at least 3 hours
- **Clinical cure:** definition may have varied in each study
- **Mortality:** 14 days, 28 days or anytime during study

Results

Primary outcomes

Outcome	Trials	N	OR	95% CI	*p*	I²	Result
Clinical cure	9	755	1.04	0.74–1.46	0.83	0%	NSS
Mortality	9	541	1.00	0.48–2.06	1.00	14.8%	NSS

Fig. 3 Mortality difference between patients who received infusion and boluses of antibiotic. OR, odds ratio; CI, confidence interval [from Jason A. Roberts, Steven Webb, David Paterson, Kwok M. Ho, Jeffrey Lipman,. A systematic review on clinical benefits of continuous administration of beta-lactam antibiotics. Crit Care Med 2009 Vol. 37, No. 6. DOI: 10.1097/CCM.0b013e3181a0054d]

Study	Infusion n/N	Bolus n/N	OR (random) 95% CI	Weight %	OR (random) 95% CI
Kojika 2005 (50)	1/5	0/5		4.22	3.67 [0.12, 113.73]
Lagast 1983 (48)	5/20	4/25		18.40	1.75 [0.40, 7.63]
Angus 2000 (45)	3/10	9/11		10.82	0.10 [0.01, 0.74]
Nicolau 2001 (49)	2/17	2/18		10.47	1.07 [0.13, 8.56]
Pedeboscq 2001 (44)	0/3	0/4			Not estimable
Georges 2005 (21)	3/25	3/23		14.55	0.91 [0.16, 5.03]
Lau 2006 (22)	3/128	1/130		8.97	3.10 [0.32, 30.16]
Rafati 2006 (23)	5/20	6/20		20.00	0.78 [0.19, 3.13]
Roberts 2007 (24)	3/29	0/28		5.41	7.53 [0.37, 152.73]
Sakka 2007 (25)	1/10	2/10		7.16	0.44 [0.03, 5.88]
Total (95% CI)	**267**	**274**		**100.0**	**1.00 [0.48, 2.06]**

Total events: 26 (Infusion), 27 (Bolus)

Test for heterogeneity: $Chi^2 = 9.39$, $df = 8$ ($P = 0.31$); $I^2 = 14.8\%$

Test for overall effect: $Z = 0.00$ ($P = 1.00$)

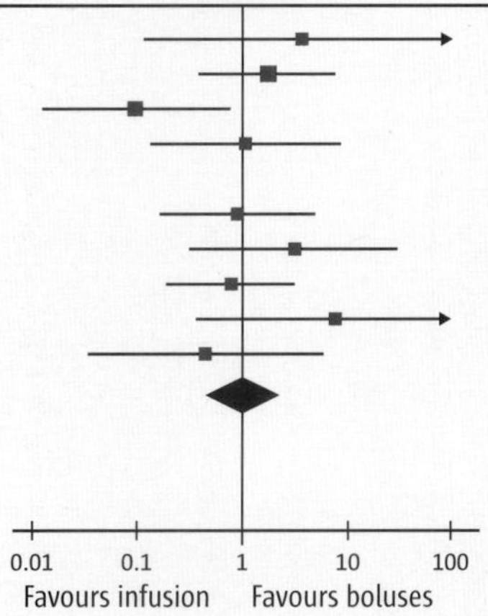

0.01 0.1 1 10 100

Favours infusion Favours boluses

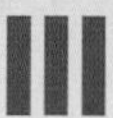

Author's conclusion

The results of the meta-analysis showed that continuous infusion of beta-lactam antibiotics was not associated with a significant improvement in clinical outcomes. However the continuous infusion arms had lower daily doses of the drug. One of the observational studies showed a significant reduction in clinical cure while the other showed a significant reduction in mortality with continuous infusions. Although these had larger numbers of patients, they were not included in the pooled analysis because they did not meet predetermined criteria.

Problems & limitations

- Most studies had very small numbers of patients, less than 30 patients in each arm, while only one study had more than 100 patients
- Very large heterogeneity of patient populations (e.g. critically ill in 6 studies only, neutropenic sepsis, COPD)
- Most studies either showed clinical cure or mortality but not both

Advantages

- Observational studies and the large confidence intervals suggest that continuous infusions may be beneficial in specific patient groups
- Both of these studies include critically ill patients with Gram-negative sepsis which is more likely to benefit from continuous infusion as beta-lactams do not have post antibiotic effects on these pathogens
- Lower drug doses with a continuous infusion may have beneficial cost implications

Expert opinion

George Dimopoulos

How valid and robust are the data?

This review found 14 RCTs and 2 observational studies (not included in the pooled analysis) conducted over a 30 years period including a total of 846 patients. Most studies had very small numbers of patients, less than 30 patients in each arm, while only one study had more than 100 patients. Very large heterogeneity of patient populations (e.g. critically ill in 6 studies only, neutropenic sepsis, COPD). Most studies either showed clinical cure or mortality but not both.

Should clinical practise be influenced by this?

This review has highlighted that continuous infusion of beta lactam antibiotics was not associated with a significant improvement in clinical outcomes. The unincluded observational studies in the pooled analysis had larger numbers of patients and large confidence intervals suggesting that critically ill patients with Gram-negative sepsis are more likely to benefit from continuous infusion as beta-lactams do not have post-antibiotic effects on these pathogens. One of these studies showed a significant reduction in clinical cure while the other showed a significant reduction in mortality with continuous infusions.

What's the next step?

I believe that the use of continuous or 'extended infusion' of antibiotics has advantages regarding the use of beta-lactams although there are no available data regarding their concentration levels ($C_{maximum}$ and trough levels). This underscores the need of performing larger RCTs.

8

Citation

Roberts JA, Webb S, Paterson D, Ho KM, Lipman J. A systematic review on clinical benefits of continuous administration of beta-lactam antibiotics. Crit Care Med 2009 Vol. 37, No. 6. DOI: 10.1097/CCM.0b013e3181a0054d

AMSTAR: methodological quality of the review

1.	Was "a priori" design provided?	Y
2.	Was study selection and data extraction adequate?	Y
3.	Was the literature search comprehensive?	Y
4.	Was 'Grey Literature' used?	Y
5.	Was a list of excluded studies provided?	N
6.	Where the characteristics of included studies provided?	Y
7.	Was the scientific quality of studies assessed & documented?	Y
8.	Was the scientific quality of studies weighted appropriately in forming conclusions?	Y
9.	Were the methods used for data synthesis appropriate?	Y
10.	Was the potential for publication bias assessed?	Y
11.	Were any conflicts of interest stated?	Y

Overall quality of trials included	Low
Overall quality of the review	High

Ventilator-associated pneumonia

Condition: ventilator-associated pneumonia (VAP)

Clinical question: Are there any factors, present on the day of admission to ICU or on diagnosis of VAP, which can be used to accurately predict the potential mortality in ICU patients with VAP?

Several studies have suggested an association between various factors such as initial treatment or pathogen isolated with mortality. However, none of these have been confirmed consistently in subsequent studies.

Review characteristics

- **Eligibility criteria**: studies which only enrolled adult patients with VAP that was microbiologically confirmed with quantitative cultures of respiratory samples and that reported on mortality
- **Exclusions**: intervention studies due to their narrow patient selection criteria
- **Number of studies**: 26 (15 prospective and 11 retrospective) observational studies
- **Number of patients**: 2,827
- **Population**: adults ventilated for at least 48 hours, in both medical and surgical ICUs
- **Study dates**: 1994–2009

Definitions

- **VAP**: clinical features that are well recognised: temperature, WCC, purulent secretions, CXR changes **plus**
- **Microbiology**: sample retrieved by tracheal aspirates, BAL or protected specimen brush or telescopic catheter. Quantitative > 10^3 colony forming units
- **Appropriate initial treatment**: if antibiotics were given within 24 hours of VAP onset
- **ALI & ARDS**: consensus definitions

Results

1. Mortality: All-cause mortality at ICU discharge or 28-day was 34% (960/2827) overall (range 16–53%)
2. Predictors of mortality in patients with VAP present on admission to ICU

Mortality	Condition	OR	95% CI
Highest	Acute respiratory Failure (c.f. non respiratory causes of ICU admission)	1.99	1.15–3.42
	Community acquired pneumonia	4.17	1.79–9.71
	Malignancy	2.20	1.10–4.40
Lowest	Trauma	0.35	0.22–0.57

8

Tab. 1 Risk factors for mortality in patients with microbiologically confirmed VAP at the day of pneumonia diagnosis [from Ilias I. Siempos, Konstantinos Z. Vardakas, Christos E. Kyriakopoulos, Theodora K. Ntaidou, and Matthew E. Falagas. Predictors of mortality in adult patients with ventilator associated pneumonia: a meta-analysis. SHOCK, Vol. 33, No. 6, pp. 590Y601, 2010 DOI: 10.1097/SHK.0b013e3181cc0418]

Type of factor	No. patients in studies reporting specific data	Pooled OR; 95% CI*	p
Inappropiate initial treatment	1314	2.92; 2.01–4.22	< 0.001
Polymicrobial infection	265	0.60; 0.34–1.04	0.07
Bacteremia	501	2.07; 1.16–3.71	0.01
ARDS/ALI	284	2.28; 1.24–4.21	0.008
Shock	1009	3.90; 2.31–6.61	< 0.001
Late-onset VAP	482	1.62; 1.01–2.59	0.05
Previous receipt of antimicrobial agents[1]	148	2.67; 0.91–7.89	0.08
Sepsis	233	4.77; 2.22–10.25	< 0.001

* All pooled ORs were calculated by using a random effects model.

[1] Before the onset of VAP.

3. Pathogens associated with higher mortality were: non-fermenting Gram-negative bacteria and A.baumannii, associated with the lowest mortality was MSSA, but only in 2 studies. The other results didn't reach statistical significance.
4. There was concordance between studies with certain continuous variables associate with higher mortality

Reported by > 5 studies	Reported by < 5 studies
Age	CPIS (clinical pulmonary infection) score
Disease severity at admission (APACHE II + SOFA II)	Serum CRP
Disease severity at VAP diagnosis (APACHE II, SOFA II & Logistic Organ Dysfunction (LOD) score)	Body temperature
SOFA score	WCC
–	PaO_2/FiO_2

Author's conclusion

The synthesized evidence allowed the calculation of the magnitude of effect between predictors and mortality, which may help clinicians devise predicting scores for patients with VAP. Furthermore, this highlighted the association between inappropriate treatment (delay in administering antibiotics or antimicrobials to which the causative organism is not sensitive) and mortality. This being a modifiable factor can be influenced to improve patient outcome.

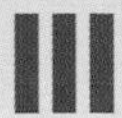

Problems & limitations

- Inadequate data to comment on the role of fungi in VAP
- Large variability in mortality rates is multifactorial but may partly be due to different definitions, criteria or causative organisms between studies
- Due to the nature of the data, only univariate analysis could be undertaken for some of the predictors, which would therefore more accurately be referred to as "associations"

Advantages

- Strict eligibility criteria for VAP ensured that all patients did have VAP however this may have excluded other patients with VAP based on qualitative cultures.
- The finding that the prognosis of VAP caused by Gram-negative bacilli is worse than that caused by Gram-positive bacteria concurs with expert opinion

Expert opinion

Jordi Rello

How valid and robust are the data?

All-cause ICU mortality is 34% consistent with mortality in standard ICUs for ventilated patients. Appropriate initial treatment has to take into consideration that organism remained susceptible to the antibiotic choice. Quantitative microbiology is considered if sample count was above 1,000 cfu. But this is only a useful breakpoint for PSB. BAL and QTA require higher thresholds. It remains unknown for which patients a tracheobronchitis was documented.

Should clinical practice be influenced by this?

It is difficult to generalize on clinical practice as reported. Factors associated with ICU mortality are related to five elements: 1. Severity of the patient at ICU admission; 2. Prior duration of hospitalization; 3. Host (Age, gender and comorbidities); 4. Appropriate use of antibiotic treatments; 5. The organism in regard to comparing MRSA, P. aeruginos, other nonfermentative GNB, Enterobacteriaceae, H. influenzae & core Gram-positive (MSSA, pneumococci, other streptococci). I disagree that GNB rods are associated with higher mortality than Gram-positive cocci. For instance, ICU mortality for MRSA is statistically higher than H. influenzae

What's the next step?

For an analysis taking in account sub-classification in the above-mentioned organisms, a comparison of potential prognostic variables is required. Moreover, the cohort has to be split into three categories, with independent analysis, depending on very high (> 50%), high (21–50%) and low (< 20%) estimated ICU mortality.

8

Citation

Siempos II, Vardakas KZ, Kyriakopoulos CE, Ntaidou TK and Falagas ME. Predictors of mortality in adult patients with ventilator associated pneumonia: a meta-analysis. SHOCK, Vol. 33, No. 6, pp. 590Y601, 2010 DOI: 10.1097/SHK.0b013e3181cc0418

AMSTAR: methodological quality of the review

1.	Was "a priori" design provided?	Y
2.	Was study selection and data extraction adequate?	Y
3.	Was the literature search comprehensive?	Y
4.	Was 'Grey Literature' used?	Y
5.	Was a list of excluded studies provided?	N
6.	Where the characteristics of included studies provided?	Y
7.	Was the scientific quality of studies assessed & documented?	NA
8.	Was the scientific quality of studies weighted appropriately in forming conclusions?	Y
9.	Were the methods used for data synthesis appropriate?	Y
10.	Was the potential for publication bias assessed?	NA
11.	Were any conflicts of interest stated?	N

Overall quality of trials included	All observational studies
Overall quality of the review	High

Selective decontamination of the digestive tract

Condition: respiratory tract infections (RTI)

Clinical question: Does antibiotic prophylaxis reduce RTI or mortality in ICU?

The incidence of pneumonia amongst ICU patients is as high as 40% and is associated with significant morbidity and mortality of up to 50%. One method that has been shown to be significantly effective in reducing the incidence of RTI in ICU is selective decontamination of the digestive tract (SDD) which involves applying topical non-absorbable antibiotics to the orophynx and digestive tract with or without systemic antibiotics. SDD has not been shown to reduce mortality and may adversely affect outcome should it result in propagation of multidrug resistant organisms.

Review characteristics

- **Eligibility criteria:** RCTs on antibiotic prophylaxis for preventing RTI and death
- **Exclusions:** studies where < 50% underwent mechanical ventilation for > 48 hours Elective oesophageal resection, cardiac or gastric surgery, liver transplant or those with acute liver failure
- **Number of studies:** 36 (17 studies used topical + systemic versus control; 14 studies used topical verses control; 5 studies used topical + systemic versus systemic ABx)
- **Number of patients:** 6,914
- **Population:** adult ICU patients (mostly general ICUs but also trauma and surgical ICUs)
- **Study dates:** 1988–2007

8

Definition

- **Intervention:** systemic and/or topical antibiotics but type was not restricted
- **Control:** no prophylaxis or placebo
- **RTI:** no restrictions on the type of RTI or the diagnostic criteria
- **Mortality:** ICU mortality for some trials, others used mortality on hospital discharge

Results

Primary outcomes

- **RTI Outcome:** statistically significant reduction in RTI in the study group
- **Mortality Outcome:** statistically significant reduction in mortality in topical +systemic ABx group but not with topical ABx
- No adverse events were recorded

Fig. 4 Comparison 1 Topical plus systemic versus no prophylaxis, Outcome 1 Overall mortality [from Liberati A, D'Amico R, Pifferi S, Torri V, Brazzi L, Parmelli E. Antibiotic prophylaxis to reduce respiratory tract infections and mortality in adults receiving intensive care. Cochrane Database of Systematic Reviews 2009, Issue 4. Art. No.: CD000022, © Cochrane Collaboration, reproduced with permission]

Review: Antibiotic prophylaxis to reduce respiratory tract infections and mortality in adults receiving intensive care
Comparison: 1 Topical plus systemic versus no prophylaxis; Outcome: 1 Overall mortality

Study or subgroup	Treatment n/N	Control n/N	Weight %	Odds Ratio M-H, Fixed, 95% CI
Abele-Horn 1997	11/58	5/30	1.2	1.17 [0.37, 3.74]
Aerdts 1991	4/28	12/60	1.5	0.67 [0.19, 2.29]
Blair 1991	24/161	32/170	6.0	0.76 [0.42, 1.35]
Boland 1991	2/32	4/32	0.8	0.47 [0.08, 2.75]
Cockerill 1992	11/75	16/75	3.1	0.63 [0.27, 1.48]
de Jonge 2003	113/466	146/468	25.0	0.71 [0.53, 0.94]
Finch 1991	15/24	10/25	0.8	2.50 [0.79, 7.90]
Jacobs 1992	14/45	23/46	3.5	0.45 [0.19, 1.06]
Kerver 1988	14/49	15/47	2.5	0.85 [0.36, 2.04]
Krueger 2002	52/265	75/262	13.7	0.61 [0.41, 0.91]
Palomar 1997	14/50	14/49	2.3	0.97 [0.41, 2.33]
Rocha 1992	27/74	40/77	5.6	0.53 [0.28, 1.02]
Sanchez-Garcia 1992	51/131	65/140	8.7	0.74 [0.45, 1.19]
Stoutenbeek 2007	42/201	44/200	7.9	0.94 [0.58, 1.51]
Ulrich 1989	22/55	33/57	4.4	0.48 [0.23, 1.03]
Verwaest 1997	47/220	40/220	7.1	1.22 [0.76, 1.96]
Winter 1992	33/91	40/92	5.7	0.74 [0.41, 1.34]
Total (95% CI)	**2025**	**2050**	**100**	**0.75 [0.65, 0.87]**

Total events: 496 (Treatment), 614 (Control)
Heterogeneity: $Chi^2 = 15.55$, $df = 16$ ($P = 0.49$); $I^2 = 0.0\%$
Test for overall effect: $Z = 3.94$ ($P = 0.000081$)

Odds Ratio M-H, Fixed, 95% CI — axis: 0.1 0.2 0.5 1 2 5 10
Favours treatment | Favours control

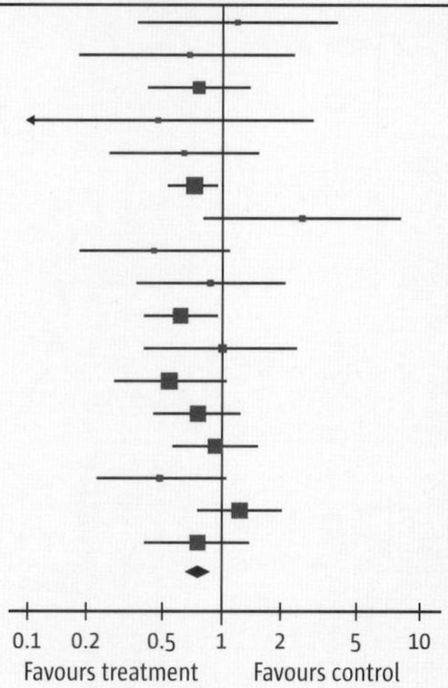

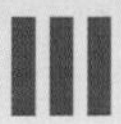

Rx Comparison for RTI	Trials/n	Study Gp RTI	Control Gp RTI	OR	95% CI	NNT
Topical + systemic versus no treatment	16 trials 3024 patients	19%	40%	0.28	0.2–0.38	4
Topical versus no treatment	18 trials 2850 patients	20%	31%	0.44	0.31–0.63	7

Rx Comparison for Mortality	Trials/n	Study Gp Mortality	Control Gp Mortality	OR	95% CI	NNT
Topical + systemic versus no treatment	17 trials 4075 patients	24%	30%	0.75	0.65–0.87	18
Topical only versus control	20 trials 3016 patients	25%	26%	0.97	0.82–1.16	-

Author's conclusion

The use of topical and systemic antibiotics significantly reduces both RTI and mortality when compared to no treatment.

Problems & limitations

- The antibiotic regimen and outcome definitions were not the same across studies
- Only 26 trials had 100% of patients in the study ventilated, in 1 trial only 59% of patients were ventilated

Advantages

- The reduction in RTI for the protocol using topical plus systemic antibiotics was consistent in all subgroup analysis regardless of study design

Expert opinion

Jordi Rello

How valid and robust are the data?

It is unclear if mortality means 28-days, ICU or hospital mortality and whether homogeneous criteria is used in the analysed studies. Introduction indicates that SDD has not been shown to reduce mortality. This is not true. A large Dutch study, led by Bonten has reported signifi cant reduction in mortality (NEJM).

Should this influence clinical practice?

Current data are difficult to generalize. Before clinical practice has to be influenced, it is required to delimitate the effect on specific subsets of patients (e.g. transplant, trauma, surgery, medical treatment, burns, etc.).

8

What's the next step?
The effect has to be assessed in relation to the quality of trials. It is expected that low-quality trials show a higher impact than high-quality trials. Moreover, a comparison with oral decontamination using chlorhexidine alone is warranted.

Citation

Liberati A, D'Amico R, Pifferi S, Torri V, Brazzi L, Parmelli E. Antibiotic prophylaxis to reduce respiratory tract infections and mortality in adults receiving intensive care. Cochrane Database of Systematic Reviews 2009, Issue 4. Art. No.: CD000022. DOI: 10.1002/14651858.CD000022.pub3

AMSTAR: methodological quality of the review

1.	Was "a priori" design provided?	Y
2.	Was study selection and data extraction adequate?	Y
3.	Was the literature search comprehensive?	Y
4.	Was 'Grey Literature' used?	Y
5.	Was a list of excluded studies provided?	Y
6.	Where the characteristics of included studies provided?	Y
7.	Was the scientific quality of studies assessed & documented?	Y
8.	Was the scientific quality of studies weighted appropriately in forming conclusions?	Y
9.	Were the methods used for data synthesis appropriate?	Y
10.	Was the potential for publication bias assessed?	Y
11.	Were any conflicts of interest stated?	Y

Overall quality of trials included	Moderate
Overall quality of the review	High

Antibiotic prophylaxis for pancreatic necrosis

Condition: pancreatic necrosis in acute pancreatitis

Clinical question: Is the use of prophylactic antibiotics in pancreatic necrosis effective and safe?

Acute severe pancreatitis is a common abdominal emergency associated with severe local and systemic inflammation resulting in multiple organ dysfunction syndromes. Pancreatic necrosis is a recognized complication of pancreatitis which if infected increases the mortality rate from approximately 5–10% to 40%. There appears to be a 2-week period during which superinfection may be preventable, although it remains unclear whether any antibiotic can penetrate necrotic tissue or if any benefit achieved is through high concentrations in surrounding tissues and the blood to inhibit the spread of the usually implicated gut organisms. The role of prophylactic antibiotics has been controversial because of the potential for encouraging the emergence of multidrug resistant organisms and opportunistic fungal infections, the incidence of which has increased dramatically since the widespread use of prophylaxis. A previous MA (2006) suggested a survival advantage with prophylaxis, 2 RCTs have been published since.

Review characteristics

- **Eligibility criteria:** RCTs comparing prophylactic antibiotics with placebo
- **Subgroup analysis:** 1. ABx regime, 2. timing of therapy, and 3. aetiology of pancreatitis were planned but 2 & 3 were not performed due to inadequate data
- **Exclusions:** trials that combined antibiotic prophylaxis with SDD or any other therapy
- **Number of studies:** 7 trials
- **Number of patients:** 404
- **Population:** patients with CT-proven necrotising acute pancreatitis
- **Study dates:** 1989–2007

8

Definitions

- **Pancreatic necrosis:** diagnosed by contrast enhanced CT according to international consensus criteria
- **Antibiotic prophylaxis:** effective therapy commenced within 7 days of onset of pancreatitis
- **Control:** placebo + best supportive care

Results

Primary outcomes

All-cause mortality: antibiotics were associated with a trend towards a decrease in mortality but this was not statistically significant.

Infected pancreatic necrosis was not significantly different between treatment and control groups.

Outcomes	Trials	Study Gp	Control Gp	RR	95% CI	p
Mortality	7	8.4%	14.4%	0.6	0.34–1.05	0.07
Infected Necrosis	7	19.7%	24.4%	0.85	0.57–1.26	0.42

Secondary outcomes	Trials	N	Result
Non-pancreatic infections	5	318	Less in treatment group but NSS
All site infections	5	318	Less in treatment group but NSS
Resistant organisms	2	158	Increased in only one study
Fungal infections	7	404	Not increased in treatment group
Operative treatment	6	348	Not decreased in the treatment group

Subgroup analysis

There was a trend towards less pancreatic infections and mortality with beta-lactams but NSS.

With imipenem there were significant reductions in all infection rates including pancreatic necrosis but no significant reduction in mortality or other secondary outcomes.

There was no difference with quinolones.

Author's conclusion

There was a general trend towards a reduction in mortality and infection rates in the groups that received antibiotic prophylaxis although this was not statistically significant. These outcomes show some concordance with previous analyses.

Problems & limitations

- Small numbers of patients
- Some studies were terminated early either due to unexpected results from interim analysis or lack of funding
- Heterogeneity between trials in duration and types of antibiotics as well as diagnostic criteria for infections

Advantages

- Strict diagnostic criteria for pancreatic necrosis clearly define the study group.
- This MA demonstrated that beta-lactams particularly imipenem were most likely to confer any clinical benefit therefore may provide direction for future studies

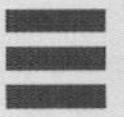

Fig. 5 Comparison 1 Antibiotics versus control, Outcome 1 Mortality [from Villatoro E, Mulla M, Larvin M. Antibiotic therapy for prophylaxis against infection of pancreatic necrosis in acute pancreatitis. Cochrane Database of Systematic Reviews 2010, Issue 5. Art.No.: CD002941, © Cochrane Collaboration, reproduced with permission]

Review: Antibiotic therapy for prophylaxis against infection of pancreatic necrosis in acute pancreatitis
Comparison: 1 Antibiotics versus control
Outcome: 1 Mortality

Study or subgroup	Antibiotics n/N	Control n/N	Risk Ratio M-H, Fixed, 95% CI	Weight %	Risk Ratio M-H, Fixed, 95% CI
Pederzoli 1993	3/41	4/33		15.1	0.60 [0.15, 2.51]
Sainio 1995	1/30	7/30		23.9	0.14 [0.02, 1.09]
Schwarz 1997	0/13	2/13		8.5	0.20 [0.01, 3.80]
Nordback 2001	2/25	5/33		14.7	0.53 [0.11, 2.50]
Isenmann 2004	3/41	4/35		14.7	0.64 [0.15, 2.67]
Dellinger 2007	6/41	5/41		17.1	1.20 [0.40, 3.62]
Rkke 2007	2/12	2/16		5.9	1.33 [0.22, 8.16]
Total (95% CI)	**203**	**201**		**100.0**	**0.60 [0.34, 1.05]**

Total events: 17 (Antibiotics), 29 (Control)
Heterogeneity: $Chi^2 = 4.75$, $df = 6$ ($P = 0.58$) $I^2 = 0.0\%$
Test for overall effect: $Z = 1.80$ ($P = 0.072$)

0.05 0.2 1 5 20
Favours treatment Favours control

Expert opinion

George Dimopoulos

How valid and robust are the data?
This review found 7 RCTs conducted over a 20-year period, heterogeneity was significant (duration and types of antibiotics as well as diagnostic criteria for infections), patient numbers are small. Strict diagnostic criteria for pancreatic necrosis clearly define the study group.

Should clinical practise be influenced by this?
This review has highlighted lack of evidence as opposed to evidence against use of antibiotic therapy for prophylaxis against infection of pancreatic necrosis in acute pancreatitis. A general trend towards a reduction in mortality and infection rates in the groups that received antibiotic prophylaxis has been observed, however without any statistical significant difference.

What's the next step?
I believe that the prophylactic use of antibiotics in patients with pancreatic necrosis in acute pancreatitis reflects a debatable issue making necessary the need for large RCTs.

Citation

Villatoro E, Mulla M, Larvin M. Antibiotic therapy for prophylaxis against infection of pancreatic necrosis in acute pancreatitis. Cochrane Database of Systematic Reviews 2010, Issue 5. Art. No.: CD002941. DOI: 10.1002/14651858.CD002941.pub3.

AMSTAR: methodological quality of the review

1.	Was "a priori" design provided?	Y
2.	Was study selection and data extraction adequate?	Y
3.	Was the literature search comprehensive?	Y
4.	Was 'Grey Literature' used?	Y
5.	Was a list of excluded studies provided?	Y
6.	Where the characteristics of included studies provided?	Y
7.	Was the scientific quality of included studies assessed & documented?	Y
8.	Was the scientific quality of studies weighted appropriately in forming conclusions?	Y
9.	Were the methods used for data synthesis appropriate?	Y
10.	Was the potential for publication bias assessed?	Y
11.	Were any conflicts of interest stated?	Y

Overall quality of trials included	Low
Overall quality of the review	High

9

Neuro-intensive care

Haemostatic drugs for TBI ____ 196
Routine ICP monitoring ____ 199
Cooling post stroke ____ 202

Also see:
Section 4: Cardiovascular dynamics
Therapeutic hypothermia

Haemostatic drugs for TBI

Condition: traumatic brain injury (TBI)
Intervention: haemostatic drugs
Clinical questions: Do haemostatic drugs reduce the disability or mortality associated with a TBI? Do haemostatic drugs increase thrombotic complications in these patients?

TBI is prevalent in a young population and is associated with significant morbidity and mortality. Secondary brain injury as a result of intracranial bleeding is common, and occurs after arrival at the hospital in approximately half of these patients making it a potentially preventable complication. There is some evidence to suggest that antifibrinolytics may prevent rebleeding in SAH and reduce death and dependency in primary intracerebral haemorrhage however, there are no data for patients with TBI.

Review characteristics

- **Eligibility criteria**: any RCT comparing haemostatic drugs with placebo, no treatment or other haemostatic drugs
- **Number of studies**: 2 RCTs included; both are trials comparing rFVIIa with placebo; 1 of these was a post-hoc analysis within a subgroup of patients from a larger trial of trauma patients
  CRASH-2 was on-going at the time
- **Number of patients**: 127
- **Population**: any patient with TBI
- **Study dates**: published 2007–2008

Definitions

- **TBI**: not specified but assumed to be consensus definition

Results

Study type/n	Primary outcomes for the study group (rFVIIa)
Post-hoc subgroup	**Mortality at 30 days**: RR 0.64 (CI 0.25–1.63)
30 patients	**Disability**: not reported
	Thrombotic Complications: RR 0.16 (CI 0.01–2.99) 2 complications in placebo arm, nil in study group
RCT	**Mortality at last follow-up**: RR 1.08 (CI 0.44–2.68)
97 patients	**Disability**: inadequate reporting, generally no difference
	Thrombotic complications: RR 2.36 (CI 0.53–10.51)

Study	Secondary outcomes for the study group (rFVIIa)
Post-hoc subgroup	None reported
RCT	Intracranial blood volume at 72 hours: mean difference −3.10 (CI 10.47–4.27)
	Brain ischaemia: 1 cerebral infarction in placebo group, nil in study group
	Neurosurgical operation: 3 in placebo group, 1 in study group Reoperation: 1 in placebo group, nil in study group
	Renal failure: not reported

Author's conclusion

There are no reliable data that haemostatic drugs reduce disability or mortality in patients with traumatic brain injury. No RCTs of antifibrinolytics in TBI were identified to include.

Problems & limitations

- Both studies were very small, furthermore, one of these was a post hoc analysis therefore no conclusions can be drawn from these results

Advantages

- This has highlighted the lack of data in this area

Citation

Perel P, Roberts I, Shakur H, Thinkhamrop B, Phuenpathom N, Yutthakasemsunt S. Haemostatic drugs for traumatic brain injury. Cochrane Database of Systematic Reviews 2010, Issue 1. Art. No.: CD007877. DOI: 10.1002/14651858.CD007877.pub2.

Additional information

CRASH-2 has been published since this review. This was a large multicentre RCT with more than 20000 patients. This showed that tranexamic acid (TXA) used early (within 1–3 hours) from injury in adult trauma patients significantly reduced the risk of death due to bleeding. Subgroup analysis by GCS suggested that TXA is likely to be effective in all groups.

Citation: Effects of tranexamic acid on death, vascular occlusive events, and blood transfusion in trauma patients with significant haemorrhage (CRASH-2): a randomised, placebo-controlled trial. CRASH-2 trial collaborators. The Lancet. July 2010; Vol 376 (9734):23–32. DOI:10.1016/S0140-6736(10)60835-5

Approximately 30% of CRASH-2 patients have a concomitant TBI, who will undergo CT imaging as standard care. The CRASH-2 Intracranial Bleeding Study (IBS) will be conducted in 300 CRASH-2 participants. The CRASH-2 IBS involves performing a second brain CT scan at 24 to 48 hours in these patients to evaluate the quantity of bleeding by using validated methods and an expert who will be blinded to the treatment allocation. Due to be reported in November 2011

A second RCT was conducted in Thailand to evaluate the effectiveness of TXA in patients with moderate to severe TBI. This should have been completed in May 2009.

The results of these trials may significantly alter the outcome of this meta-analysis.

AMSTAR: methodological quality of the review

1.	Was "a priori" design provided?	Y
2.	Was study selection and data extraction adequate?	Y
3.	Was the literature search comprehensive?	Y
4.	Was 'Grey Literature' used?	P
5.	Was a list of excluded studies provided?	Y
6.	Were the characteristics of included studies provided?	Y
7.	Was the scientific quality of studies assessed & documented?	Y
8.	Was the scientific quality of studies weighted appropriately in forming conclusions?	NA
9.	Were the methods used for data synthesis appropriate?	NA
10.	Was the potential for publication bias assessed?	Y
11.	Were any conflicts of interest stated?	Y

Overall quality of trials included	Low
Overall quality of the review	High

9

Routine ICP monitoring

Condition: raised intracranial pressure (ICP)

Diagnostic: ICP monitoring

Clinical question: Does routine ICP monitoring in all acute cases of coma reduce the risk of mortality or severe disability?

It is now well recognised that brain injury does not exclusively result from the primary insult but also as a result of secondary hypoxic-ischaemic injury. This process continues while the patient is in hospital and is therefore potentially reversible. Non randomised trials have suggested that mortality and morbidity after TBI can be reduced by prompt resuscitation and meticulous management of intracranial pressure. More recently the focus has shifted from management of ICP to that of cerebral perfusion pressure. Real-time ICP monitoring would allow clinicians to target treatment appropriate to the severity of the problem. Although benefits of ICP monitoring may be limited to conditions where an appropriate clinical response exists such as haematoma evacuation after TBI compared to medical causes of coma such as meningoencephalitis.

Invasive means of measuring ICP are not in themselves without risk, infection and bleeding are recognised complications of probe placement. Non-invasive techniques of measuring ICP are still in the experimental phase.

Review characteristics

- **Eligibility criteria:** RCTs of ICP monitoring in all causes of acute coma versus no ICP monitoring
- **Exclusion:** indirect estimations by imaging techniques e.g. CT or Doppler USS
- **Number of studies:** 8 RCTs found: all excluded as criteria were not met
- **For further information:** see original article – characteristics of excluded trials
- **Number of patients:** NA
- **Population:** patients with acute severe coma of traumatic or non-traumatic aetiology

9

Definitions

- **ICP Monitoring:** any invasive or semi-invasive means
- **Acute severe coma:** admission GCS < 8

Main findings

There were no RCTs that fitted the criteria

Primary outcomes would have been mortality and severe disability as or persistent vegetative state as defined by the Glasgow Outcome Score (GOS)

Secondary outcomes would have been complications: infection and haemorrhage

Author's conclusion

There is lack of RCT evidence of the role of ICP monitoring in either traumatic or non-traumatic causes of coma. The use of ICP monitoring thus remains controversial with wide international variability in clinical practice.

Expert opinion

Mauro Oddo

How valid and robust are the data?
No studies were included in this meta-analysis, due to lack of RCT comparing ICP versus no-ICP monitoring in patients with severe brain injury, including those with traumatic brain injury (TBI).

Should clinical practise be influenced by this?
No, clinical practice should not be influenced by this review. Guidelines for the indications of ICP monitoring exist, particularly for TBI patients (see 2007 Guidelines for severe TBI, Brain Trauma Foundation) and clinical practice should therefore be directed by available international expert recommendations.

What's the next step?
To compare standard ICP monitoring versus advanced brain physiologic (e.g. ICP plus brain tissue oxygen) monitoring in the management of patients with acute coma who are at risk of developing secondary intracranial hypertension, based on structural lesions on admission head CT scan. While awaiting such trials, and in view of the lack of valid alternative non-invasive tools, direct ICP monitoring should continue to guide ICU clinicians in the management of secondary brain oedema.

Citation

Forsyth RJ, Wolny S, Rodrigues B. Routine intracranial pressure monitoring in acute coma. Cochrane Database of Systematic Reviews 2010, Issue 2. Art. No.: CD002043. DOI: 10.1002/14651858.CD002043.pub2.

AMSTAR: methodological quality of the review

1.	Was "a priori" design provided?	Y
2.	Was study selection and data extraction adequate?	Y
3.	Was the literature search comprehensive?	Y
4.	Was 'Grey Literature' used?	Y
5.	Was a list of excluded studies provided?	Y
6.	Were the characteristics of included studies provided?	NA
7.	Was the scientific quality of studies assessed & documented?	NA
8.	Was the scientific quality of studies weighted appropriately in forming conclusions?	NA
9.	Were the methods used for data synthesis appropriate?	NA
10.	Was the potential for publication bias assessed?	NA
11.	Were any conflicts of interest stated?	Y

Overall quality of trials included	NA
Overall quality of the review	High

Cooling post stroke

Condition: acute stroke

Intervention: cooling

Clinical questions: Does temperature lowering therapy reduce the risk of death or disability in acute stroke? What is the risk of haemorrhagic or infective complications with this therapy?

The incidence of stroke is rising as the population ages. It is currently the second leading cause of death world-wide and the main cause of disability in the developed world. Treatment of ischaemic strokes was largely supportive until recently. Aspirin administered within 48 hours after onset reduces the risk of death or disability by 1%. Both intravenous thrombolysis and direct intra-arterial thrombolysis reduce these risks by 10% however the treatment window is 3 and 6 hours respectively. Intravenous thrombolysis may not be available at all hospitals, whereas the availability of intra-arterial thrombolysis is limited to centres with neuroradiology/neurosurgery.

Up to 25% of patients with acute stroke have a rise in body temperature which has been associated with a worse outcome in observational studies. Furthermore, animal studies have shown that temperature reduction to below 35°C reduces both infarct size (by a third) and disability, but best results were seen with temperatures below 32°C. Therapeutic hypothermia has been shown to be beneficial in cardiac surgery and following cardiac arrest but not so in traumatic brain injury.

Review characteristics

- **Eligibility criteria**: all RCTs and non-randomised controlled clinical trials (CCT) of temperature lowering therapy versus control in patients with stroke
- **Number of studies**: 8 trials – 6 RCTs and 2 CCTs. (5 pharmacological and 3 physical temperature reduction techniques)
- **Number of patients**: 423 (trial range 19–77)
- **Population**: adults within 24 hours of ischaemic or haemorrhagic stroke
- **Study dates**: 2000–2003

9

Definitions

- **Control**: placebo or open label
- **Intervention**: any physical method of cooling, pharmacological cooling including NSAIDs or both
- **Pharmacological cooling**: 3 trials used paracetamol, 1 used paracetamol or ibuprofen and 1 used metamizole
- **Physical cooling**: forced air surface cooling for 6 hours, ice for 12–72 hours, endovascular cooling for 24 hours
- **Functional outcome at**: death or dependency measured by the modified Rankin scale (mRS), Barthel Index (BI) or other method of assessing ADLs

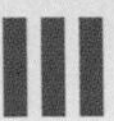

Results

Primary outcome: poor outcome at 1–3 months (varied between trials)

Pooled analysis of 7 trials showed no difference in death and disability

Subgroup analysis	no heterogeneity between trials that used pharmacological cooling. High heterogeneity between trials that used physical cooling
Pharmacological cooling based on agent and duration	no difference
Physical cooling	based on trial quality: no difference

Secondary outcomes

Outcomes	Trials	Result	I^2
Death	All	No difference	0%
Temperature	3 Pharmacological	Temperature was 0.2°C lower in the active treatment group	
Haemorrhage	1 Pharmacological	1 haemorrhagic transformation in treatment group	
	1 Physical	2 haemorrhagic transformation in treatment group	
Infection	All	More infections in treatment group but NSS (OR 1.5, 95% CI 0.8–2.6)	0%
Arrhythmias	1	3/20 in intervention versus 2/20 in control	
Hypotension	1 Physical	4/10 intervention group versus 1/9 control	
DVT	1 Physical	7/20 intervention group versus 4/20 control	
None of the adverse events resulted in trial termination			

Author's conclusion

The results showed no difference between pharmacological or physical cooling in terms of outcomes; therefore cooling cannot currently be recommended. There are insufficient data to suggest maximum time window to treatment, optimal target temperature or duration of therapy. The method of temperature measurement needs to be considered as the trials used various techniques such as tympanic, rectal, bladder and oesophageal probes but brain temperature is 1–2°C higher with larger differences in pyrexial patients. However this treatment option is promising and results of large RCTs are awaited.

Fig. 1 Comparison 1 Temperature reduction versus control, Outcome 1 Death or dependency mRS ≥ 3 [from Den Hertog HM, van der Worp HB, Tseng MC, Dippel DWJ. Cooling therapy for acute stroke. Cochrane Database of Systematic Reviews 2009, Issue 1. Art. No.: CD001247, © Cochrane Collaboration, reproduced with permission]

Review: Cooling therapy for acute stroke; Comparison: 1 Temperature reduction versus control; Outcome: 1 Death or dependency mRS ≥ 3

Study or subgroup	Body temperature lowering n/N	Control n/N	Odds Ratio M-H, Fixed, 95% CI	Weight	Odds Ratio M-H, Fixed, 95% CI
1 Pharmacological temperature reduction					
Castillo 2003	15/31	14/29		17.9%	1.00 [0.36, 2.77]
Dippel 2001a	17/26	6/12		6.8%	1.89 [0.47, 7.59]
Dippel 2001b	13/25	6/12		9.3%	1.08 [0.27, 4.29]
Dippel 2003a	13/26	6/13		9.6%	1.17 [0.31, 4.43]
Dippel 2003b	9/24	6/12		12.0%	0.60 [0.15, 2.44]
Kasner 2002	14/20	13/19		9.6%	1.08 [0.28, 4.20]
Koennecke 2001	5/20	10/22		17.1%	0.40 [0.11, 1.49]
Subtotal (95% CI)	**172**	**119**		**82.2%**	**0.93 [0.57, 1.50[**
Total events: 86 (Body temperature lowering), 61 (Control)					
Heterogeneity: $Chi^2 = 3.18$, df = 6 (P = 0.79); $I^2 = 0.0\%$					
Test for overall effect: Z = 0.30 (P = 0.77)					
2 Physical temperature reduction					
De Georgia 2004	13/18	13/22		7.8%	1.80 [0.47, 6.85]
Krieger 2001	5/10	8/9		10.1%	0.13 [0.01, 1.41]
Subtotal (95% CI)	**28**	**31**		**17.8%**	**0.85 [0.30, 2.45]**
Total events: 18 (Body temperature lowering), 21 (Control)					
Heterogeneity: $Chi^2 = 3.62$, df = 1 (P = 0.06); $I^2 = 72\%$					
Test for overall effect: Z = 0.29 (P = 0.77)					
Total (95% CI)	**200**	**150**		**100.0%**	**0.92 [0.59, 1.42]**
Total events: 104 (Body temperature lowering), 82 (Control)					
Heterogeneity: $Chi^2 = 6.77$, df = 8 (P = 0.56); $I^2 = 0.0\%$					
Test for overall effect: Z = 0.39 (P = 0.69)					

0.01 0.1 1 10 100

Favours experimental Favours control

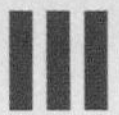

Problems & limitations

- Only two trials included haemorrhagic stroke patients
- 3 trials were still on-going and 1 awaiting assessment
- A long time interval was allowed between stroke symptoms and intervention
- Patient numbers were small
- There was a small temperature difference between intervention and control in trials that used pharmacological cooling
- Missing important data such as whether or not patients were ventilated or the temperature achieved in the trials that used physical cooling

Advantages

- Variability in-patient characteristics between trials was low
- All patients were assessed with CT or MRI prior to randomisation.
- Low incidence of loss to follow up

Expert opinion

Pedro Navarrete-Navarro

How valid and robust are the data?

This review did not find any large RCTs conducted over the last 10 years, about hypothermia in acute stroke and included cohort studies. A vast literature on an experimental level exists in this field.

Regarding hyperthermia and fever control in acute brain injury, recent meta-analyses, series of cases and cohort studies were analysed.

Should clinical practise be influenced by this?

There is no scientific evidence today that support the routine use of hypothermia in acute ischemic stroke. At experimental level, hypothermia is a robust neuroprotectant against a variety of brain injuries, its efficacy includes, the duration of cooling, the time when cooling begins and reperfusion of occluded vessels.

Hyperthermia, in the acute clinical setting after ischemic stroke, has a negative impact on morbidity and mortality. Although normothermia is recommended, there are no prospective RCTs demonstrating the benefit of fever control in these patients.

What's the next step?

Hypothermia is useful reducing ICP and brain oedema secondary to acute ischemic stroke in humans. Large RCTs are needed to move from biological to clinical level.

Prospective RCTs are needed to determinate if the beneficial impact of hyperthermia prevention is outweighed by the potential risks of prolonged fever prevention.

Citation

Den Hertog HM, van der Worp HB, Tseng MC, Dippel DWJ. Cooling therapy for acute stroke. Cochrane Database of Systematic Reviews 2009, Issue 1. Art. No.: CD001247. DOI: 10.1002/14651858.CD001247.pub2.

Additional information

The following studies were on-going at the time of the review

- Hemmen TM et al. Intravenous thrombolysis plus hypothermia for acute ischemic stroke (ICTuS-L). Stroke 2010 Oct; 41 (10): 2265–70. Epub 2010 Aug 19
  A multicentre RCT that enrolled 59 patients. This showed no difference in mortality or Rankin Scale score after 3 months but the incidence of pneumonia was significantly higher in the hypothermia group.
- Van Breda et al. PAIS. Paracetamol (Acetaminophen) In Stroke) ISCRTN 7718480
  A multicentre double blind placebo controlled trial of high dose (6g/day) acetaminophen that aims to enrol 2500 patients.

AMSTAR: methodological quality of the review

1.	Was "a priori" design provided?	Y
2.	Was study selection and data extraction adequate?	Y
3.	Was the literature search comprehensive?	Y
4.	Was 'Grey Literature' used?	Y
5.	Was a list of excluded studies provided?	Y
6.	Were the characteristics of included studies provided?	Y
7.	Was the scientific quality of studies assessed & documented?	Y
8.	Was the scientific quality of studies weighted appropriately in forming conclusions?	Y
9.	Were the methods used for data synthesis appropriate?	Y
10.	Was the potential for publication bias assessed?	Y
11.	Were any conflicts of interest stated?	Y

Overall quality of trials included	4 moderate, 4 low
Overall quality of the review	High

10

Nutrition and metabolism

Early enteral nutrition 208
Nutrition in pancreatitis 212
Enteral versus parenteral nutrition in pancreatitis 216
Glucose-insulin-potassium infusion 223

Also see:
Section 12: Paediatric intensive care
Nutritional support for critically ill children

Early enteral nutrition

Intervention: early enteral nutrition (EN)

Clinical question: Does early standard enteral nutrition confer any benefit for critically ill patients?

Many guidelines recommend that EN is commenced within 24 hours of ICU admission for patients expected to stay 2 or more days; however observational studies suggest that up to 60% receive no EN for 48 hours which may be justified by the absence of convincing evidence to support these recommendations in the ICU population.

What is the rationale for early feeding?

It has been proposed that the intestinal system may provide the 'substrate' for MODS in ICU patients as the gut's integrity and immune function become compromised by critical illness allowing for bacterial translocation and resulting in cytokine 'storming'.

There is evidence to suggest that EN may ameliorate these damaging gut mucosal changes thereby reducing MODS and mortality.

Review characteristics

- **Eligibility criteria:** RCTs of standard EN within 24 h versus standard care
- **Exclusions:** trials with major methodological flaws such as pseudo-randomisation (failure to conserve allocation concealment) and loss to follow-up > 10% were excluded
- **Population:** ventilated medical and surgical ICU patients including burns, pancreatitis, peritonitis and trauma patients
- **Number of studies:** 6 RCTs
- **Number of patients:** 234 patients
- **Study dates:** 1990–2008

Definitions

- **Enteral:** any feeding tube route
- **Standard formula:** any formula NOT supplemented with immune-enhancing ingredients such as glutamine or arginine

Results

Primary outcomes

Outcome	Trials/n	Result
Mortality	6/234	Statistically significant reduction in mortality, $p < 0.02$
QOL		Not reported by any of the trials
Physical function		Not reported by any of the trials

Fig. 1 Primary analysis: Mortality [With kind permission from Springer Science+Business Media: Intensive Care Medicine, Early enteral nutrition provided, provided within 24 h of injury or intensive care unit admission, significantly reduces mortality in critically ill patients: a meta-analysis of randomised controlled trials, 35 (12), 2009, 2018–2027, Doig GS, Heighes PT, Simpson F, Sweetman EA and Davies AR., Figure 2]

Review: Early EN (<24h) vs. Control (Primary Analysis)
Comparison: 01 early EN vs. Control
Outcome: 01 Mortality, intention to treat analysis

Study or sub-category	Early EN (<24 h) n/N	Control n/N	OR (fixed) 95% CI	Weight %	OR (fixed) 95% CI
Chiarelli 1990	0/10	0/10			Not estimable
Kompan 1999	0/17	2/19		13.40	0.20 [0.01, 4.47]
Kompan 2004	0/27	1/25		8.89	0.30 [0.01, 7.63]
Nguyen 2008	6/14	6/14		19.95	1.00 [0.22, 4.47]
Chuntrasakul 1996	1/21	3/17		18.38	0.23 [0.02, 2.48]
Pupelis 2001	1/30	7/30		39.38	0.11 [0.01, 0.99]
Total (95% CI)	**119**	**115**		**100**	**0.34 [0.14, 0.85]**

Total events: 8 (early EN (<24 h)), 19 (Control)
Test for heterogeneity: $Chi^2 = 3.20$, df = 4 (P = 0.52); $I^2 = 0.0\%$
Test for overall effect: Z = 2.31 (P = 0.02)

0.1 0.2 0.5 1 2 5 10
Favours EN Favours control

10

Secondary outcomes

Outcome	Trials/n	Result
Vomiting	1/10	No difference in burns patients
Pneumonia	2/80	Significant reduction in pneumonia in study group, $p < 0.01$
Bacteraemia	1/10	No significant difference
Sepsis	0	Not reported
MODS	2/96	No difference but possible trend towards fewer organ failures in study group in 1 trial

Authors' conclusion

Reduction in mortality and pneumonia is concordant with results of other meta-analyses of early EN in non-critically ill patients which showed a reduction in mortality and infectious complications. The sensitivity and simulation exercise both support the primary results.

The previous MA on early enteral feed extended the definition of early to 60 or 72 hours which explains why their results only showed a trend towards reduced mortality.

Problems & limitations

- Small number of trials
- Small sized trials
- Non standardised control ranged from EN commenced after 24 hours; iv 5% dextrose and TPN although these groups were not statistically heterogeneous.
- Critically ill was not clearly defined in terms of APACHE II or SOFA scores
- Will it be possible to convince the critical care community that 24 hours can really make a difference as based on this data?

10

Advantages

- No evidence of statistical heterogeneity across the studies
- Results agree with scientific hypothesis. No contradictions
- Sensitivity analysis confirmed primary analysis outcome

Expert opinion

David Noble

How valid and robust are the data?

The conduct of the study is meticulous. However, the numbers of patients are small and the clinical heterogeneity of patients substantial. Patient populations studied in 5 of 6 studies may not reflect case-mix in many ICUs-trauma (3), pancreatitis/peritonitis (1), or thermal injury (1). Robust and valid conclusions for general ICU populations cannot be made under these circumstances.

Should clinical practice be influenced by this?
The evidence is insufficiently robust to drive practice in general or medical intensive care units.

What's the next step?
The signal of potential benefit is sufficiently strong that a large pragmatic randomised trial is warranted to better guide clinical practice.

Citation

Early enteral nutrition provided, provided within 24 h of injury or intensive care unit admission, significantly reduces mortality in critically ill patients: a meta-analysis of randomised controlled trials. Doig GS, Heighes PT, Simpson F, Sweetman EA and Davies AR. Intensive Care Medicine 2009; 35 (12): 2018–2027

AMSTAR: methodological quality of the review

1.	Was "a priori" design provided?	Y
2.	Was study selection and data extraction adequate?	Y
3.	Was the literature search comprehensive?	Y
4.	Was 'Grey Literature' used?	Y
5	Was a list of excluded studies provided?	N
6	Where the characteristics of included studies provided?	Y
7.	Was the scientific quality of studies assessed & documented?	Y
8.	Was the scientific quality of studies weighted appropriately in forming conclusions?	Y
9.	Were the methods used for data synthesis appropriate?	Y
10.	Was the potential for publication bias assessed?	Y
11.	Were any conflicts of interest stated?	Y

Overall quality of trials included	Low
Overall quality of the review	High

Nutrition in pancreatitis

Condition: severe acute pancreatitis (SAP)
Intervention: nutrition
Clinical question: What is the evidence for various nutritional strategies in acute pancreatitis?

Pancreatitis is common, the latest reported incidence of acute pancreatitis is 56.5 per 100,000, with 20% of those cases being severe attacks. Severe pancreatitis results in systemic inflammation and multiple organ failure particularly if pancreatic necrosis becomes infected when mortality can be as high as 40%. Ileus and duodenal compression precluded oral intake and thus traditionally patients were kept 'nil-by-mouth' in order to minimise pancreatic stimulation. This changed in 1974 following a paper by Feller et al. which showed reduced mortality and complications in those who were fed parenterally (PN) compared to those who were fasted. Gut disuse is associated with intestinal ischaemia and decrease in gut mucosal barrier thus facilitating bacterial translocation and exacerbating systemic inflammation as well as promoting the transition of pancreatic necrosis to infected pancreatic necrosis. To avoid both pancreatic stimulation and gut ischaemia, post-pyloric naso-jejunal enteral feeding (NJ-EN) was explored.

Review characteristics

- **Eligibility criteria:** all studies of nutrition in patients with pancreatitis
- **Population:** patients with pancreatitis mild or severe in most trials
- **Number of studies and patients:**
  - **NJ-EN versus PN:** 7 studies (n = 431) + 1 meta-analysis (n = 291)
  - **NG versus NJ:** 2 studies, 1 of these is an RCT (n = 50) & 1 systematic review of the 2 studies (n = 92)
  - **Probiotics:** 1 RCT (n = 296) + 1 meta-analysis of 4 trials
  - **Combination immune-nutrition:** 3 studies & 1 meta-analysis (n = 78)
  - **Anti-oxidant supplementation:** 2 studies, 1 of these is a cohort (n = 46)
  - **Study dates:** 1998–2008

Definitions

- **Severe acute pancreatitis:** varied between studies Glasgow score > 3, Ranson score > 3 or APACHE II score > 5 or > 8

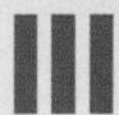

Results

Types of nutrition	Evidence
Naso-jejunal enteral nutrition compared with parenteral nutrition	Level 1
Since 1998 several studies of NJ-EN compared with PN in a population that included SAP showed reduced infectious complications, markers of inflammation, organ failure, LOS and radiological changes of pancreatitis. This effect was greatest with the sickest cohort of patients (APACHE II > 13). There was no detectable difference in mortality.	
Naso-jejunal enteral feeding is safe when started immediately (within 6 hours)	Level 3
Naso-gastric (NG) feeding is equivalent to naso-jeunal feeding	Level 3
NG feeding appears to be equivalent in terms of safety and outcomes and is more practical than NJ feeding as the feeding tube does not need to be endoscopically or radiologically placed.	
Probiotic feed supplementation is not beneficial	Level 1
The theory was that probiotics maintained normal bacterial colonisation in a group that was frequently treated with broad spectrum antibiotics.	
Probiotic feed supplementation may cause harm and increase mortality	Level 2?
1 RCT (n = 296) Mortality in the probiotic group was 16% compared to 6% (placebo). 8 patients in the probiotic group developed fatal gut ischaemia compared to none in the placebo group (RR 2.53, 95% CI 1.22–5.25, $p = 0.004$). This mortality difference was not supported by the meta-analysis.	
There is no evidence to support combination immune-nutrition	Level 2
No evidence exits to confirm the benefit of prokinetics in SAP	
Neostigmine reduces ileus in critically ill patients with pseudo-obstruction but has not been examined in SAP. Metoclopramide, erythromycin and neostigmine may inhibit the normal neuroendocrine response after colorectal surgery and prolong ileus.	
Intravenous supplementation of anti-oxidants is not supported.	Level 2

Grading of evidence

- **Level 1**: multiple RCTs or meta-analysis
- **Level 2**: adequately powered single RCT
- **Level 3**: experimental non-randomised data
- **Level 4**: quasi-experimental design e.g. cohort study

Author's conclusion

The largest therapeutic benefits have been derived from the recognition of SAP as a multi-system inflammatory process and the role of bacterial translocation in the transition to infected necrosis. There is good evidence for NJ-EN although differences in mortality have not been demonstrated; entry criteria heterogeneity may have resulted in underestimation of treatment effect. The benefit from enteral feeding is certain; however many other facets of nutritional management remain to be elucidated.

Problems & limitations

- Several scoring systems are used to predict SAP therefore no consistency between studies
- Predicting SAP is not synonymous with actually having SAP and pancreatic necrosis
- In some studies mortality data were not available but also studies were small and therefore underpowered to detect differences in mortality

Advantages

- The one trial that used CT to confirm pancreatic necrosis showed the greatest treatment effect.
- There are consistent treatment effects between studies of NJ-EN versus PN

Expert opinion

Daren K. Heyland

How valid and robust are the data?
The methods are inadequately described so the reader has no sense of the adequacy of the search process and the reproducibility of the data abstraction. No quality assessment of the individual study was reported and no meta-analyses were performed (whereas these do exist in other reviews). Moreover, the authors were limited to review to studies published to English.

Should clinical practice be influenced by this?
This review has highlighted the clinical trials examining various aspects of the nutritional management of severe pancreatitis. All of the stated conclusions are consistent with best practices' statements done from other reviews with the following exceptions: 1) These authors do not comment on the role of IV glutamine. When PN is used in pancreatitis, it should be supplemented with IV glutamine. 2) Although there is no evidence for motility agents in pancreatitis specifically, there is no reason not to apply the studies of motility agents conducted in critically ill patients (which may have included patients' pancreatitis). Thus, metoclopramide and erythromycin could be recommended in managing high gastric residual volumes in this patient population. 3) The conclusions about the role of antioxidants are inaccurate. There are numerous randomized trials of critically ill patients, some in patients with pancreatitis specifically and many such patients were included in these studies which show a reduction in mortality. These nutrients should be recommended to patients with severe acute pancreatitis.

What is the next step?
Clearly more research is needed because the evidentiary basis informing the nutritional management is small and of low quality. However, this paper represents a summary of best practice based on the current evidence (with the exceptions noted above).

Citation

Ahmad Al Samaraee, Iain JD McCallum, Peter E. Coyne, Keith Seymour. Nutritional strategies in acute severe pancreatitis: a systematic review of the evidence. The Surgeon 8 (2010) 105–110 Doi: 10.1016/j.surge.2009.10.006

Additional information

Go to the next review summary on EN versus PN in acute pancreatitis

AMSTAR: methodological quality of the review

1.	Was "a priori" design provided?	Y
2.	Was study selection and data extraction adequate?	Y
3.	Was the literature search comprehensive?	Y
4.	Was 'Grey Literature' used?	P
5	Was a list of excluded studies provided?	N
6.	Where the characteristics of included studies provided?	P
7.	Was the scientific quality of studies assessed & documented?	N
8.	Was the scientific quality of studies weighted appropriately in forming conclusions?	U
9.	Were the methods used for data synthesis appropriate?	NA
10.	Was the potential for publication bias assessed?	N
11.	Were any conflicts of interest stated?	N

Overall quality of trials included	Unclear
Overall quality of the review	Low

Despite the low AMSTAR score, this review represents a very important topic and provides a useful summary of some of the available data.

Enteral versus parenteral nutrition in pancreatitis

Condition: acute pancreatitis

Intervention: nutrition

Clinical question: Is there any difference in mortality, morbidity or LOS in patients with acute pancreatitis that receive enteral nutrition (EN) compared to those that receive total parenteral nutrition (TPN)?

Acute pancreatitis creates a hypermetabolic, hyperdynamic, catabolic stress state associated with systemic inflammation and nutritional deterioration. In severe acute pancreatitis (SAP) increased caloric requirements and protein loss combined with inadequate oral intake as a result of anorexia, nausea, vomiting and ileus results in a negative protein balance that may be associated with higher mortality. Acute pancreatitis causes increased gut permeability; furthermore a metabolically deprived gut absorbs various bacterial products such as endotoxin, leading to exacerbation of inflammation and the development of nosocomial infections. TPN was the traditional mode of nutritional support however over the last 10–15 years the role of enteral nutrition in the management of patients with pancreatitis has been established. EN can maintain the integrity and function of intestinal mucosa; however stimulation of the pancreas should and can be avoided if EN is delivered to the small intestine. While TPN avoids pancreatic stimulation it has been associated with the risk of catheter sepsis, metabolic and electrolyte disturbances and is expensive.

Review characteristics

- **Eligibility criteria:** RCTS that compared TPN with EN in acute pancreatitis
- **Population:** adults (above 16 years) with acute pancreatitis
- **Number of studies:** 8 RCTs
- **Number of patients:** 348
- **Study dates:** 1997–2007

Definition

- **Acute pancreatitis:** clinical presentation + elevated serum amylase and one of the following scoring systems Ranson's, APACHE II, Imrie and Balthazar CT score or CRP
- **TPN:** delivered through a central or peripheral line
- **EN:** delivered through a naso-jejunal feeding tube placed endoscopically or under fluoroscopy

Main findings for EN compared to PN

Outcome	Trials	N	RR	95% CI	GRADE
Mortality	8	348	0.5	0.28–0.91	Low
Mortality*	7	295	0.39	0.2–0.77	-
Mortality in SAP**	3	136	0.18	0.06–0.58	-
MOF	6	278	0.55	0.37–0.81	Moderate
Operative intervention	7	316	0.46	0.26–0.82	Moderate
Systemic inflammation	7	259	0.39	0.23–0.65	Moderate
Local septic complications	5	246	0.74	0.4–1.35	Moderate
Hospital mortality	4	145	Reduced by MD 2.37 days 95% CI 7.18–2.44		

* Mortality is the pooled mortality with one study excluded where a number of deaths occurred after resolution of pancreatitis and were due to unrelated causes

** Mortality in SAP Sub group analysis

Gut mucosa barrier protection: 2 studies only which reported different parameters

Measured parameter	Result in EN	Result in PN	Significance
Alpha-TNF	+++	–	NSS
IL-6	– – –	– – –	NSS
Glutamine	–	+	NSS
TBARS	++	++++	NSS
IgG	– –	+	NSS
IgM	–	++	NSS

+ Denotes increase. – Denotes decrease.

Relative magnitude of change in EN versus PN group is indicated by the number of + or –.

TBARS: thiobarbituric acid-reactive substances

Fig. 2 Forest plot of comparison: 1 Enteral versus parenteral nutrition for acute pancreatitis, outcome: 1.1 Mortality [Al-Omran N, Al Balawa ZH, Tashkandi MF, Al-Ansari LA. Enteral versus parenteral nutrition for acute pancreatitis. Cochrane database of systematic reviews 2010, Issue 1. Art No.: CD002837, © Cochrane Collaboration, reproduced with permission]

Study or subgroup	Favours EN Events	Favours EN Total	TPN Events	TPN Total	Weight %	Risk Ratio M-H, Fixed, 95% CI	Year
Kalfarentzos 1997	1	18	2	20	6.6	0.56 [0.05, 5.62]	1997
McClave 1997	0	16	0	16		Not estimable	1997
Olah 2002	2	41	4	48	12.8	0.59 [0.11, 3.03]	2002
Abou-Assi 2002	8	26	6	27	20.5	1.38 [0.56, 3.44]	2002
Gupta 2003	0	8	0	9		Not estimable	2003
Louie 2005	0	10	3	18	8.9	0.25 [0.01, 4.35]	2005
Petrov 2006	2	35	12	34	42.4	0.16 [0.04, 0.67]	2006
Casas 2007	0	11	2	11	8.7	0.20 [0.01, 3.74]	2007
Total (95% CI)		**165**		**183**	**100**	**0.50 [0.28, 0.91]**	

Total events: 13 (EN), 29 (TPN)
Heterogeneity: $Chi^2 = 7.84$, df = 5 (P = 0.17); $I^2 = 36.0\%$
Test for overall effect: Z = 2.28 (P = 0.02)

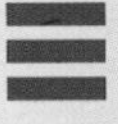

Fig. 3 Forest plot of comparison: 1 Enteral versus parenteral nutrition for acute pancreatitis, outcome: 1.2 Mortality in patients with acute pancreatitis excluding those from (Kalfarentzos 1997) in which death resulted after resolution of acute pancreatitis and was attributed to other causes; cardiac surgery, cancer of the liver, squamous cell carcinoma of the pharynx and intracerebral haemorrhage. [Al-Omran N, Al Balawa ZH, Tashkandi MF, Al-Ansari LA. Enteral versus parenteral nutrition for acute pancreatitis. Cochrane database of systematic reviews 2010, Issue 1. Art No.: CD002837, © Cochrane Collaboration, reproduced with permission]

Study or subgroup	Favours EN		TPN		Weight	Risk Ratio	Year
	Events	Total	Events	Total	%	M-H, Fixed, 95% CI	
Kalfarentzos 1997	[illegible]	18	2	20	7.1	0.56 [0.05, 5.62]	1997
McClave 1997	0	16	0	16		Not estimable	1997
Abou-Assi 2002	[illegible]	26	4	27	14.7	1.04 [0.29, 3.72]	2002
Olah 2002	[illegible]	41	4	48	13.8	0.59 [0.11, 3.03]	2002
Gupta 2003	0	8	0	9		Not estimable	2003
Louie 2005	0	10	3	18	9.6	0.25 [0.01, 4.35]	2005
Petrov 2006	[illegible]	35	12	34	45.5	0.16 [0.04, 0.67]	2006
Casas 2007	0	11	2	11	9.3	0.20 [0.01, 3.74]	2007
Total (95% CI)		**165**		**183**	**100**	**0.39 [0.20, 0.77]**	

Total events: 9 (EN), 27 (TPN)
Heterogeneity: $Chi^2 = 4.36$, $df = 5$ ($P = 0.50$); $I^2 = 0\%$
Test for overall effect: $Z = 2.70$ ($P = 0.007$)

Fig. 4 Forest plot of comparison: 1 Enteral versus parenteral nutrition for acute pancreatitis, outcome: 1.2 Mortality in patients with severe acute pancreatitis (SAP). [Al-Omran N, Al Balawa ZH, Tashkandi MF, Al-Ansari LA. Enteral versus parenteral nutrition for acute pancreatitis. Cochrane database of systematic reviews 2010, Issue 1. Art No.: CD002837, © Cochrane Collaboration, reproduced with permission]

Study or subgroup	Favours EN		TPN		Weight	Risk Ratio	Year
	Events	Total	Events	Total	%	M-H, Fixed, 95% CI	
Gupta 2003	0	8	0	9		Not estimable	2003
Louie 2005	0	10	3	18	14.9	0.25 [0.01, 4.35]	2005
Petrov 2006	2	35	12	34	70.6	0.16 [0.04, 0.67]	2006
Casas 2007	0	11	2	11	14.5	0.20 [0.01, 3.74]	2007
Total (95% CI)		**64**		**72**	**100**	**0.18 [0.06, 0.58]**	

Total events: 2 (EN), 17 (TPN)
Heterogeneity: $Chi^2 = 0.07$, df = 2 (P = 0.96); $I^2 = 0\%$
Test for overall effect: Z = 2.89 (P = 0.004)

Risk Ratio
M-H, Fixed, 95% CI
0.01 0.1 1 10 100
Favours experimental Favours control

Authors' conclusion

In patients with acute pancreatitis enteral feeding significantly reduces mortality, systemic infections, multiple organ failure and the need for operative intervention compared to TPN. There was also a trend towards less local septic and other complications and hospital LOS. In the subgroup analysis the results for patients with SAP showed even more significant reduction in mortality and systemic infections.

Problems & limitations

- Blinding for such trials is impossible
- A small number of patients was used and therefore the majority of studies were underpowered

Advantages

- Finding in all trials favoured EN

Expert opinion

Daren K. Heyland

How valid and robust are the data?
The methods are well described and done according to current standards. Thus, readers can have confidence in the results. However, please note that the number of studies and number of patients studied is very small so the estimates of treatment effect are not very stable.

Should clinical practice be influenced by this?
There is an overwhelming signal that EN is preferred to PN in patients with severe acute pancreatitis. There is no rationale for practitioners starting initial nutrition therapy with PN. Early EN should be initiated via nasogastric or naso-jejunal route and PN could be considered if EN is not well tolerated after several days of attempting to maximize EN delivery (using motility agents and small bowel tubes).

What is the next step?
Published audits of practice still demonstrate early use of PN in this population. The next step is to work on knowledge translation strategies to ensure great compliance with this nutritional practice.

Citation

Al-Omran N, Al Balawa ZH, Tashkandi MF, Al-Ansari LA. Enteral versus parenteral nutrition for acute pancreatitis. Cochrane database of systematic reviews 2010, Issue 1. Art No.: CD002837. DOI: 10.1002/14651858.CD002837.Pub2.

10

Additional information

- Go to the previous review summary on "Nutritional Strategies in severe acute pancreatitis"
- 5 of the studies were included in both reviews
- This review did not examine the effect of EN delivered via a naso-gastric tube but acknowledges 2 trials which concluded that EN via the stomach was safe and effective

AMSTAR: methodological quality of the review

1.	Was "a priori" design provided?	Y
2.	Was study selection and data extraction adequate?	Y
3.	Was the literature search comprehensive?	Y
4.	Was 'Grey Literature' used?	Y
5.	Was a list of excluded studies provided?	Y
6.	Where the characteristics of included studies provided?	Y
7.	Was the scientific quality of studies assessed & documented?	Y
8.	Was the scientific quality of studies weighted appropriately in forming conclusions?	Y
9.	Were the methods used for data synthesis appropriate?	Y
10.	Was the potential for publication bias assessed? Funnel plot would have been used if 10 or more studies were included	N
11.	Were any conflicts of interest stated?	Y

Overall quality of trials included	Moderate
Overall quality of the review	High

Glucose-insulin-potassium infusion

Condition: circulatory shock

Intervention: glucose-insulin-potassium (GIK) infusion

Clinical question: Does the use of GIK infusions in critically ill patients with septic and other forms of shock improve mortality?

GIK infusions have been used in patients with cardiovascular disease since the 1960's. The rationale behind this therapy in acute myocardial infarction (AMI) is that GIK supresses both circulating levels and myocardial uptake of free fatty acids; exogenous glucose provides for more efficient myocardial energy production and the potassium promotes electrical stability. Some advocate the use of GIK in critical illness as metabolic and inotropic therapy. In sepsis and shock states, the heart develops insulin resistance as a result of excessive pyruvate dehydrogenase de-activation. Insulin reactivates this complex to allow optimal glucose and lactate oxidation by the myocardium and thus improving inotropy.

Review characteristics

- **Eligibility criteria**: RCTs which compared a continuous infusion of GIK with standard therapy or placebo
- **Exclusions**: 6 studies of GIK in sepsis because they were not RCTs
- **Population**: adults with critical illness either in ICU or operating theatre; or who were in a group with a mortality rate of 15% or more
- **A priori**: subgroup analysis of 1) High-quality studies 2) Patients with septic shock 3) Patients with other forms of shock
- **Post Hoc**: subgroup analysis 1) Patients with AMI 2) Patients undergoing cardiac surgery
- **Number of studies**: 23 studies
- **Number of patients**: 22,525 [range 8–10,088 (Mehta)]
- **Study dates**: 1968 x 1; 1970's x 3; 1980's x 4; the rest 1997–2008

Definition

- **Mortality**: varied as authors' end of time frame mortality was used (mostly in-hospital mortality, 30-day in 4 studies, 60-day in 1 study and 1-year in 1 study)
- **GIK**: formulation varied. Duration of infusion varied from 6 hours to 48 hours but was 168 hours in 1 study

Results

Primary outcome: pooled OR for mortality

Trials	N	OR	95% CI
All 23	22525	1.02	0.93–1.11
4 high-quality studies	20694	1.04	0.95–1.14
AMI only: 10 studies	21461	0.98	0.81–1.19
Cardiac surgery only : 13 studies	1104	0.7	0.29–1.72

Fig. 5 Forest plot of all included studies. Odds ratios with 95% confidence intervals are shown on the right and the corresponding study is shown on the left. *Studies which were excluded from the summary odds ratio calculation because there were no occurrences of the primary outcome in the study [Michael A. Puskarich, Michael S. Runyon, Stephen Trzeciak, Jeffrey A. Kline and Alan E. Jones. Effect of Glucose-Insulin-Potassium Infusion on Mortality in Critical Care Settings: A Systematic. J Clin Pharmacol 49: 758–767, © 2009 by Copyright Clearance Cenoriginally, reprinted by Permission of SAGE Publications]

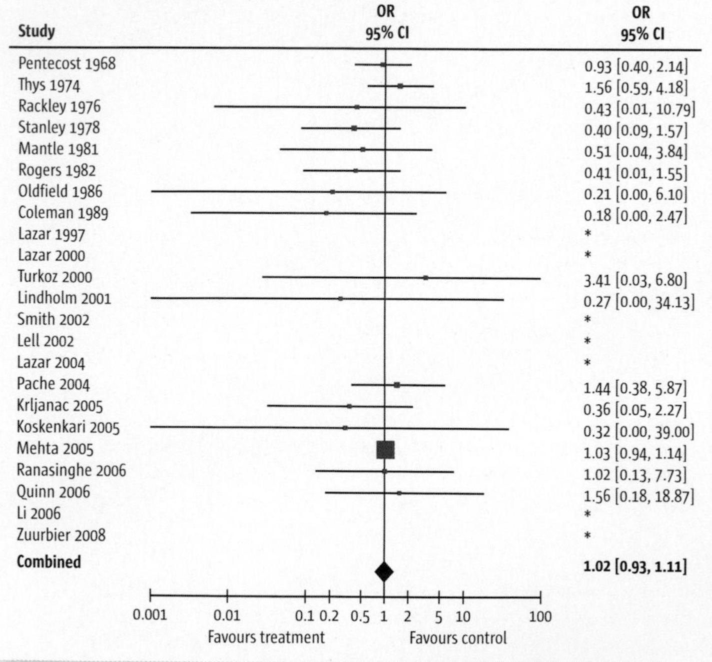

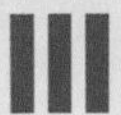

Adverse effects

Event	Trials	Result
Hypoglycaemia	6	0.5% in the GIK group versus 0.1% in the control group
Hyperkalaemia	4	4.3% in the GIK group versus 1.6% in the control group

Authors' conclusion

There is no significant effect of GIK therapy in patients with acute myocardial infarction or cardiac surgery however there is no evidence from which to draw any conclusion in populations with septic shock and other forms of circulatory shock.

Problems & limitations

- 89.7% of the patients came from a single multicentre study (Mehta) of 20,195 patients
- There were no RCTs in patients with septic shock

Advantages

- There was a large number of patients from a high-quality multicentre RCT
- The results didn't change with various statistical analyses or with excluding the largest trial

Expert opinion

David Noble

How valid and robust are the data?
The data are robust in the context of postoperative cardiac surgical patients and patients who have had acute myocardial infarcts. There are no data relevant to other types of ICU patients.

Should clinical practice be influenced by this?
Currently there are no patient-centred outcome data to support use of GIK infusions in the intensive care setting.

What is the next step?
Large scale clinical trials of more representative ICU patients are not warranted unless new small explanatory trials indicate potential benefit for general or specific ICU populations.

Citation

Michael A. Puskarich, Michael S. Runyon, Stephen Trzeciak, Jeffrey A. Kline and Alan E. Jones. Effect of Glucose-Insulin-Potassium Infusion on Mortality in Critical Care Settings: A Systematic. J Clin Pharmacol 2009 49: 758 originally published online 5 May 2009, DOI: 10.1177/0091270009334375

AMSTAR: methodological quality of the review

1.	Was "a priori" design provided?	Y
2.	Was study selection and data extraction adequate?	Y
3.	Was the literature search comprehensive?	Y
4.	Was 'Grey Literature' used?	Y
5.	Was a list of excluded studies provided?	Y
6.	Where the characteristics of included studies provided?	Y
7.	Was the scientific quality of studies assessed & documented?	N
8.	Was the scientific quality of studies weighted appropriately in forming conclusions?	U
9.	Were the methods used for data synthesis appropriate?	Y
10.	Was the potential for publication bias assessed?	Y
11.	Were any conflicts of interest stated?	Y

Overall quality of trials included	Only 4 were high-quality
Overall quality of the review	High

11

Outcomes

Off-hours admission and mortality 228
Risk of readmission to ICU 232
Quality of life after ICU 236
Long-term mortality after ICU 241
Health insurance in the USA 245

Off-hours admission and mortality

Condition: critical illness
Subject area: off-hours or out-of-hours admissions
Clinical question: Does "off-hours" admission to ICU have any impact on mortality?

Patients are likely to be most unstable in the first few hours after admission to critical care. At the time of admission they require intensive resuscitation measures; diagnostic investigations to establish the underlying cause of their illness and specific therapy. Most intensive care units do not maintain the same level of staffing during "off-hours" (night time, weekends and holidays). A large body of literature has shown decreased complications, length of stay or mortality in units with mandatory intensivist consultation, 24 hours intensivist coverage and increased levels of nursing staff. However one large retrospective study showed higher odds of death in critically ill patients treated by critical care physicians compared to those who were not. Studies examining the impact of admission timing on outcomes have also had inconsistent results.

Studies examining the impact of admission timing in other conditions such as the acute epiglottitis, abdominal aortic aneurysm, pulmonary embolism, intracerebral haemorrhage and trauma have found an increased risk of death during off-hours.

Review characteristics

- **Eligibility criteria**: studies evaluating the association between "off-hours" admission and mortality that adjusted for disease severity
- **Exclusions**: studies where the setting was not ICU e.g. emergency department
- **Population**: adults admitted to intensive care units
- **Number of studies**: 10 Cohort studies. 3 prospective and 7 retrospective
  - 4 in North America, 4 in Europe and 2 in Asia
  - 3 single centre studies, 7 multicentre of which one study included 102 ICUs in the UK (Wunsch 2004)
  - 8 studies evaluated night-time admission and 6 evaluated weekend admission
- **Number of patients**: night-time admissions n = 135,220, weekends n = 180,600
- **Study dates**: 2002–2009

Definitions

- **Off-hours**: night-time or weekends
- **Reference group**: Patients admitted during the day were compared to those admitted at night. Patients admitted during weekdays were compared to those admitted at the weekend
- **Intensivist**: not specifically defined but presumed consultant intensivist. For 1 study it was an in-training intensivist with more than 52 on-site night shifts of experience

Main findings: pooled results

Organisational structure

2 studies – intensivists were present at night time

5 studies – no intensivist was present at night

1 study – an intensivists was present 24 hours a day

4 studies – an intensivist was present part of the day

4 studies – resident physicians or fellows were present during off-hours

Night-time admission and mortality

Mortality was 21.4% for daytime admissions and 20.8% for night-time admissions

There was no difference in the adjusted odds of death between these

(OR 1.0, 95% 0.87–1.17, $p = 9.56$)

Subgroup analysis:

No night-time intensivists (OR 1.0, 95% CI 0.79–1.41, $p = 0.73$)

With a night-time intensivist (0.93, 95% CI 0.87–0.99, $p = 0.02$)

Weekend admission and mortality

Mortality was 11.1% for weekday admissions and 15.5% for weekend admissions

The adjusted odds of death were significantly higher for the patients admitted over the weekend

(OR 1.08, 95% CI 1.04–1.13, $p < 0.001$)

Subgroup analysis:

No intensivist on-site (OR 1.07, 95% CI 0.99–1.15, $p = 0.081$)

Intensivist on-site (OR 1.03, 95% 0.61–1.73, $p = 0.916$)

Author's conclusion

Night-time admissions were not associated with a worse outcome. Patients admitted to an ICU during the weekend appear to have an 8% higher risk of death (adjusted for severity of illness) compared with patients admitted during weekdays. This result should be interpreted with caution because the meta-analysis was dominated by one study (Barnett 2002). Increased mortality at the weekend can be explained by a number of factors including lower physician-to-patient ratio and difficulties in obtaining diagnostic tests. The absence of increased night-time risk may be related to the shorter "down-time" before daytime activities resume. Patients admitted during the day remain critically ill or deteriorate during off-hours and may still then receive substandard care which may have caused an underestimate in the impact of off-hours care.

Problems & limitations

- The studies did not explore the contribution of changes in nurse staffing levels during off-hours which may have a profound impact
- There was significant heterogeneity between the studies evaluating night-time admissions

Fig. 1 Adjusted effect of weekend admission to the ICU on mortality. Weight is the relative contribution of each study to the overall OR (random effects model with 95% CI) [from Rodrigo Cavallazzi, Paul E. Marik, Amyn Hirani, Monvasi Pachinburavan, Tajender S. Vasu and Benjamin E. Leiby. Association between time of admission to ICU and Mortality: A systematic Review and Metaanalysis. Chest 2010;138;68–75. Reproduced with permission from the American College of Chest Physicians]

Author	Year	Odds Ratio (95% CI)	Weight %
Barnett	2002	1.09 [1.04, 1.15]	63.66
Uusaro	2003	1.20 [1.01, 1.43]	5.32
Ensminger	2004	1.06 [0.96, 1.18]	14.83
Sheu	2007	0.79 [0.50, 1.25]	0.77
Laupland	2008	1.05 [0.95, 1.17]	14.83
Lee	2008	1.03 [0.61, 1.73]	0.59
Overall (I^2 = 0%, p = 0.585)		**1.08 [1.04, 1.13]**	**100.00**

Note: Weights are from random effects analysis

Advantages

- Several multicentre studies and large numbers of patients were included
- Included studies were all performed within the last decade
- Statistically analysis did not show any evidence of publication bias

Expert opinion

Maurizia Capuzzo

How valid and robust are the data?

This review found 10 studies comparing patients' daytime and night-time admissions to ICU (8 of them considering hospital mortality and 2 ICU mortality) and 8 studies comparing week and weekend admissions to ICU. Definitions were not homogeneous, and significant heterogeneity was present for the former but not for the latter. The higher mortality of patients admitted at the weekend was confirmed after excluding the widest study contributing to 64% of the pooled Odd Ratio. Therefore, this result appears quite robust.

11

Should clinical practice be influenced by this?

This review concerns the organization. Therefore, ICU directors, general hospital management, politicians and policy makers should be aware of the findings of this review. Each of them could play their role, the ICU directors increasing the presence of an expert intensivist in the weekends, hospital management guaranteeing appropriate (diagnostic and therapeutic) support, and the politicians providing the money required.

What is the next step?

There were many differences in the organizational structure of the ICUs where the studies reviewed were performed (including the type of physician staff, resident or fellow, intensivist or non intensivist) do not allow us to look at the causes of the increased mortality of night-time admissions. These and other points at hospital level should be the object of a large multicentre worldwide research.

Citation

Cavallazzi R, Marik PE, Hirani A, Pachinburavan M, Vasu TS, Leiby BE. Association between time of admission to ICU and Mortality: A systematic Review and Metaanalysis. Chest 2010;138; 68–75. DOI 10.1378/chest.09-3018

AMSTAR: methodological quality of the review

1.	Was "a priori" design provided?	Y
2.	Was study selection and data extraction adequate?	Y
3.	Was the literature search comprehensive?	Y
4.	Was 'Grey Literature' used?	Y
5.	Was a list of excluded studies provided?	P
6.	Where the characteristics of included studies provided?	Y
7.	Was the scientific quality of studies assessed & documented?	Y
8.	Was the scientific quality of studies weighted appropriately in forming conclusions?	Y
9.	Were the methods used for data synthesis appropriate?	Y
10.	Was the potential for publication bias assessed?	Y
11.	Were any conflicts of interest stated?	Y

Overall quality of trials included	High quality
Overall quality of the review	High

Risk of readmission to ICU

Condition: critical illness

Subject area: ICU readmissions

Clinical question: Is there any association between severity of illness and readmission to ICU during the same hospitalisation?

Approximately 10% of patients discharged from ICU are readmitted at some point during the same hospitalization. This may be due to inappropriately early discharge from ICU, inadequate level of care on the general wards or a combination. Readmission to ICU is associated with adverse events and is regarded as a potential marker of quality of care. It is important to be able to identify these patients so that appropriate management decisions can be made, for example ICU outreach after discharge.

Review characteristics

- **Eligibility criteria:** studies that used a valid severity of illness index
- **Exclusions:** review articles
- **Population:** adult patients readmitted to ICU during the same hospitalisation. Patients were from both teaching and community hospitals; and from general, medical, surgical and cardiothoracic ICUs
- **Number of studies:** 11 (9 retrospective cohort studies, 2 case-control studies)
- **Number of patients:** 220,866 (range 130–103,984)
- **Study dates:** 1993–2008

Definitions

- **Severity of illness scores used in the studies:** APACHE II, APACHE III, SAPS and SAPS II

Results

11

The patients readmitted to ICU had higher severity of illness scores compared to those who were not readmitted (SMD = 0.35, 95% CI 0.23–0.48). This means that readmitted patients had severity of illness scores that were approximately one third of a standard deviation higher.

Each standard deviation increase in illness severity was calculated to give a summary estimate of 43% increase in readmission risk

This result was consistent irrespective of the time at which illness severity was measured

At admission (SMD = 0.35, 95% CI 0.23–0.48, $p < 0.001$)

At discharge (SMD = 0.36, 95% CI 0.27–0.45, $p < 0.001$)

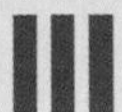

Fig. 2 Forest plots of standardised mean difference (SMD) (including 95% confidence intervals) in severity of illness between readmissions and non-readmissions to ICU. Severity of illness at admission panel (A) and discharge panel (B). The area of the blue squares reflects the weight each study contributes to the meta-analysis (inverse variance). The diamond at the bottom of the graph is the summary estimate (SMD) and 95% confidence interval from a random effects model (REM). TH = teaching hospital, CH = community hospital; ap2 and ap3 = Acute Physiology and Chronic Health Evaluation II and III, respectively: SAPS = Simplified Acute Physiology Score. Line of no-difference and summary effect lines added [Reprinted from Severity of illness and risk of readmission to intensive care: A meta-analysis. Steven A. Frost, Evan Alexandrou, Tony Bogdanovski, Yenna Salamonson, Patricia M. Davidson, Michael J. Parr, Ken M. Hillman. Resuscitation 80 (2009) 505–510, with permission from Elsevier]

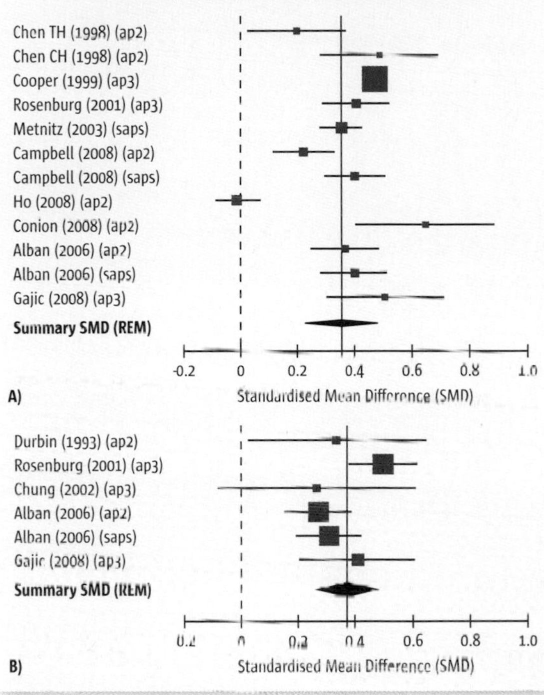

Author's conclusion

The meta-analysis shows that there's an association between severity of illness score and readmission to ICU risk and that this effect was consistent regardless of which illness severity score was used.

The SWIFT (the Stability and Workload Index For Transfer) score is a tool that was developed to identify patients who are at risk of readmission to ICU and has been shown to be a better discriminator than APACHE II plus characteristics of illness such as ICU LOS, duration of mechanical ventilation and days to ICU admission. [Gajic O, Malinchoc M, Comfere TB, Harris MR, Achouitic A, Yilmaz M, et al. The Stability and

Workload Index For Transfer score predicts unplanned intensive care unit patient readmission: initial development and validation. Crit Care Med 2008; 36: 676–82]

Problems & limitations

- All included studies were either observational and/or susceptible to bias

Advantages

- The results agree with a previous review which identified severity of illness as a predictor or ICU readmission
- This has highlighted the need to develop mechanisms to recognize detrimental events in patients at risk and specific interventions that might reduce the risk of deterioration and readmission

Expert opinion

Maurizia Capuzzo

How valid and robust are the data?
This review found 11 articles involving different number of patients (range 130–103,984) of worldwide ICUs. The studies did not show relevant heterogeneity and the final sample was wide. The data are robust.

Should clinical practice be influenced by this?
This review cannot really influence the daily clinical practice because the relationship between severity of illness and risk of ICU readmission is an information lacking specificity. It would not be wise for intensivists to prolong the ICU stay of a patient that has improved enough to be discharged when a new patient needing organ support is at the door of the ICU.

What is the next step?
Next step may be to identify the specific clinical predictors of ICU readmission in the light of the reasons for unplanned ICU readmissions. At present clinicians can only speculate on possible solutions, which can range from discharge to intermediate care or high dependency units (where present), to follow-up former ICU patients after discharge to general ward. Considering that the matter does not allow RCT, real world future studies are indicated to compare the efficacy and the costs of possible solutions.

Citation

Frost SA, Alexandrou E, Bogdanovski T, Salamonson Y, Davidson PM, Parr MJ, Hillman KM. Severity of illness and risk of readmission to intensive care: A meta-analysis. Resuscitation 80 (2009) 505–510 doi:10.1016/j.resuscitation.2009.02.015

AMSTAR: methodological quality of the review

1.	Was "a priori" design provided?	Y
2.	Was study selection and data extraction adequate?	Y
3.	Was the literature search comprehensive?	Y
4.	Was 'Grey Literature' used?	Y
5.	Was a list of excluded studies provided?	N
6.	Where the characteristics of included studies provided?	Y
7.	Was the scientific quality of studies assessed & documented?	NA
8.	Was the scientific quality of studies weighted appropriately in forming conclusions?	Y
9.	Were the methods used for data synthesis appropriate?	Y
10.	Was the potential for publication bias assessed?	Y
11.	Were any conflicts of interest stated?	Y

Overall quality of trials included	NA
Overall quality of the review	High

Quality of life after ICU

Condition: critical illness

Outcome: quality of life (QOL)

Clinical question: What impact does critical illness have on long-term health status and quality of life?

Advances in diagnostic, therapeutic and supportive care in intensive have improved survival from critical illness. Most studies assess mortality or survival however quality of life is also an important outcome but is rarely included in study data. Measuring QOL requires the use of validated assessment tools, is labour-intensive, time consuming and may be ambiguous. It has been shown that in patients admitted to ICU, the pre-admission QOL is low compared to the general population and that poor baseline QOL is associated with a poor outcome, it is therefore important that studies assess pre-ICU admission QOL so that the relative influence of pre-morbid condition compared to the acute critical illness can be determined.

Review characteristics

- **Eligibility criteria**: studies published between 1999 and 2009 that assessed QOL after at least 12 months from ICU discharge using one of the four QOL assessment tools detailed below
- **Exclusions**: studies with less than 50 patients, articles with exclusively cardiac or thoracic surgery patients, case reports and literature reviews.
- **Population**: survivors of critical illness
- **Number of studies**: 53 studies: 10 multicentre, 36 in Europe (15 in Scandinavian countries), 13 in the USA, 4 in Canada
- **Number of patients**: 10,165
- **Study dates**: 1999–2009

Definitions

- **Long-term**: 12 months or more
- **ARDS/Sepsis/Severe trauma/Elderly**: not specified, presumed author or consensus definitions

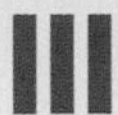

Results

Study characteristics

Diagnostic Category
11 studies concerned ARDS patients
3 studies of patients requiring prolonged mechanical ventilation
8 trauma studies
6 article about patients suffering cardiac arrest
6 studies of elderly patients
2 pancreatitis studies
3 sepsis studies
4 studies of various topics
10 studies were of critically ill patients in general
Follow-up (FU)
8 studies had FU at 1 year
15 studies had ranges within their FU time
12 studies evaluated QOL at strict time points
8 studies had median FU times of 5 years
Assessment tools
55% of studies used SF-36
21% used EQ-5D
9% used NHP
8% used RAND-36
8% used a combination
Postal surveys were used in 42%, telephone interviews in 26%, face-to-face interviews in 23%
9% used a combination of techniques
Response rates
Less than 50% in 3 studies
50–79% in 24 studies
80% or more in 26 studies

Quality of life

Survivors of ARDS, prolonged mechanical ventilation, severe trauma and sepsis had significant impairment in QOL.

Physical aspects improved over time but mental and emotional state was static or declined.

In ARDS or prolonged MV the factors associated with decrements in QOL were:

1. impaired respiratory function
2. weakness
3. Cognitive disorders
4. Post-traumatic stress disorder

Trauma patient were usually young and healthy before ICU admission and thus QOL declined substantially.

Factors that were negatively associated with QOL were:

1. Severity of injury
2. Degree of brain damage
3. Female gender

Survivors of cardiac arrest, pancreatitis, AKI and oesophagectomy had a good QOL that was equivalent or better than the age and gender matched general population

---

Elderly patients had a reduced QOL particularly with regard to the physical domains

Perceived QOL was good reflecting good adaptions to their limitations

---

At 1 year general ICU patients had reduced QOL compared to an age and gender matched population

This was predominantly in the physical domains

This improved over time such that after several years it was comparable to the general population

---

In the general ICU studies, there were conflicting results about the influence of age on long-term QOL

Only 9 studies measured pre-admission QOL

5 studies assessed patients' pre-ICU QOL a long time after their ICU admission which exposes results to recall bias.

Pre-ICU QOL assessment by proxy is the alternative which tends to slightly underestimate the patient's QOL but is generally reliable

In 2 studies, poor preadmission QOL was associated with a prolonged reduction in QOL after ICU discharge

---

Assessment tools

1. Medical Outcomes Study 36-item Short Form Health Survey (SF-36)
   Uses 36 items to measure 8 domains: physical functioning, role limitation due to physical problems, bodily pain, general health perceptions, energy/vitality, social functioning, role limitation due to emotional problems and mental health
2. RAND 36-Item Health Survey (RAND-36)
   This was developed from the SF-36, the counting system differs but the questions and final results are almost identical

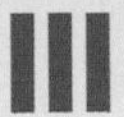

3. Euro-Qol-5D (EQ-5D)
This is a questionnaire comprised of three parts. A descriptive 5 item questionnaire for: mobility, self-care, usual activities, pain/discomfort and anxiety/depression; each item is answered "no problem", "moderate problem " or "severe problem" and thus patients can be categorised into 1 of 243 (3^5) states. Each of these health states can be converted into one single summary index or utility. The EQ-VAS (visual analogue scale) is a self-rated health scale from 0 to 100. This is less validated in critically ill populations than the SF-36
4. Nottingham Health Profile (NHP)
This is a two part questionnaire. 38 questions assess 6 domains: physical mobility, pain, sleep, energy, emotional reactions and social isolation. Part 2 list 7 activities of daily living: occupation, house work, social activity, home life, sex life, hobbies, and holidays. Consistency and sensitivity to change are better with SF-36 and RAND-36 than the NHP

Author's conclusion

Survivors of critical illness have a lower QOL than an age and gender-matched normal population, specifically long-term QOL appears to be largely dependent on diagnostic category. Patients with ARDS, prolonged MV, severe trauma and severe sepsis have the most significant reductions in QOL that last a long time. Good QOL despite persisting symptoms may reflect acclimatisation to disease, and is highest in elderly patients with good socioeconomic status. QOL did improve slowly over a long period of time.

Factors that could be presumed to worsen QOL such as age and ICU LOS may not necessarily be indictors of poor overall QOL, and psychological and emotional factors may have a less tangible influence than physical impairments. At 1 year physical problems tended to dominate but at longer follow-up emotional problems seemed more relevant.

Problems & limitations

- Difference in study design, patient populations, QOL assessment tools, follow-up time and response rates preclude one overall conclusion
- Four QOL assessment tools were included but generic instruments are less sensitive in specific conditions which may have targeted assessment tools
- A better method of QOL assessment is to ascertain how QOL has changed since critical illness but only 9 studies measure pre-ICU admission QOL
- Only 49% of studies had a response rate of 80% which is considered acceptable. Lack of response to such surveys can be for a variety of reasons: death, severe disability, PTSD therefore responders may represent a healthier sample and bias results

11

Advantages

- The SF-36 and RAND-36 which are the generic instruments of choice in critically ill patients was used in 63% of the studies
- The changes in QOL over time have highlighted the importance of assessment at various time intervals and the need for pre-ICU QOL assessment for future studies

Citation

Oeyen SG, Vandijck DM, Benoit DD, Annemans L, Decruyenaere JM. Quality of life after intensive care: A systematic review of the literature. Crit Care Med 2010 Vol. 38, No. 12 DOI: 10.1097/CCM.0b013e3181f3dec

AMSTAR: methodological quality of the review

1.	Was "a priori" design provided?	Y
2.	Was study selection and data extraction adequate?	Y
3.	Was the literature search comprehensive?	Y
4.	Was 'Grey Literature' used? Limited to English language	P
5.	Was a list of excluded studies provided?	N
6.	Where the characteristics of included studies provided?	Y
7.	Was the scientific quality of studies assessed & documented?	Y
8.	Was the scientific quality of studies weighted appropriately in forming conclusions?	Y
9.	Were the methods used for data synthesis appropriate?	NA
10.	Was the potential for publication bias assessed?	NA
11.	Were any conflicts of interest stated?	Y

Overall quality of trials included	40% moderate (4 studies were high quality)
Overall quality of the review	High

11

Long-term mortality after ICU

Condition: sepsis, severe sepsis and septic shock
Outcomes: mortality and quality of life
Clinical question: What is the impact of sepsis on mortality and long-term outcomes?

Sepsis syndrome is both a common reason for admission to ICU and a common complication in ICU patients admitted with other illnesses. Despite improvement in antimicrobial therapy and supportive care, mortality from sepsis remains high. Patients with sepsis have complications that may have long-term sequelae e.g. acute kidney injury, acute lung injury, critical illness polyneuromyopathy and delirium such that 28-day mortality which is reported in most clinical studies may significantly underestimate morbidity and mortality. Furthermore, the pathogenetic mechanism of the infecting organism as well as the host's responses may have unappreciated effects on organ systems particularly the central nervous system.

Review characteristics

- **Eligibility criteria:** studies (observational and controlled trials) that included quantitative reporting of validated quality of life (QOL) or mortality data at least 90 days after ICU discharge
- **Exclusions:** Studies of other ICU populations were only included if they reported QOL or mortality data for the sepsis population
- **Population:** adults (> 18 years) with sepsis, severe sepsis or septic shock. Mixed population: medical, surgical, hospital wide or ICU patients as well as HIV patients in 1 study
- **Number of studies:** 30 studies. (1 multicentre, 13 from USA, 2 from Canada, 10 from European countries, 3 from South America and Asia). 17 observational studies
- **Number of patients:** Total 36,889 (range 24–16,019) RCTs = 4,593 patients
- **Study dates:** 1994–2009

Definitions

- **Long-term:** more than 3 months
- **Euro-Qol-5D (EQ-5D)**
- **Uses a 5-item questionnaire for:** mobility, self-care, usual activities, pain/discomfort and anxiety/depression (answers are "no", "some" or "extreme"). The EQ-VAS (visual analogue scale) is a self-rated health scale from 0 to 10
- **Medical Outcomes Study's 36-item short form general health survey (SF-36)**
- **Uses 36 items to measure 8 domains:** physical functioning, role limitation due to physical problems, bodily pain, general health perceptions, energy/vitality, social functioning, role limitation due to emotional problems and mental health

Results

Study characteristics

Populations

13 studies compared septic patients to control population

3 studies were RCTs in which controls were septic patients that didn't receive additional therapy e.g. activated protein C, antilipopolysaccharide

Study design

4 studies controlled for confounding variables by randomisation, statistical adjustment and by comparison to a matched population

Matched controls were the normal population in 14 studies

16 articles did not attempt to adjust for confounders

Follow-up

FU ranged from 3 months to 10 years

8 studies reported end points of 3–6 months

11 studies used 1 year end points

7 studies reported end points of more than 1 year

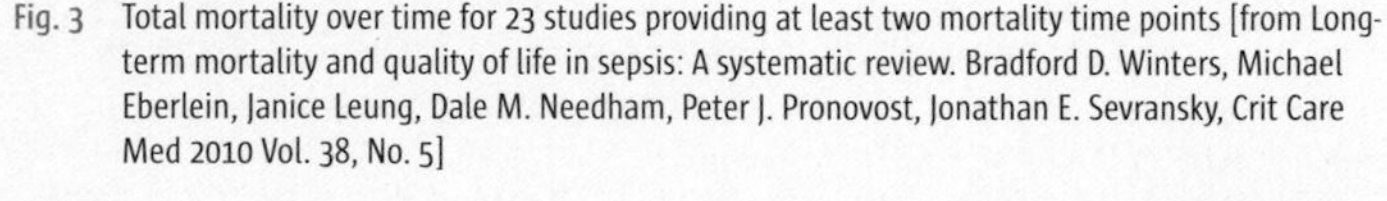

Fig. 3 Total mortality over time for 23 studies providing at least two mortality time points [from Long-term mortality and quality of life in sepsis: A systematic review. Bradford D. Winters, Michael Eberlein, Janice Leung, Dale M. Needham, Peter J. Pronovost, Jonathan E. Sevransky, Crit Care Med 2010 Vol. 38, No. 5]

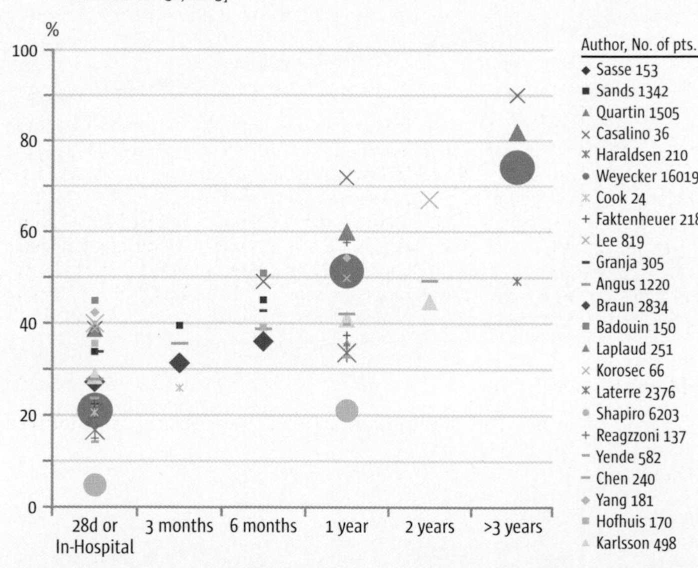

Outcomes

Mortality
26 studies provide mortality data, 23 of these used at least 2 time points
Total 1 year mortality ranged from 21.5% to 71.9%
17 studies reported additional mortality after hospital discharge at 1 year of 7% to 43%
Mortality after hospital discharge in 4 controlled studies that compared septic patients to various non-septic populations showed 1 year mortality of between 7% and 25.6% in the septic patients and in non-septic patients mortality was between 2% and 13.2%
2 RCTs of APC showed similar 1 year after hospital discharge mortality rates of 15% and 17% without any difference between the APC and placebo groups.
1 cohort study showed similar mortality rates between septic and non-septic groups at 6 months of 9% and 8% respectively
3 studies provided mortality at 3–5 years after hospital discharge which ranged from 21% to 54%
6 observational studies provided shorter mortality end points after hospital discharge of: 5% at 3 months, 11.3% at 5 months and between 3% and 12% at 6 months.
Quality of life (QOL)
12 studies provide QOL data
3 used EQ-5D (2 compared septic cohort to non-septic and 1 compared a septic cohort to the general population), 6 used SF-36 and 4 used multiple scores
All studies that used EQ-5D and 5 that used SF-36 found decrement in QOL over the long term
2 studies found a significantly decreased baseline QOL in the septic patients compared to the general population

Author's conclusion

Patients with all degrees of sepsis have an increased mortality compared to non-septic patients or the normal population which continues over a number of years after hospital discharge. Certain co-morbidities such as diabetes, immunodeficiency and haematological malignancy both increase the risk of sepsis and are associated with increased mortality, it is difficult to ascertain the relative contribution to mortality of the sepsis syndrome and underlying disease. Septic patients also had decrements in QOL measures over the long-term, similar to patients with ALI. Again because of the overlap in syndromes between sepsis and ALI, it is difficult to ascertain the relative contribution of each condition to the deficits.

Problems & limitations

- Limited study quality due to inadequate control groups and insufficient adjustment for confounding variables
- Only a qualitative not quantitative analysis is provided

Advantages

- Large number of patients in several different continents
- Results were consistent in most studies, in different countries, in different patient populations and across varying severity of illness
- Results agree with previous studies that showed persistent function disability at 2 years in survivors of ALI, of which sepsis is the most common cause

Citation

Winters BD, Eberlein M, Leung J, Needham DM, Pronovost PJ, Sevransky JE. Long-term mortality and quality of life in sepsis: A systematic review. Crit Care Med 2010 Vol. 38, No. 5 DOI: 10.1097/CCM.0b013e3181d8cc1d

AMSTAR: methodological quality of the review

1.	Was "a priori" design provided?	Y
2.	Was study selection and data extraction adequate?	Y
3.	Was the literature search comprehensive?	Y
4.	Was 'Grey Literature' used?	Y
5.	Was a list of excluded studies provided?	N
6.	Where the characteristics of included studies provided?	Y
7.	Was the scientific quality of studies assessed & documented?	Y
8.	Was the scientific quality of studies weighted appropriately in forming conclusions?	Y
9.	Were the methods used for data synthesis appropriate?	NA
10.	Was the potential for publication bias assessed?	NA
11.	Were any conflicts of interest stated?	Y

Overall quality of trials included	Low to moderate quality
Overall quality of the review	High

Health insurance in the USA

Subject area: health insurance

Clinical question: Does health insurance status in the USA have any impact on access to and delivery of critical care services?

The structure of health services in the USA differs to those in Europe in that many healthcare facilities and service provision are controlled by the private sector. Although most US citizens over 65 years and those under 65 who have permanent physical disabilities or meet other special criteria are eligible for government run social insurance programs which cover 80% of medical costs, others require some form of private health insurance in order to procure health services. Although US legislation prohibits hospitals from refusing emergency care to patients who are inadequately insured, this practice may still occur. Lack of insurance is associated with reduced access to primary and out-patient care; worse outcomes in certain chronic disorders and from accidental injury. One third of Americans under the age of 65 do not have health insurance during some portion of the year, yet discrepancies in care may not only apply to the uninsured. Differences in healthcare systems, insurance coverage and enrolment in managed care programs which have different policies to traditional indemnity insurance may also affect care access and delivery.

Review characteristics

- **Eligibility criteria:** studies from both medical and non-medical literature that compared two or more payment methods or insurance states and reported healthcare access, care delivery or outcomes for critically ill patients (at least 50% of the cohort must have been critically ill)
- **Exclusions:** case series and narrative reviews
- **Population:** pre-hospitalised and in-hospital critically ill patients, children and adults
- **Number of studies:** 29 observational cohort studies. 18 studies examined differences between the insured and uninsured, 8 studies compared managed care programs to traditional insurance. 4 studies examined "before and after" trends after the Medicare program switched to a prospective payment system for hospital reimbursement in 1984
- **Number of patients:** range 118–47.1 million. 10 studies had > 10,000, 4 studies had > 100,000
- **Study dates:** 1987–2008

Definitions

- **Critically ill:**
  a) admitted to a medical-surgical ICU,
  b) ventilated or on inotropes/vasopressors; with respiratory failure or ARDS; shock or severe sepsis or
  c) admitted to areas other than ICU with trauma and a high injury severity score
- **Insured category:** private/commercial insurance either managed care or non-managed care

- **Uninsured:** no insurance or classified as self-pay or charity
- **Managed care systems:** insurance programs with cost management and resource utilisation techniques aimed at reducing healthcare costs e.g. incentives for physicians and patients to choose less costly care; limiting services deemed unnecessary and improving the quality of care
- **Potentially ineffective care:** the highest quartile of costs divided by mortality at 100 days

Results: uninsured versus insured critically ill patients

Access to critical care
The uninsured were much less likely to receive critical care services (OR 0.56, 95% CI 0.55–0.56)
The uninsured were more likely to be admitted to or require ICU after they were hospitalised but NSS
The uninsured traumatically injured were less likely to be admitted to hospital (OR 0.63, 95% CI 0.62–0.65)
There was no difference in transfer times to the hospital
1 study showed that the uninsured were less likely to get an ambulance whereas another study showed that this difference was attenuated after better adjustment for confounding variables.
Care delivery in ICU
The uninsured were less likely to have invasive procedures (RR 0.92, 95% CI 0.89–0.94)
The uninsured were more likely to have life support withdrawn (OR 2.80, 95% CI 1.12–7.02)
There were more delays in hospital discharge for the uninsured (OR 4.51, 95% CI 1.46–13.93)
NSS trend that the uninsured were more likely to have mechanical ventilation withdrawn, and less likely to receive physical and occupational therapy
Mortality
5 studies: the uninsured had a higher hospital mortality (OR 1.16, 95% CI 1.01–1.33)
Sensitivity analysis showed that the uninsured had a higher independent risk of death (OR 1.25, 95% CI 1.02–1.53)

11

Association between managed care systems (MCS) compared to traditional insurance

Critical care delivery
Patients with MCS underwent 14.3% fewer procedures
MCS patients were less likely to receive "potentially ineffective care" (OR 0.75, 95% CI 0.65–0.87)
Clinical outcomes
5 studies: There was no difference in ICU and hospital LOS
4 studies: MCS unadjusted mortality was lower (OR 0.64, 95% CI 0.48–0.85) but this was of borderline significance once adjusted for confounding variables (OR 0.80, 95% CI 0.64–1.00)

Fig. 4 Hospital mortality rates for uninsured versus insured critically ill patients. (A) Unadjusted mortality rates. (B) Adjusted mortality rates [from Fowler RA, Noyahr L-A, Thornton JD, Pinto R, Kahn JM, Adhikari NKJ et al., on behalf of the American Thoracic Society Disparities in Healthcare Group. An Official American Thoracic Society Systematic Review: The Association between Health Insurance Status and Access, Care Delivery, and Outcomes for Patients Who Are Critically Ill. Am J Respir Crit Care Med Vol 181. pp 1003–1011, 2010. Reprinted with permission of the American Thoracic Society. Copyright ©American Thoracic Society]

Study	Odds Ratio 95% CI	Weight %
Curtis 1998	0.84 [0.51, 1.38]	2.4
Schnitzler 1998	0.90 [0.81, 1.00]	21.5
Durairaj 2003	0.91 [0.71, 1.17]	7.6
Danis 2006	1.15 [1.10, 1.19]	33.3
O'Brien 2008	1.17 [1.15, 1.19]	35.2
Overall	**1.07 (0.99, 1.16]**	**100**

Overall effect: p = 0.09; Heterogeneity: I^2 = 86.2%

0.5 1.0 2.0

Favours Uninsured Favours Insured

A)

Study	Odds Ratio 95% CI	Weight %
Schnitzler 1998	0.93 [0.84, 1.03]	25.8
Durairaj 2003	1.11 [0.87, 1.42]	15.1
Danis 2006	1.22 [1.18, 1.27]	29.7
O'Brien 2008	1.37 [1.31, 1.43]	29.4
Overall	**1.16 (1.01, 1.33]**	**100**

Overall effect: p = 0.03; Heterogeneity: I^2 = 94.1%

0.5 1.0 2.0

Favours Uninsured Favours Insured

B)

There was no difference in ICU admissions in the USA before and after the introduction of the prospective payment system compared to the fee-for-service system.

Author's conclusion

Overall the uninsured receive fewer critical care services; they are more likely to have life support withdrawn and may have a higher risk of death. Interestingly once hospitalised the uninsured are more likely to be admitted to critical care. Restricted access to healthcare resulting in more advanced illness at presentation may explain this finding. Hospitals are obliged to provide emergency care for the uninsured but not continuing care once the patient's condition has been stabilised, this leads to increased unnecessary inter-hospital transfers but also delays in discharge due to difficulties finding facilities willing to accept care for these patients. No significant differences in outcomes were found between Medicaid and private/commercial insurance however Managed Care Systems did lead to fewer invasive procedures and less use of potentially ineffective care.

Problems & limitations

- All studies were observational and therefore more susceptible to bias
- Clinical and statistical heterogeneity between studies with regards to design, populations and duration
- Heterogeneity limited the ability to combine point estimates of effect to specific outcomes

Advantages

- Large numbers of patients included
- Three quarters of the studies that adjusted for confounding variable found increased estimate of mortality amongst the uninsured critically ill
- This has highlighted the need to explore options to reduce such inequalities

Expert opinion

Maurizia Capuzzo

How valid and robust are the data?

This study found 29 observational studies suitable for analysis. A publication bias cannot be excluded and the potentially confounders were not included in all studies. The heterogeneity of studies was so wide that it was impossible to quantitatively combine for measures of delivery of care. Heterogeneity remained relevant for the comparison of hospital mortality rates of uninsured versus insured critically ill patients, and with managed versus non managed care. Therefore data are not really robust.

Should clinical practice be influenced by this?

This review cannot influence the clinical practice of any physicians honouring professional ethics. The politicians must be aware of the possible effects of the lack of insurance coverage on the outcome of critically ill citizens.

What is the next step?

If the aim of a national government is the common good (including the well-being of all citizens); politicians should organize a randomized controlled trial, clustering States with similar characteristics to the usual health insurance present in the USA, or introduce a public health insurance. Epidemiologists, physicians and statisticians should help the society in such a tremendous effort.

Citation

Fowler RA, Noyahr L-A, Thornton JD, Pinto R, Kahn JM, Adhikari NKJ et al., on behalf of the American Thoracic Society Disparities in Healthcare Group. An Official American Thoracic Society Systematic Review: The Association between Health Insurance Status and Access, Care Delivery, and Outcomes for Patients Who Are Critically Ill. Am J Respir Crit Care Med Vol 181. pp 1003–1011, 2010 DOI: 10.1164/rccm.200902-0281ST

More details are available in the online supplement from this issues table of contents at www.atsjournals.org

Additional information

President Barack Obama introduced a Healthcare reform bill in 2010 detailing many changes to healthcare provision to take place over the next 4 years. These include changes to insurance provision, incentives for businesses to provide healthcare benefits and a tax penalty for those who fail to obtain health insurance.

AMSTAR: methodological quality of the review

1.	Was "a priori" design provided?	Y
2.	Was study selection and data extraction adequate?	Y
3.	Was the literature search comprehensive?	Y
4.	Was 'Grey Literature' used?	Y
5.	Was a list of excluded studies provided?	Y
6.	Where the characteristics of included studies provided?	Y
7.	Was the scientific quality of studies assessed & documented?	Y
8.	Was the scientific quality of studies weighted appropriately in forming conclusions?	Y
9.	Were the methods used for data synthesis appropriate?	Y
10.	Was the potential for publication bias assessed?	NA
11.	Were any conflicts of Interest stated?	Y

Overall quality of trials included	NA
Overall quality of the review	High

12

Paediatric intensive care

Continuous negative extrathoracic pressure ____ 252
Heliox for croup ____ 255
Bacterial meningitis ____ 258
Nutritional support for critically ill children ____ 263
Other relevant reviews ____ 265

Continuous negative extrathoracic pressure

Condition: acute hypoxaemic respiratory failure (AHRF) of non-cardiogenic origin
Intervention: continuous negative extrathoracic pressure (CNEP)
Clinical question: Does the use of continuous negative extrathoracic pressure or non-invasive continuous positive pressure ventilation (NiCPAP) reduce morbidity or mortality in AHRF?

The high morbidity and mortality associated with AHRF in children depends upon the aetiology and the severity of illness. Supportive measures such as oxygen therapy, CPAP and mechanical ventilation are the mainstay of therapy until the underlying cause has been treated. Mechanical ventilation needs to be delivered via an endotracheal tube. Intubation and invasive ventilation itself is associated with various complications such as sub-glottic stenosis and infection. The use of negative pressure or non-invasive ventilation would minimise such concerns. CNEP has been shown to improve oxygenation in several animal models and uncontrolled studies have shown similar results in neonates.

Review characteristics

- **Eligibility criteria:** all RCTs or quasi-randomised trials comparing CNEP or NiCPAP with standard therapy in AHRF
- **Exclusions:** further 10 studies either were not randomised or patients did not meet the criteria for AHRF
- **Population:** infants under 1 year old with bronchiolitis and oxygen requirement of 40% or more to maintain saturations between 96–99%
- **Number of studies:** only 1 RCT identified of infants under 1-year old with bronchiolitis and oxygen requirement of 40% or more to maintain saturations between 96–99%
- **Number of patients:** 33 (15 received CNEP and 18 were controls)
- **Study date:** 1994

Definitions

- Standard therapy: including PPV with endotracheal intubation
- Control: management was not clear

12

Results

Only 1 study with 33 infants has assessed the efficacy of this intervention
Oxygen requirements: reduced to less than 30% in 4 infants in the CNEP group within 1 hour. No infants in the control group had such an improvement (RR 10.7, 95% CI 0.6–183.9, RD 0.27, 95% CI 0.02–0.51)
None of the patients in the CNEP group required assisted ventilation, whereas 1 infant in control group with nasal CPAP did require assisted ventilation.
Median duration of CNEP was 5 days, range 1 to 7 days
No complications have been reported

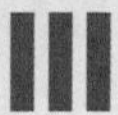

Author's conclusion

No recommendations can be made give the lack of evidence for non-invasive ventilation modes in infants and children with AHRF. The uncontrolled evidence available that suggests improvements in oxygenation, avoidance of intubation and reductions in hospital stay needs to be validated by large controlled trials

Problems & limitations

- Only 1 RCT and 33 patients

Advantages

- Highlights the lack of evidence for a potentially useful intervention

Expert opinion

Juan Balcells Ramírez

How valid and robust are the data?
This review found only one eligible study involving 33 infants with a clinical diagnosis of bronchiolitis requiring a high fraction of Inspired oxygen. The randomization procedure of the study was not reported, blinding of intervention was not possible and information regarding masking of assessment of outcome was not certain. Therefore, this is a review based on a single, small, low quality study. Validity of the review should be questioned as it is based on weak data.

Should clinical practice be influenced by this?
By no means should clinical practice be influenced by data that can be considered anecdotal in terms of scientific evidence. Although continuous negative extrathoracic pressure may seem a potentially useful intervention, this review only highlights the lack of evidence supporting its use in clinical practice.

What's the next step?
Properly designed and sized clinical trials focused on specific populations should be carried out before continuous negative extrathoracic pressure may be considered a useful therapy for acute hypoxemic respiratory failure in children.

Citation

Shah PS, Ohlsson A, Shah JP. Continuous negative extrathoracic pressure or continuous positive airway pressure for acute hypoxemic respiratory failure in children. Cochrane Database of Systematic Reviews 2008, Issue 1. Art. No.: CD003699. DOI: 10.1002/14651858.CD003699.pub3.

AMSTAR: methodological quality of the review

1.	Was "a priori" design provided?	Y
2.	Was study selection and data extraction adequate?	Y
3.	Was the literature search comprehensive?	Y
4.	Was 'Grey Literature' used?	Y
5.	Was a list of excluded studies provided?	Y
6.	Were the characteristics of included studies provided?	Y
7.	Was the scientific quality of studies assessed & documented?	Y
8.	Was the scientific quality of studies weighted appropriately in forming conclusions?	NA
9.	Were the methods used for data synthesis appropriate?	NA
10.	Was the potential for publication bias assessed?	Y
11.	Were any conflicts of interest stated?	Y

Overall quality of trials included	Low
Overall quality of the review	High

12

Heliox for croup

Condition: croup
Intervention: heliox
Clinical question: Does heliox relieve the distressful symptoms of croup?

Croup or larygnotracheobronchitis triggered by a variety of viral infections affects children up to the age of 6 years old. Symptoms occur as a result of inflammation and oedema of the subglottic mucosa causing airway narrowing and respiratory distress. Significant airway narrowing leads to increased work of breathing, fatigue and eventually respiratory failure necessitating intubation and ventilation. Corticosteroids have been shown to improve the symptoms of croup however they take time to work. Supportive treatment consists of supplemental oxygen and nebulised adrenaline in the more severe cases.

Helium is an inert very low density gas, such than when mixed with oxygen results in heliox which is 3 fold less dense than air. Reducing the density of inhaled gas results in more laminar flow with less resistance and may thus reduce the work of breathing.

Review characteristics

- **Eligibility criteria:** RCTs or quasi-RCTs comparing heliox with placebo or active treatment
- **Exclusions:** other causes of airway obstruction such as epiglottitis, or inhaled foreign body
- **Population:** children with a clinical diagnosis of croup (aged 6 months to 4 years)
- **Number of studies:** 2 RCTs
- **Number of patients:** 44 (15 & 29)
- **Study dates:** 1998 & 2001

Definition

- **Croup score:** each study used a different scoring system: Westley 1978 and Taussig 1975
- **Intervention:** heliox (70% helium/30% oxygen)
- **Control:** humidified oxygen in one study and oxygen + nebulised adrenaline in the other study

12

Results

Primary outcome: change in croup score

Combined analysis was not possible. Both studies showed an improvement in croup score in the heliox group however this was either not statistically significant or transient.

Secondary outcomes

There were no differences in symptoms of severity such as heart rate, respiratory rate or oxygen saturations.

No adverse events were reported.

Author's conclusion

There is insufficient evidence to make any recommendation regarding the use of heliox in croup. A greater reduction in croup score was observed in both studies although this didn't reach statistical significance in 1 study (n = 15) it is likely that this study was underpowered resulting in a type 2 error; the apparent statistical significance of this result in the second study (n = 29) cannot be evaluated due to lack of data.

Problems & limitations

- Participant numbers were extremely small
- Significant clinical heterogeneity between studies: 1 study used heliox versus humidified oxygen and no other treatment, whereas the other compared heliox to oxygen and nebulised adrenaline and both groups had received intramuscular dexamethasone
- Duration and method of delivery of heliox also varied considerably and may have been suboptimal
- 1 study excluded children with severe croup which is the group that may benefit most; and the other excluded those who required rescue nebulisation

Advantages

- Heliox (70% helium/30% oxygen) was used in both studies

Citation

Vorwerk C, Coats T. Heliox for croup in children. Cochrane Database of Systematic Reviews 2010, Issue 2. Art.No.:CD006822. DOI: 10.1002/14651858.CD006822.pub2.

Additional information

Resistance to flow depends upon both physical dimensions of the airway lumen and characteristics of the fluid which flow through it. Flow in the respiratory tract is principally laminar, which is associated with lower resistance. Laminar flow is more likely to occur in a short wide lumen through which a fluid of lower density and higher viscosity flows. [Laminar flow in physics is described by the Hagen-Poiseuille principle]

Turbulence, which is associated with higher resistance and is more likely to occur in a narrower lumen, where kinks, bends or irregularities occur and where fluid density and velocity are high such as during forced inspiration. [The likelihood of turbulence to occur is described by a dimensionless number known as Raynold's Number]

AMSTAR: methodological quality of the review

1.	Was "a priori" design provided?	Y
2.	Was study selection and data extraction adequate?	Y
3.	Was the literature search comprehensive?	Y
4.	Was 'Grey Literature' used?	Y
5.	Was a list of excluded studies provided?	Y
6.	Were the characteristics of included studies provided?	Y
7.	Was the scientific quality of studies assessed & documented?	Y
8.	Was the scientific quality of studies weighted appropriately in forming conclusions?	Y
9.	Were the methods used for data synthesis appropriate?	NA
10.	Was the potential for publication bias assessed?	Y
11.	Were any conflicts of interest stated?	Y

Overall quality of trials included	Low
Overall quality of the review	High

Bacterial meningitis

Condition: bacterial meningitis
Intervention: antibiotics
Clinical question: Is a short course of antibiotic treatment safe?

Community-acquired bacterial meningitis is common in children particularly in developing countries; and is associated with significant morbidity and mortality. Current recommendations are based on observational studies and recommend 7 days antibiotic therapy for Neisseria meningitidis and 7–14 days for Haemophilus influenzae or Streptococcus pneumoniae. Reducing the duration of therapy will have a beneficial impact on healthcare resources especially in countries where these resources are limited.

Review characteristics

- **Eligibility criteria:** RCTs comparing short versus long course of antibiotics for community-acquired bacterial meningitis that used the same antibiotic, dose and route of administration in both groups
- **Population:** children aged 3 weeks up to age 16 years
- **Number of studies:** 5 RCTs (in 5 different countries)
- **Number of patients:** 383 (range 52–119)
- **Study dates:** 1985–2002

Definitions

- **Short course:** up to 7 days
- **Long course:** at least 2 days longer than the short course
- **Bacterial meningitis:** clinical manifestations (fever, headache, altered mental state or meningeal irritation) + evidence of bacterial aetiology (positive CSF Gram stain, culture or LAT) or positive BC + CSF abnormality (increased neutrophils, and protein with reduced glucose)
- **Clinical success:** complete recovery or substantial improvement in symptoms and signs
- **Clinical outcomes:** were determined at the end of therapy (therefore shorter time in the group receiving a short course of ABx)

Results

Primary outcome

Outcome	Trials	N	Result
Clinical success	5	383	No difference

Fig. 1 Meta-analysis of the end-of-therapy clinical success in patients with bacterial meningitis treated with short-course versus long-course antibiotic regimens. Horizontal lines, 95% CI; squares, point-estimates; size of the squares, weight of the study in the meta-analysis; diamond, pooled odds ratio (OR) plus 95% CI; vertical line, "no difference' line between compared treatments; area to the right of the vertical line indicates higher clinical success for short-course regimens [reproduced from Karageorgopoulos DE, Valkimadi PE, Kapaskelis A, Rafailidis PI, Falagas ME. Short versus long duration of antibiotic therapy for bacterial meningitis: a meta-analysis of randomised controlled trials in children. Arch Dis Child 2009;94:607–614. doi:10.1136/adc.2008.151563, with permission from BMJ Publishing Group Ltd]

Study & year	Short course n/N	Long course n/N	OR (fixed) 95% CI	Weight (%)	OR (fixed) 95% CI
Lin et al. 1985	31/35	29/35		13.63	1.60 (0.41, 6.26)
Kavaliotis et al. 1989	23/26	25/26		11.86	0.31 (0.03, 3.16)
Martin et al. 1990	39/47	37/45		26.46	1.05 (0.36, 3.10)
Roine et al. 2000	46/53	35/47		20.15	2.25 (0.80, 6.31)
Singhi et al. 2002	26/35	26/34		27.89	0.89 (0.30, 2.66)
Total (95% CI)	**196**	**187**		**100.00**	**1.24 (0.73, 2.11)**

Total events: 165 (short course), 152 (long course)

Test for heterogeneity: $\chi^2 = 3.25$, df = 4 ($p = 0.52$); $I^2 = 0\%$

Test for overall effect: $Z = 0.78$ ($p = 0.44$)

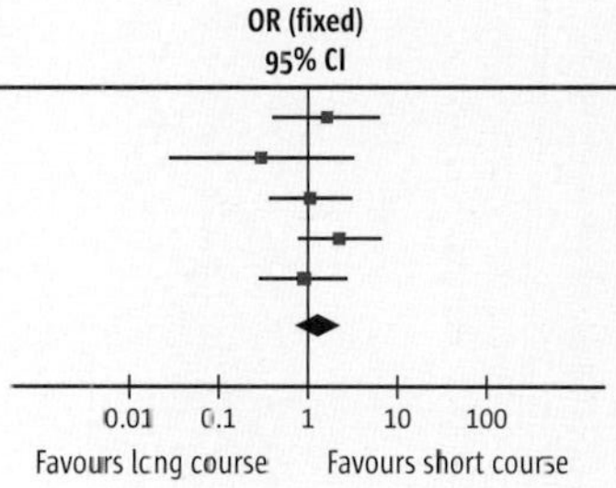

0.01 0.1 1 10 100

Favours long course Favours short course

12

Secondary outcomes

Outcome	Trials	N	Result
Mortality	2	153	Only 2 deaths reported
Abnormal CSF	1	52	Persistently abnormal CSF in 5 patients who received a short course of ABx versus 1 who received a long course
Hospitalisation	2	137	Significantly shorter in those receiving a short course of ABx (FEM WMD −2.17 days, 95% CI −3.85 to −0.50)
Adverse events	2	122	No difference
Secondary infection	2	139	No difference
Hearing impairment	4	241	No difference
Neurological impairment	5	367	No difference

Sensitivity analysis for studies with low versus high methodological quality did not change the results.

Author's conclusion

There was no difference in clinical outcomes between those receiving either a short or long course of antibiotics. Shorter antibiotic regimes did however significantly reduce the duration of hospitalization. Overall, the data quality and quantity is not enough to strongly adhere to these findings. Several other trials (not included here) have also found no difference between short and long courses of antibiotic therapy but most of these related to patients with meningococcal meningitis.

Problems & limitations

- 3 of the studies were open-label
- In 2 studies randomization was after the initial course of antibiotics: 1 study only randomised patients with rapid initial recovery; in the other study those with positive CSF culture after 15 hours of treatment were excluded, therefore patients with severe disease or potentially resistant organisms are under-represented
- In 1 trial (n = 102) most patients received intravenous dexamethasone
- Follow up timing varied from day of discharge to 6 months post discharge

Advantages

- All the trials used intravenous ceftriaxone and used short courses of 4–7 days versus long courses 7–14 days
- Most RCTs included N meningitidis, S pneumoniae and H influenzae; only one did not include patients with N meningitidis
- Statistical between-studies heterogeneity of outcomes was very low

Expert opinion

Joan Balcells Ramírez

How valid and robust are the data?

This review and meta-analysis found 5 open-label RCTs involving children conducted over a 17-year period in five different countries. All the trials were on community-acquired bacterial meningitis treated with the same antibiotic in the same daily dosage, being the duration of therapy the only difference in the intervention. In addition, statistical between-studies heterogeneity of outcomes was very low. Thus, the data should be considered valid.

Should clinical practise be influenced by this?

This review supports the concept that short course treatment for bacterial meningitis can be used without compromising relevant outcomes such as: clinical success and hearing or neurological impairment. Nevertheless, between-studies differences in patient selection for short course antibiotics and differences in dexamethasone use as well as the inability to analyse data by causative organism should warn against routine applicability of the study findings in medical practice.

What's the next step?

Morbidity and/or mortality related to inappropriate courses of antibiotic treatment should be considered unacceptable. Properly designed RCTs should address the issues of precise criteria for adequate patient selection in relation to specific causative organism.

Citation

Karageorgopoulos DE, Valkimadi PE, Kapaskelis A, Rafailidis PI, Falagas ME (2009) Short versus long duration of antibiotic therapy for bacterial meningitis: a meta-analysis of randomised controlled trials in children. Arch Dis Child;94:607–614. doi:10.1136/adc.2008.151563

Additional information

An international multicentre RCT sponsored by WHO is underway to evaluate 5 versus 10 days of ceftriaxone treatment for bacterial meningitis in children. ISRCTN38717320.

12

AMSTAR: methodological quality of the review

1.	Was "a priori" design provided?	Y
2.	Was study selection and data extraction adequate?	Y
3.	Was the literature search comprehensive?	Y
4.	Was 'Grey Literature' used? Limited to English and fully published articles	P
5.	Was a list of excluded studies provided?	N
6.	Were the characteristics of included studies provided?	Y
7.	Was the scientific quality of studies assessed & documented?	Y
8.	Was the scientific quality of studies weighted appropriately in forming conclusions?	Y
9.	Were the methods used for data synthesis appropriate?	Y
10.	Was the potential for publication bias assessed?	Y
11.	Were any conflicts of interest stated?	N

Overall quality of trials included	2 low and 3 high (Jadad score)
Overall quality of the review	Moderate-high

Nutritional support for critically ill children

Condition: critical illness
Intervention: nutrition
Clinical question: What is the impact of enteral nutrition (EN) and parenteral nutrition (PN) given in the first week of critical illness on mortality?

Administration of nutrition in critically ill children is often considered a priority however this has been questioned because metabolic requirements change. The measured metabolic rate for critically ill children is often at or below basal metabolic rate; not higher as was previously thought. Overfeeding is not without its risks; carbohydrates can impede ventilator weaning, protein does not completely prevent catabolism, and high calorific intake can increase fat deposition in the liver and worsen inflammation. Both animal and human studies have suggested that underfeeding in critical illness may improve survival. Nutritional support improves immune function, wound healing and measured proteins; and malnutrition is associated with poor outcomes. Whether nutritional support during the first week of critical illness improves clinically meaningful outcomes is unclear. "The point at which 'safe' starvation ends and malnutrition related complications begin has yet to be defined" (Preiser 2003).

Review characteristics

- **Eligibility criteria:** RCTs where EN or PN where administered within 7 days. In the only study included, EN within 24 hours of admission was compared to standard care
- **Exclusions:** studies that did not specify predetermined outcomes; studies examining immunonutrition or routes of EN delivery. Studies of premature or low birth weight neonates
- **Population:** critically ill children in PICU
- **Number of studies:** 1 RCT
- **Number of patients:** 72 (with > 25% BSA burns)
- **Study date:** published 2002 (data collected over 10 years)

Definition

- **Standard Care:** no tube feeding or oral diet for at least 48 hours

12

Results

Primary outcome: 30 day mortality

No statistically significant difference.

Secondary outcomes

No statistically significant difference in any other outcomes such as sepsis, ventilator days, length of stay or adverse events.

Author's conclusion

It seems intuitive that nutritional support early during critical illness would be beneficial but there is limited data upon which to form any opinion. Critically ill children do not experience hypermetabolism; furthermore metabolism and mitochondrial function are altered.

Problems & limitations

- Lack of trials addressing this question

Advantages

- 1 trial identified during the search comparing gastric versus small-bowel feeding found that more calories were provide to the small-bowel feeding group and they showed a trend towards increased mortality, ventilator days and LOS supporting the hypothesis that feeding may in fact be harmful in certain circumstances

Citation

Joffe A, Anton N, Lequier L, Vandermeer B, Tjosvold L, Larsen B, Hartling L. Nutritional support for critically ill children. Cochrane Database of Systematic Reviews 2009, Issue 2. Art. No.: CD005144. DOI: 10.1002/14651858.CD005144.pub2.

Additional information

See Section 10: Early enteral nutrition: Early EN provided within 24 hours of injury or ICU admission significantly reduces mortality in critically ill patients.

The nutritional needs of children and adults with critical illness may be different in many ways: in terms of responses to critical illness; underlying co-morbidities; pre-existing energy reserves and metabolic demands.

AMSTAR: methodological quality of the review

1.	Was "a priori" design provided?	Y
2.	Was study selection and data extraction adequate?	Y
3.	Was the literature search comprehensive?	Y
4.	Was 'Grey Literature' used?	Y
5.	Was a list of excluded studies provided?	Y
6.	Were the characteristics of included studies provided?	Y
7.	Was the scientific quality of studies assessed & documented?	Y
8.	Was the scientific quality of studies weighted appropriately in forming conclusions?	NA
9.	Were the methods used for data synthesis appropriate?	NA
10.	Was the potential for publication bias assessed?	Y
11.	Were any conflicts of interest stated?	Y

Overall quality of trials included	1 RCT: Low quality on Jadad scale
Overall quality of the review	High

Other relevant reviews

The following reviews also included paediatric populations

Section 2: Acute respiratory failure (ARF) – Acute respiratory distress syndrome (ARDS)
Inhaled nitric oxide
Aerosolized prostacyclin

Section 3: Acute respiratory failure – Non-ARDS
Corticosteroids for pneumonia
Corticosteroids to prevent and treat post extubation stridor
Corticosteroids to prevent extubation failure
Heated humidification versus HME

Section 4: Cardiovascular dynamics
Vasopressin for vasodilatory shock

Section 5: Ethics
Organ donation

Section 8: Infection
Procalcitonin

Section 13. Sepsis
Albumin for fluid resuscitation

13

Sepsis

Early versus late broad spectrum antibiotics 268
Combination antibiotics 270
De-escalation of antibiotics 275
Albumin for fluid resuscitation 278
Corticosteroids for severe sepsis & septic shock 283
Granulocyte & granulocyte-macrophage colony stimulating factor 292

Also see:
Section 4: Cardiovascular dynamics
Vasopressin for vasodilatory shock
Section 8: Infection

Early versus late broad spectrum antibiotics

Condition: severe sepsis

Intervention: early antibiotic therapy

Clinical question: Is there any evidence to support the use of early antibiotics in patients with severe sepsis who are bound for ICU?

The recommendations in the surviving sepsis guidelines reinforce that antibiotics should be given within 1–3 hours (sepsis resuscitation bundle) in adults with severe sepsis seen in the emergency department.

Review characteristics

- **Eligibility criteria:** RCTs
- **Population:** adults with severe sepsis bound for ICU
- **Number of studies:** 0
- **Number of patients:** 0

Definitions

- **Severe sepsis:** according to SCCM criteria of SIRS plus organ failure or haemodynamic instability
- **Early:** within 1 hour of ED admission
- **Late:** greater than 1 hour after ED admission

Main findings

- There were no studies that fulfilled the inclusion criteria
- **Primary Outcomes would have been:** mortality at 28 and hospital LOS
- **Secondary Outcomes would have been:** development of MOF and ICU LOS

Authors' conclusion

There is no level 1 evidence for the use of early antibiotics in severe sepsis; however, there are a number of trials that support early antibiotic administration in similar groups. A major challenge is the accurate diagnosis of sepsis or SIRS, thus the use of antibiotics too early may lead to unnecessary administration in other disease states that can mimic sepsis such as MI or PE, furthermore, antibiotic selection is often random.

Problems & limitations

- It is very difficult and indeed unethical to conduct a trial that knowingly provides the control group with inferior therapy such as placebo or even late antibiotics when the general consensus is that early and targeted antibiotics result in better outcomes
- This review has not considered observational studies which although not ideal, nevertheless do contribute significantly to our understanding of disease and its management

Advantages

- Good review of the other literature pertaining to sepsis and septic shock

Expert opinion

Jordi Rello

How valid and robust are the data?
There were no RCTs, and observational studies were not considered. Septic shock was considered to be an exclusion criterion. This is a severe limitation that might influence findings. Early antibiotic therapy is defined as one started within 1 hour. This is very strict. The surviving sepsis campaign defines it as within three hours of arrival to ED.

Should clinical practice be influenced by this?
No

What's the next step in the management of these patients? What's next in general?
In severe sepsis antibiotics should be administered early. A more relevant topic for RCTs is the duration of antibiotic therapy.

Citation

Early versus late pre-intensive care unit admission broad spectrum antibiotics for severe sepsis in adults. Cochrane Database of Systematic Reviews 2010, Issue 10. Art. No.: CD007081. DOI. 10.1002/14651858.CD007081.pub2.

AMSTAR: methodological quality of the review

1.	Was "a priori" design provided?	Y
2.	Was study selection and data extraction adequate?	NA
3.	Was the literature search comprehensive?	Y
4.	Was 'Grey Literature' used?	NA
5.	Was a list of excluded studies provided?	NA
6.	Where the characteristics of included studies provided?	NA
7.	Was the scientific quality of studies assessed & documented?	NA
8.	Was the scientific quality of studies weighted appropriately in forming conclusions?	NA
9.	Were the methods used for data synthesis appropriate?	NA
10.	Was the potential for publication bias assessed?	NA
11.	Were any conflicts of interest stated?	Y

Overall quality of trials	NA
Overall quality of review	High

Combination antibiotics

Condition: sepsis or septic shock
Intervention: combination antibiotics
Clinical question: Should combination antibiotics be used for all cases of sepsis or only the most severe cases i.e. those with septic shock?

It is common practice to use combination antibiotic therapy to treat patients with sepsis and septic shock. The rational for this is to increase the spectrum of coverage, however many of the antibiotics in current use inherently have broad cover. Some studies do support combination therapy in specific conditions such as endocarditis and neutropenic sepsis but generally if an organism is susceptible to one agent, any benefit of a second drug is questionable. Efficacy of some treatments such as immunomodulatory therapy of sepsis has been identified as contingent on the severity of illness and risk of death and this may apply also to combination antibiotic therapy.

Review characteristics

- **Eligibility criteria**: randomized and observational studies, all aetiologies of bacterial sepsis or septic shock, comparing single versus combination therapy
- **Exclusions**: Studies of endocarditis or meningitis because mechanism of death in these is not primarily sepsis. Studies where a 'superior' agent was compared with a combination that included an 'inferior' agent
- **Population**: sepsis and septic shock
- **Number of studies**: 50 studies (13 RCTs, 33 retrospective cohort studies, 14 prospective observational studies)
  Data from 12 studies were split into mutually exclusive groups according to presence of shock or severity of illness giving 62 datasets
- **Number of patients**: 8504 (4553 monotherapy, 3951 combination therapy) Range 16–1111
- **Study dates**: 1 from 1974, the rest between 1982–2007

Definition

- **Combination therapy**: two or more bactericidal antibiotics of different antimicrobial class and mechanism of action; causative organism had to be sensitive to both

Results

Primary outcome: pooled OR for mortality/clinical failure

No significant advantage to combination therapy but stratification of datasets by monotherapy mortality changes these results

When monotherapy mortality < 15%: favours monotherapy

When monotherapy mortality 15–25%: no difference between mono or combination therapy

When monotherapy mortality > 25%: significant advantage of combination therapy

(OR 0.54; 95% CI 0.45– 0.66; $p < 0.0001$; $I^2 = 0\%$)

Stratification by presence or absence of each of critical illness and shock showed a significant advantage to combination therapy in the more ill group.

Consolidation of combined shock and critically ill datasets gave similar results (OR 0.51; 95% CI 0.36–0.72; $p < 0.0002$; $I^2 = 0\%$)

Further analysis

There was statistically significant heterogeneity among eligible datasets

However, stratification of datasets in terms of mortality resulted in a marked decrease in heterogeneity as illustrated by the results above where $I^2 = 0\%$

No other stratification resulted in reduced heterogeneity in all strata

Observational studies: high heterogeneity and no benefit to combination therapy shown

RCTs: low heterogeneity and no benefit to combination therapy shown

Exploratory subgroup analysis by date for studies before and after 1993 when more potent antibiotics became widely available showed no difference

Stratification by antimicrobial class or clinical syndrome e.g. CAP versus VAP showed no difference

Meta regression results support all these findings.

Author's conclusion

Combination antibiotic therapy reduces mortality in those with serious bacterial sepsis but only in the group that are at the highest risk of death such as those with septic shock and therefore presumably a higher pathogen burden. Antibiotic combinations particularly beta-lactams with aminoglycosides, fluoroquinolones and macrolides can act synergistically to accelerate pathogen clearance. Combination therapy however, may be detrimental to low-risk patients (those with < 15% mortality risk with monotherapy). The mechanism for this survival disadvantage is unclear and appears most likely related to drug toxicity in low risk patients.

Fig. 1 Subset analysis comparing combination antibiotic therapy with monotherapy for reducing mortality of life-threatening infections associated with sepsis in shock/critically ill and non-shock/non-critically ill patient datasets (derived from 12 studies in which groups could be separated), [with kind permission from Anand Kumar, Nasia Safdar, Shravan Kethireddy, Dan Chateau. A survival benefit of combination antibiotic therapy for serious infections associated with sepsis and septic shock is contingent only on the risk of death: A meta-analytic/meta-regression study. Crit Care Med 2010 Vol. 38, No. 8 1651]

Group	Monotherapy Mortality (%)	Combination Therapy Mortality (%)	Odds ratio	I^2 (%)	P-value
Non-shock	86/680 (12.6)	96/666 (14.4)	1.06 [0.73–1.52]	13.7	.7721
Shock	96/188 (51.1)	177/422 (41.9)	0.56 [0.39–0.83]	0.8	.0043
Non-critically ill	23/313 (7.3)	35/339 (10.3)	1.10 [0.46–2.60]	45.3	.8321
Critically ill	32/64 (50.0)	34/128 (26.6)	0.33 [0.15–0.74]	0	.0067
Non-shock/Non-critically ill	109/993 (11.0)	131/1005 (13.0)	1.06 [0.76–1.47]	19.1	.7178
Shock/Critically ill	128/252 (50.1)	211/550 (38.4)	0.51 [0.36–0.72]	0	.0002
Overall	**237/1245 (19.0)**	**342/1555 (22.0)**	**0.76 [0.57–1.02]**	**33.8**	**.0622**

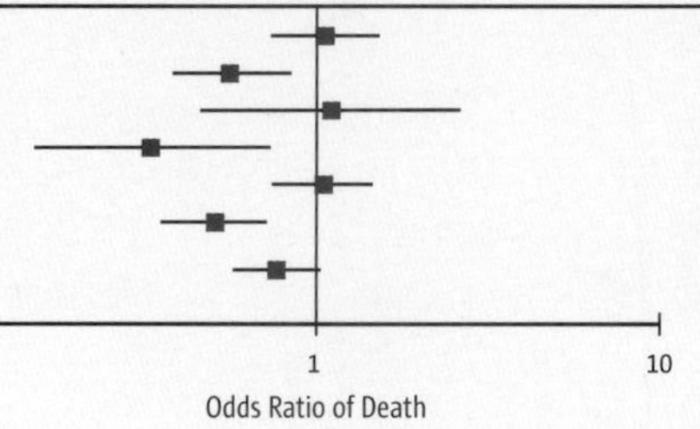

0.1 1 10

Odds Ratio of Death

Problems & limitations

- Large number of observational studies, particularly retrospective studies
- In 14 studies (19 datasets) the microbiological sensitivities of organisms was inferred, not confirmed, however exclusion of those datasets involving inferred rather than confirmed (i.e. proven) microbiological sensitivity did not alter the findings

Advantages

- Datasets were split into mutually exclusive groups according to severity of illness, which differed to previous meta-analyses which focused on specific clinical syndromes such as community acquired pneumonia
- Statistical analysis of stratified datasets consistently gave the same results

Expert opinion

George Dimopoulos

How valid and robust are the data?
Data we have to keep in mind but without strong evidence for our clinical practice.

Should clinical practice be influenced by this?
No.

What is the next step?
An RCT in order to answer the question of whether or not antibiotic combinations indicate superiority compared to monotherapy.

Citation

Anand Kumar, Nasia Safdar, Shravan Kethireddy, Dan Chateau. A survival benefit of combination antibiotic therapy for serious infections associated with sepsis and septic shock is contingent only on the risk of death. A meta-analytic/meta-regression study. Crit Care Med 2010 Vol. 38, No. 8 1651 DOI: 10.1097/CCM.0b013e3181e96b91

AMSTAR: methodological quality of the review

1.	Was "a priori" design provided?	Y
2.	Was study selection and data extraction adequate?	Y
3.	Was the literature search comprehensive?	Y
4.	Was 'Grey Literature' used?	Y
5.	Was a list of excluded studies provided?	Y
6.	Where the characteristics of included studies provided?	Y
7.	Was the scientific quality of studies assessed & documented?	N
8.	Was the scientific quality of studies weighted appropriately in forming conclusions?	U
9.	Were the methods used for data synthesis appropriate?	Y
10.	Was the potential for publication bias assessed?	Y
11.	Were any conflicts of interest stated?	Y

Overall quality of trials included	Unclear/Variable
Overall quality of the review	High

De-escalation of antibiotics

Condition: sepsis, severe sepsis or septic shock

Clinical question: Is de-escalation of antimicrobial therapy safe?

Severe sepsis and septic shock are associated with mortality rates of 27% and 54% respectively in European countries and may be higher in developing countries. The most prevalent pathogen species implicated are: *Staphylococcus; Escherichia Coli; Candida; Pseudomonas; Acinetobacter; Streptococcus; Klebsiella; Enterococcus.; Enterobacter* and *Proteus*. In order to identify the pathogen causing sepsis, it is standard practice is to take appropriate cultures before commencing antibiotics. In severe sepsis this should not delay treatment administration; however it is important to be aware that blood cultures will become sterile within hours of antibiotic administration. Broad spectrum antibiotics are often used initially to ensure adequate cover for probable infections. Once the organism is identified and sensitivities are known, surviving sepsis guidelines recommend de-escalation: changing the antibiotic regimen to a narrower spectrum therapy by changing the antimicrobial agent or discontinuing a combination. The purpose of de-escalation is to reduce the problems associated with antimicrobial overuse such as emerging pathogen resistance and adverse events.

Review characteristics

- **Eligibility criteria:** RCTs or quasi-randomized trials comparing
- **Exclusions:** studies where patients were treated with empirical but inadequate antimicrobial therapy
- **Population:** adult patients with sepsis, severe sepsis or septic shock
- **Number of studies:** There were no eligible studies

Because of the lack of studies, non-randomized studies that expressed the idea of a 'more restrictive' or 'rational' use of antimicrobials or of adjustment of initial empirical therapy were considered. 42 references were identified, most of which were narratives. 12 were cohort studies but their interventions were not of interest.

Definitions in this review

- **De-escalation:** changing appropriate broad-spectrum antibiotic therapy to a narrower-spectrum one (by either changing the antimicrobial agent or discontinuing an eventual antimicrobial combination or both) according to culture results or shortening the time course of therapy
- **Standard therapy:** maintenance of initial broad-spectrum empirical treatment

13

Author's conclusion

There is no direct evidence as to whether de-escalation is effective or safe for patients with sepsis, severe sepsis or septic shock.

Expert opinion

Ricard Ferrer

How valid and robust are the data?
There were no randomized controlled trials testing de-escalation antimicrobial treatment for adult patients diagnosed with sepsis, severe sepsis or septic shock could be included in the meta-analysis.

Should clinical practice be influenced by this?
The current recommendation is to de-escalate empirical antimicrobial therapy on the basis of culture results and elimination of redundant combination therapy, because one can more effectively target the causative pathogen, resulting in decreased antimicrobial exposure and substantial cost savings. Despite the fact that this recommendation is not based on randomized controlled trials, there is enough rationale to maintain it.

What is the next step?
It is necessary to establish the real impact of de-escalation on antimicrobial resistance development, its true cost-effectiveness profile, and whether it genuinely does improve clinical outcomes. Significant work needs to be done to establish the most effective tools to implement de-escalation, particularly in terms of providing clear guidelines to clinicians to enable them to be confident in applying this manoeuver.

See also

Review summary on Combination Antibiotic therapy for serious infections associated with sepsis and septic shock.

Citation

Gomes Silva BN, Andriolo RB, Atallah ÁN, Salomão R. De-escalation of antimicrobial treatment for adults with sepsis, severe sepsis or septic shock. Cochrane Database of Systematic Reviews 2010, Issue 12. Art. No.: CD007934. DOI: 10.1002/14651858.CD007934.pub2

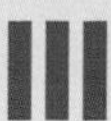

AMSTAR: methodological quality of the review

1.	Was "a priori" design provided?	Y
2.	Was study selection and data extraction adequate?	Y
3.	Was the literature search comprehensive?	Y
4.	Was 'Grey Literature' used?	NA
5.	Was a list of excluded studies provided?	Y
6.	Where the characteristics of included studies provided?	NA
7.	Was the scientific quality of studies assessed & documented?	NA
8.	Was the scientific quality of studies weighted appropriately in forming conclusions?	NA
9.	Were the methods used for data synthesis appropriate?	NA
10.	Was the potential for publication bias assessed?	NA
11.	Were any conflicts of interest stated? No conflicts	Y

Overall quality of trials included	NA
Overall quality of the review	High

Albumin for fluid resuscitation

Intervention: albumin

Clinical question: Does resuscitation with albumin containing solutions compared to other fluids improve outcome in patients with sepsis?

Fluid resuscitation is one of the fundamental components of treating patients with sepsis as demonstrated by goal directed therapy. The Surviving Sepsis Guidelines recommend the use of crystalloid or colloid for early resuscitation in sepsis. These are largely based on the SAFE study which showed no difference in mortality in a mixed population of intensive care patients between those resuscitated with 4% human albumin and 0.9% saline. While the limitations of subgroup analysis are well recognised; subgroup analysis of patients with severe sepsis suggested that albumin may be beneficial.

Review characteristics

- **Eligibility criteria**: RCTs that compared fluid resuscitation with albumin containing fluids compared to other fluid regimens. Including studies where the group with sepsis was a subgroup within a larger population
- **Exclusions**: studies where mortality data were not available
- **Population**: children or adults with sepsis, severe sepsis or septic shock. 1 study of patients with ARDS, 1 study included all patients who required fluid resuscitation (SAFE); and 1 study included septic and non-septic patients that required fluid resuscitation
- **Number of studies**: 17 studies (8 primarily conducted on a population with sepsis; 9 where patients with sepsis were a subgroup of a larger population)
  8 studies (n = 383) used 20% albumin; 9 studies (n = 1594) that use 4%, 4.5% or 5% albumin
- **Number of patients**: 1977 (range 26–150)
- **Study dates**: 1983–2009

Definition

- **Sepsis**: presumed consensus definition

Results

Primary outcome: pooled OR for all-cause mortality for patient resuscitated with albumin versus other fluids

Trials	OR	95% CI	p	I^2
All studies	0.82	0.67–1.0	0.047	0%
With SAFE study removed	0.84	0.59–1.18	0.31	–
Random effects model to pool all studies	0.84	0.69–1.02	0.08	–
Studies that used 20% albumin	1.08	0.7–1.68	0.73	–
Studies that used more dilute albumin	0.76	0.61–0.95	0.02	–
15 adult studies (n = 1729)	0.87	0.71–1.07	0.18	–
3 Paediatric studies (n = 248)	0.29	0.12–0.72	0.008	–

Tab. 1 Pooled estimates of the effect of resuscitation fluid regimens compared with albumin in patients with sepsis [with kind permission from Anthony P. Delaney, Arina Dan, John McCaffrey, Simon Finfer. The role of albumin as a resuscitation fluid for patients with sepsis: A systematic review and meta-analysis. Crit Care Med 2011; 39:386–391]

Fluid	Number of Studies	Total Participants	I^2	Estimate of Odds Ratio	95% Confidence Limits	p
Crystalloid	7	1441	0%	0.78	0.62–0.99	.04
Starch	12	463	0%	1.04	0.7–1.54	.84
Gelofusine	2	100	40.1%	0.27	0.06–1.14	.08

Author's conclusion

The statistically significant primary analysis result suggests that resuscitation with albumin may result in lower mortality compared with other fluids. This may be explained by the important physiological role of albumin in the circulation as a drug binder and transporter of active molecules; as a free radical scavenger; as an inhibitor of platelet aggregation and in maintenance of colloid osmotic pressure.

Problems & limitations

- Many included studies had patients with sepsis as subgroups
- Further analyses did not give statistically significant results
- There were no data on other outcomes or potential adverse effects

Advantages

- There was no evidence of statistically significant heterogeneity
- Results did not change when the largest study (SAFE) was removed or with other sensitivity analysis

Fig. 2 Forest plot showing the pooled estimate of the effect of resuscitation with albumin-containing solutions on mortality for patients with sepsis. OR, odds ratio; CI, confidence limit [from Anthony P. Delaney, Arina Dan, John McCaffrey, Simon Finfer. The role of albumin as a resuscitation fluid for patients with sepsis: A systematic review and meta-analysis. Crit Care Med 2011; 39:386–391]

Study ID	OR 95% CI	Events, Albumin	Events, Control	Weight %
Rackow et al. (32)	2.08 [0.28, 15.77]	5/7	6/11	0.61
Metildi et al. (31)	0.45 [0.04, 5.81]	10/12	11/12	0.84
Rackow et al. (33)	1.00 [0.17, 5.77]	5/10	5/10	1.14
Boldt et al. (20)	1.00 [0.22, 4.56]	5/15	5/15	1.52
Boldt et al. (19)	0.73 [0.15, 3.49]	4/15	5/15	1.67
Boldt et al. (21)	1.33 [0.30, 5.91]	7/14	6/14	1.37
Boldt et al. (22)	0.72 [0.15, 3.54]	4/14	5/14	1.63
Boldt et al. (23)	1.88 [0.39, 9.01]	6/14	4/14	1.04
Boldt et al. (24)	1.29 [0.64, 2.58]	25/75	21/75	6.38
The SAFE study investigators (4)	0.81 [0.64, 1.03]	185/603	217/615	67.91
Veneman et al. (35)	1.31 [0.26, 6.72]	5/8	14/25	1.16
Maitland et al. (29)	1.19 [0.23, 6.11]	4/23	3/20	1.21
Maitland et al. (30)	0.17 [0.04, 0.80]	2/56	11/61	4.63
Akech et al. (26)	0.12 [0.01, 1.05]	1/44	7/44	3.12
Friedman et al. (28)	0.85 [0.23, 3.21]	5/15	10/27	2.17
van der Heijden et al. (34)	0.79 [0.11, 5.49]	2/6	7/18	1.06
Dolecek et al. (27)	0.51 [0.13, 2.07]	4/30	6/26	2.54
Overall (I^2 = 0.0%; P = 0.728)	**0.82 [0.67, 1.00]**	**279/961**	**343/1016**	**100**

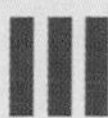

Expert opinion

Christiane Hartog

This is a well-performed, high-quality systematic review and meta-analysis which investigated all cause mortality for patients with severe sepsis who were resuscitated with regimens that included albumin solutions. The methodology of this analysis was flawless, including an adequate search strategy, validity assessment of included studies and appropriate statistical approaches to combine findings. Authors of primary studies were approached for missing information. Findings until April 2010 were included.

Seventeen studies that randomized 1977 participants were included. 8 studies included only patients with sepsis and in 9 studies patients with sepsis were a subgroup of the study population. There was no evidence of heterogeneity, $I^2 = 0\%$ ($I^2 > 50\%$ indicating heterogeneity). The use of albumin for resuscitation of patients with sepsis was associated with a reduction in mortality with the pooled estimate of the odds ratio of 0.82 (95% confidence limits 0.67–1.0, p = .047). Importantly, when 5 retracted studies by Boldt et al. were excluded, the findings remained unchanged (OR 0.76, 95% CI 0.62 to 0.95, p = .015).

The authors conclude that since the use of albumin-containing solutions for the resuscitation of patients with sepsis was associated with lower mortality compared with other fluid resuscitation regimens in this meta-analysis, clinicians should consider the use of albumin-containing solutions for the resuscitation of patients with sepsis until the results of on-going randomized controlled trials are known.

How valid and robust are the data?
The methodological quality of included studies was often not optimal. Two-thirds of the included patients came from a subgroup of the SAFE trial which, on the other hand, provided highest-quality data without major methodological limitations. Therefore, some doubt is cast on the robustness of these data.

Should clinical practice be influenced by this?
According to the authors' conclusions, clinicians may consider using albumin in patients with sepsis until the results of on-going RCTs are available. However, the considerably higher costs of albumin have to be weighed against its potential benefits. It is also unclear whether hyperoncotic albumin performs differently from albumin 4% or 5%. Observational data suggest that hyperoncotic albumin may be harmful (Schortgen F et al. The risk associated with hyperoncotic colloids in patients with shock. Intensive Care Med. 2008;34(12):2157–2168). Furthermore, there are unpublished data from a recent trial that investigated the effects of human albumin 20% in severe sepsis patients and could not demonstrate a beneficial effect.

What is the next step?
We should wait for the results from on-going trials to have evidence of higher quality on this important issue.

13

Citation

Anthony P. Delaney, Arina Dan, John McCaffrey, Simon Finfer. The role of albumin as a resuscitation fluid for patients with sepsis: A systematic review and meta-analysis. Crit Care Med 2011;39:386–391 DOI: 10.1097/CCM.0b013e3181ffe217

Additional information

The 3 trials of albumin in patients with sepsis that were on-going trials at the time of this review:

- The Efficacy of Albumin Administration for Volume Replacement in Patients with severe Sepsis and Septic Shock – the ALBumin Italian Outcome Sepsis Study (NCT00707122). Planned to enrol 1350 patients and should have finished in May 2010
- The Multicentre, Early Albumin Resuscitation During Septic Shock study (NCT00327704). This study recruited 794 patients in 27 ICUs in France and was completed in January 2011.
- The Five Percent Albumin versus Normal Saline as Fluid Resuscitation Strategies for the Management of Early Suspected Septic Shock (NCT00819416). This study recruited 47 patients and was completed in February 2010

AMSTAR: methodological quality of the review

1.	Was "a priori" design provided?	Y
2.	Was study selection and data extraction adequate?	Y
3.	Was the literature search comprehensive?	Y
4.	Was 'Grey Literature' used?	Y
5.	Was a list of excluded studies provided?	NA
6.	Where the characteristics of included studies provided?	Y
7.	Was the scientific quality of studies assessed & documented?	Y
8.	Was the scientific quality of studies weighted appropriately in forming conclusions?	Y
9.	Were the methods used for data synthesis appropriate?	Y
10.	Was the potential for publication bias assessed?	Y
11.	Were any conflicts of interest stated?	Y

Overall quality of trials included	Many suboptimal
Overall quality of the review	High

Corticosteroids for severe sepsis & septic shock

Condition: severe sepsis and septic shock
Intervention: corticosteroids (CS)
Clinical questions:
1. Does the use of corticosteroids in severe sepsis and septic shock improve short term mortality?
2. Does the dose and or duration of corticosteroids administration make any difference?

The current incidence of severe sepsis in industrialised countries ranges from 50 to 100 cases per 100,000 population, with a short term mortality of 20% to 50%. Death results from hypotension or progressive organ failure. In sepsis, the hypothalamic-pituitary gland hormonal pathway to the adrenal glands stimulates corticosteroid production. These hormones affect inflammation through the white blood cells, cytokines, and nitric oxide production. In septic shock, cytokines may suppress the cortisol response to adrenocorticotropin hormone and in almost half of patients this causes poor adrenal activity. Body tissues possibly become resistant to corticosteroids through fewer corticosteroid receptors or receptors with lower affinity.

Previous reviews have not identified any benefit of high dose corticosteroids however low dose regimes have shown promising results in several studies. Low dose corticosteroids can improve haemodynamics and organ function, modulated the inflammatory response favourably, and prolonged survival. Short courses of corticosteroids can cause rebound inflammation therefore it is postulated that not only the dose but also the duration of therapy may differentially affect patient response to treatment.

Review characteristics

- **Eligibility Criteria:** RCTs, quasi-randomized trials +/– blinding, ALI & ARDS trials if separate data on sepsis were available using any type of iv corticosteroid preparation
- **Population:** patients with severe sepsis and septic shock
- **Number of studies:** 22 RCTs included, 6 of these multicentre, 1 multinational (CORTICUS at 52 centres, n = 499); 12 excluded; and 10 on-going
- **Number of patients:** 2384
- **Study dates:** on low dose CS: 1998–2008; on high dose CS: 1971–1988

Population characteristics

- **7 trials:** severe sepsis + septic shock
- **2 trials:** severe sepsis
- **1 trial:** early ARDS + data for severe sepsis & septic shock
- **2 trials:** septic shock patients with adrenal insufficiency
- **10 trials:** vasopressor dependent shock (5 conducted corticotrophin tests)
- **9 trials:** prolonged/low dose of corticosteroid
- **5 trials:** prolonged/low dose + other corticosteroid e.g. fludrocortisone
- **1 trial:** hydrocortisone 50 mg qds for 3 versus 7 days (excluded for pooled outcome measures)

13

- **7 trials:** high dose methylpred. Dexamethasone or betamethasone

Definitions

- **Severe sepsis & Septic shock:** adequate in 21/22 trials. Inadequate in 1/22
- **Control:** standard intervention (fluids, antibiotics, vasopressors) or placebo
- **Short term mortality:** mortality at 28-day or at 14-day, at ICU or hospital discharge
- **Low dose corticosteroid:** total daily dose of 300 mg or less hydrocortisone or equivalent
- **Long course/prolonged course of corticosteroid:** full dose of treatment for at least 5 days

Results

Primary outcome: 28-day all mortality where data were available

20 trials were used for pooled outcome measures.

Trials	n	Study Gp mortality (mean)	Control Gp mortality (mean)	RR	95% CI	*p*	I²
17 RCTs	2138	35.5%	38.5%	0.84	0.71–1.00	0.05	53%
3 Quasi	246	23.1%	19.2%	1.05	0.69–1.58	0.83	-
Long dose/ Short course CS 12 RCTs	1228	37.5%	44.1%	0.84	0.72–0.97	0.02	15%
11 RCTs*	1182			0.87	0.77–0.98	0.02	1%
Short course/ high dose CS 7 Trials	1043	33.2 %	31.5 %	0.94	0.69–1.30	-	68%

*Results with the study on community acquired pneumonia removed

Primary outcomes: if no 28-day mortality data was available, 14-day or hospital mortality was used to compute the pooled analysis on 28 day mortality

Sub-group analysis: to identify heterogeneity; subjected to strict criteria; GRADE approach applied to evaluate the evidence. Justification: Older trial used high doses (as anti-inflammatory) and short courses, newer trials used low doses for longer as physiological replacement

13

Meta-regression: relationship between steroid dose and magnitude of effect:

- Confirmed lower RR of dying with prolonged treatment at full dose ($p = 0.02$) and with lower dose of corticosteroid ($p = 0.02$)

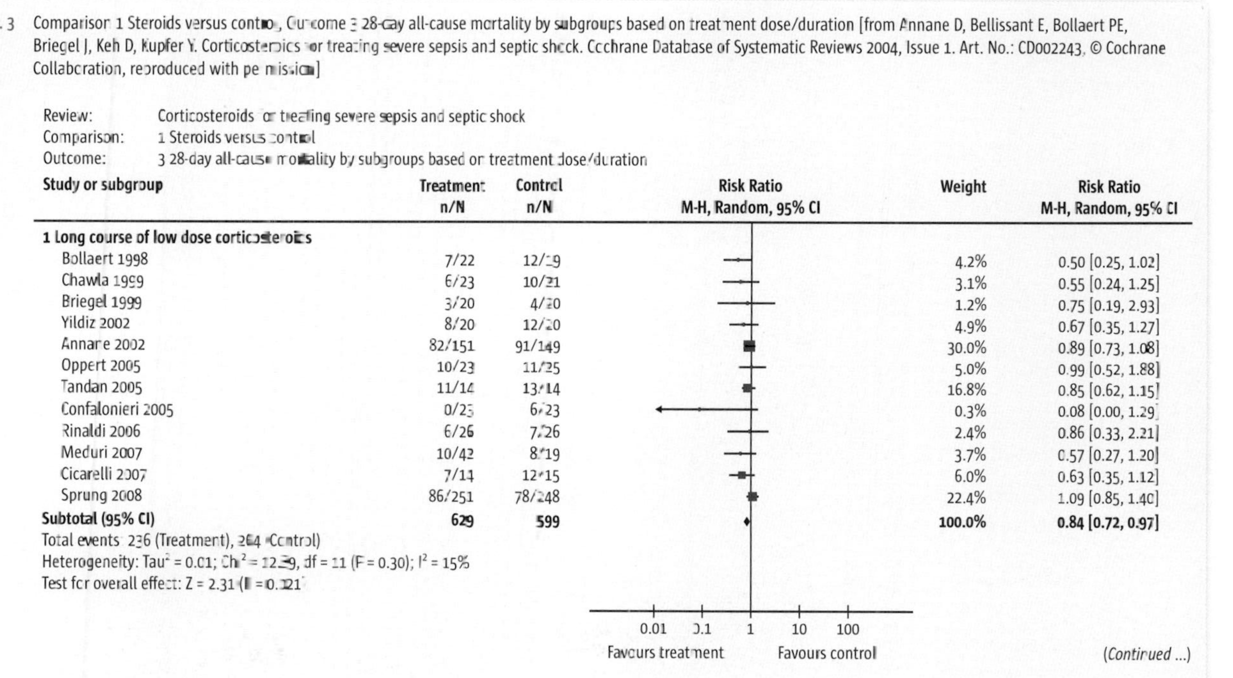

Fig. 3 Comparison 1 Steroids versus control, Outcome 3 28-day all-cause mortality by subgroups based on treatment dose/duration [from Annane D, Bellissant E, Bollaert PE, Briegel J, Keh D, Kupfer Y. Corticosteroids for treating severe sepsis and septic shock. Cochrane Database of Systematic Reviews 2004, Issue 1. Art. No.: CD002243, © Cochrane Collaboration, reproduced with permission]

Review: Corticosteroids for treating severe sepsis and septic shock
Comparison: 1 Steroids versus control
Outcome: 3 28-day all-cause mortality by subgroups based on treatment dose/duration

Study or subgroup	Treatment n/N	Control n/N	Risk Ratio M-H, Random, 95% CI	Weight	Risk Ratio M-H, Random, 95% CI
1 Long course of low dose corticosteroids					
Bollaert 1998	7/22	12/19		4.2%	0.50 [0.25, 1.02]
Chawla 1999	6/23	10/21		3.1%	0.55 [0.24, 1.25]
Briegel 1999	3/20	4/20		1.2%	0.75 [0.19, 2.93]
Yildiz 2002	8/20	12/20		4.9%	0.67 [0.35, 1.27]
Annane 2002	82/151	91/149		30.0%	0.89 [0.73, 1.08]
Oppert 2005	10/23	11/25		5.0%	0.99 [0.52, 1.88]
Tandan 2005	11/14	13/14		16.8%	0.85 [0.62, 1.15]
Confalonieri 2005	0/23	6/23		0.3%	0.08 [0.00, 1.29]
Rinaldi 2006	6/26	7/26		2.4%	0.86 [0.33, 2.21]
Meduri 2007	10/42	8/19		3.7%	0.57 [0.27, 1.20]
Cicarelli 2007	7/14	12/15		6.0%	0.63 [0.35, 1.12]
Sprung 2008	86/251	78/248		22.4%	1.09 [0.85, 1.40]
Subtotal (95% CI)	**629**	**599**		**100.0%**	**0.84 [0.72, 0.97]**

Total events: 236 (Treatment), 264 (Control)
Heterogeneity: $Tau^2 = 0.01$; $Chi^2 = 12.89$, $df = 11$ ($P = 0.30$); $I^2 = 15\%$
Test for overall effect: $Z = 2.31$ ($P = 0.021$)

(Continued ...)

(... Continued)

Study or subgroup	Treatment n/N	Control n/N	Risk Ratio M-H, Random, 95% CI	Weight	Risk Ratio M-H, Random, 95% CI
2 Short course of high dose corticosteroids					
Klastersky 1971	22/46	18/39		15.5%	1.04 [0.66, 1.63]
Schumer 1976	9/86	33/86		11.2%	0.27 [0.14, 0.53]
Lucas 1984	5/23	5/25		6.1%	1.09 [0.36, 3.27]
Sprung 1984	33/43	11/16		17.4%	1.12 [0.77, 1.61]
VASSCSG 1987	23/112	24/111		14.4%	0.95 [0.57, 1.58]
Bone 1987	65/191	48/190		18.6%	1.35 [0.98, 1.84]
Luce 1988	22/38	20/37		16.7%	1.07 [0.72, 1.60]
Subtotal (95% CI)	**539**	**504**		**100.0%**	**0.94 [0.69, 1.30]**

Total events: 179 (Treatment), 159 (Control)
Heterogeneity: $Tau^2 = 0.11$; $Chi^2 = 18.63$, df = 6 (P = 0.005); $I^2 = 68\%$
Test for overall effect: Z = 0.35 (P = 0.73)

0.01 0.1 1 10 100
Favours treatment Favours control

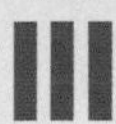

Secondary outcomes

Outcome	Trials	n	Study Gp (mean)	Control Gp (mean)	RR	95% CI	*p*	I^2
ICU Mortality	8	1048	40.5%	45.6%	0.81	0.63–1.04	0.10	46%
Hospital Mortality	15	1672	39.7%	44.0%	0.83	0.68–1.00	0.05	50%
Hospital Mortality Trials on low dose CS	10	1148	44.4%	50.4%	0.85	0.72–1.00	0.05	28%
Hospital Mortality Trials on high dose CS	5	439	38.6%	42.9%	0.84	0.52–1.36	0.47	76%
ICU LOS	8	622	WMD -4.47			-7.04 to -1.94	< 0.001	0%
Shock Reversal day 7	8	1268	63.5%	51.6%	1.29	1.06–1.58	0.01	67%
Shock Reversal day 28	6	952	66.9%	58.6%	1.12	1.02–1.23	0.02	4%

Authors' conclusion

Overall there was no significant effect of corticosteroid treatment on 28-day mortality, intensive care or hospital mortality however, the sub group analysis did show that the study group receiving a prolonged course of low dose corticosteroid did have significantly reduced 28 day all cause mortality and hospital mortality. This should be acceptable as the dose/duration relationship was a priori defined; the treatment effect was large and was confirmed by meta-regression analysis. The lower doses of corticosteroids used in the newer trials reflect acknowledgement of the role that corticosteroids play in improving immunity in sepsis rather than suppressing it.

Prolonged corticosteroid therapy significantly reduced shock duration and did not increase the risk of GI bleeding, superinfection or acquired neuromuscular weakness.

Problems & limitations

- 1 of the 2 larger trials on low dose corticosteroids did not find a survival benefit
- No standardised therapy for the control group, 4 trials did not consistently use placebo
- Neuromuscular weakness was not specifically screen for therefore may have been under-reported

Advantages

- Adequate number of patients upon which to base some conclusion

Fig. 4 Comparison 1 steroid versus control Analysis 8 Number of patients with shock reversal [from Annane D, Bellissant E, Bollaert PE, Briegel J, Keh D, Kupfer Y. Corticosteroids for treating severe sepsis and septic shock. Cochrane Database of Systematic Reviews 2004, Issue 1. Art. No.: CD002243, © Cochrane Collaboration, reproduced with permission]

Review: Corticosteroids for treating severe sepsis and septic shock
Comparison: 1 Steroids versus control
Outcome: 8 Number of patients with shock reversal

Study or subgroup	Treatment n/N	Control n/N	Risk Ratio M-H, Random, 95% CI	Weight	Risk Ratio M-H, Random, 95% CI
1 Shock reversal at day 7					
Sprung 1984	25/43	6/16		6.3%	1.55 [0.78, 3.06]
Bone 1987	85/130	83/114		20.2%	0.90 [0.76, 1.06]
Bollaert 1998	15/22	4/19		4.0%	3.24 [1.30, 8.10]
Briegel 1999	17/20	12/20		12.1%	1.42 [0.95, 2.12]
Chawla 1999	16/23	9/21		8.3%	1.62 [0.92, 2.85]
Annane 2002	60/151	40/149		14.4%	1.48 [1.06, 2.06]
Oppert 2005	14/18	16/23		13.2%	1.12 [0.78, 1.61]
Sprung 2008	186/251	145/248		21.5%	1.27 [1.12, 1.44]
Subtotal (95% CI)	**658**	**610**		**100.0%**	**1.29 [1.06, 1.58]**
Total events: 418 (Treatment), 315 (Control)					
Heterogeneity: $Tau^2 = 0.04$; $Chi^2 = 21.48$, df = 7 (P = 0.003); $I^2 = 67\%$					
Test for overall effect: Z = 2.51 (P = 0.012)					
2 Shock reversal at day 7 in trials on long course of low dose corticosteroids					
Bollaert 1998	15/22	4/19		2.6%	3.24 [1.30, 8.10]
Briegel 1999	17/20	12/20		11.8%	1.42 [0.95, 2.12]
Chawla 1999	16/23	9/21		6.5%	1.62 [0.92, 2.85]
Annane 2002	60/151	40/149		16.3%	1.48 [1.06, 2.06]

0.2 0.5 1 2 5
Favours control Favours treatment

(Continued ...)

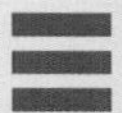

(... *Continued*)

Study or subgroup	Treatment n/N	Control n/N	Weight	Risk Ratio M-H, Random, 95% CI
Oppert 2005	14/18	16/23	13.8%	1.12 [0.78, 1.61]
Sprung 2008	[illegible]36/251	145/248	48.9%	1.27 [1.12, 1.44]
Subtotal (95% CI)	**485**	**480**	**100.0%**	**1.35 [1.16, 1.57]**
Total events: 308 (Treatment), 226 (Control)				
Heterogeneity: $Tau^2 = 0.01$; $Chi^2 = 6.3$[illegible], df = 5 (P = 0.28); $I^2 = 21\%$				
Test for overall effect: Z = 3.89 (P = 0.0[illegible]010)				
3 Shock reversal at day 28				
Bollaert 1998	15/22	7/19	2.1%	1.85 [0.96, 3.56]
Briegel 1999	18/20	15/20	12.3%	1.13 [0.86, 1.46]
Chawla 1999	17/23	10/21	3.4%	1.55 [0.93, 2.58]
Annane 2002	67/151	57/149	11.6%	1.16 [0.88, 1.52]
Tandan 2005	5/14	3/14	0.6%	1.67 [0.49, 5.67]
Sprung 2008	[illegible]00/251	183/248	70.0%	1.08 [0.98, 1.19]
Subtotal (95% CI)	**481**	**471**	**100.0%**	**1.12 [1.02, 1.23]**
Total events: 322 (Treatment), 276 (Control)				
Heterogeneity: $Tau^2 = 0.00$; $Chi^2 = 5.1$[illegible], df = 5 (P = 0.39); $I^2 = 4\%$				
Test for overall effect: Z = 2.4[illegible] (P = 0.[illegible]16)				

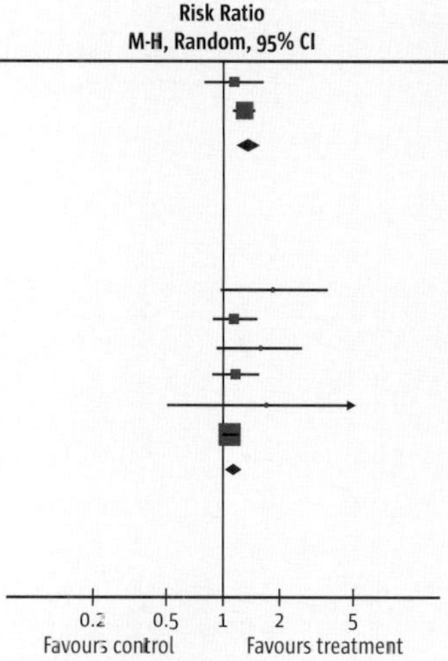

Risk Ratio M-H, Random, 95% CI

0.2 0.5 1 2 5

Favours control Favours treatment

Expert opinion

Charles Sprung

How valid and robust are the data?

This review found 20 RCTs conducted over a 53 years period with significant heterogeneity. The use of corticosteroids for patients with severe sepsis and septic shock has been controversial for decades. Two large prospective, randomized, double-blind, controlled trials (1, 2) along with five recent meta-analyses (3–7) and the present review were published to help resolve this controversy. The Annane and Sprung studies of different patient populations demonstrated different results and came to different conclusions (1, 2). Although meta-analyses may provide pooled data for answers to clinical questions and help make decisions, meta-analyses have problems. Meta-analyses do not avoid subjectivity, identify variability sources in studies or replace clinical reasoning. The recent meta-analyses of sepsis included or excluded patients differently, included different studies (patients with severe sepsis and septic shock or only septic shock) and developed conflicting conclusions (3–7). Most analyses found that steroids did not decrease mortality, reversed septic shock and did not produce major adverse events. Readers should note that the lower mortality found in patients treated with low-doses of steroids has potential publication bias as a disproportionately large number of small studies showed a beneficial corticosteroid effect (3). In addition, it is important to keep in mind that studies were not adequately powered to observe significant differences in adverse events which may be the explanation why they were not found (8).

Should clinical practice be influenced by this?

The fact that the two largest studies (1, 2) and several recent meta-analyses (3–7) of corticosteroid treatment for patients with severe sepsis and septic shock have different results and conclusions indicates that the controversy has not finished or has resolved.

What's the next step?

More studies of the role of a long course of low dose corticosteroids for patients with septic shock (especially less severely ill septic shock patients) in adults and more studies of the role of a long course of low dose corticosteroids for treating patients with severe sepsis. These studies should look into issues of mortality, morbidity, timing, tapering and adverse events.

References

1. Annane D, Sebille V, Charpentier C, et al. Effect of treatment with low doses of hydrocortisone and fludrocortisone on mortality in patients with septic shock. JAMA 2002;288:862–71.
2. Sprung CL, Annane D, Keh D, et al. for the Corticus study group. The Corticus Randomized double-blind, placebo controlled study of hydrocortisone therapy in patients with septic shock. N Engl J Med 2008; 358: 111–124.
3. Minneci PC, Deans KJ, Eichacker PQ, Natanson C. The effects of steroids during sepsis depend on dose and severity of illness: an updated meta-analysis. Clin Microbiol Infect. 2009; 15:308–18.
4. Sligl WI, Milner DA Jr, Sundar S, Mphatswe W, Majumdar SR. Safety and efficacy of corticosteroids for the treatment of septic shock: A systematic review and meta-analysis. Clin Infect Dis. 2009;49:93–101
5. Marik PE, Pastores SM, Annane D et al; American College of Critical Care Medicine. Recommendations for the diagnosis and management of corticosteroid insufficiency in critically ill adult patients: consensus statements from an international task force by the American College of Critical Care Medicine Crit Care Med. 2008;36:1937–49.

6. Annane D, Bellissant E, Bollaert PE et al. Corticosteroids in the treatment of severe sepsis and septic shock in adults: a systematic review. JAMA. 2009;301:2362–75.
7. Kalil AC, Junfeng S. Low-dose steroids for septic shock and severe sepsis: the use of Bayesian statistics to resolve clinical controversies. Int Care Med. 2011;37:420–429.
8. Sprung CL, Brezis M, Goodman S, Weiss YG. Corticosteroid therapy for patients in septic shock: Some progress in a difficult decision. Crit Care Med. 2011;39:571–4.

Recommendation

Prolonged low-dose corticosteroids should be given to patients with vasopressor - dependent septic shock: GRADE 2B.

There isn't enough evidence to determine whether corticosteroid cessation should be abrupt or gradual although the meta-regression analysis suggests that corticosteroids should be given for at least 100 hours before weaning is beneficial.

Citation

Annane D, Bellissant E, Bollaert PE, Briegel J, Keh D, Kupfer Y. Corticosteroids for treating severe sepsis and septic shock. Cochrane Database of Systematic Reviews 2004, Issue 1. Art. No.: CD002243. DOI: 10.1002/14651858.CD002243.pub2; JAMA 2009; 301(22): 2362–2375 DOI: 10.1001/jama.2009.815

AMSTAR: methodological quality of the review

1.	Was "a priori" design provided?	Y
2.	Was study selection and data extraction adequate?	Y
3.	Was the literature search comprehensive?	Y
4.	Was 'Grey Literature' used?	Y
5.	Was a list of excluded studies provided?	Y
6.	Where the characteristics of included studies provided?	Y
7.	Was the scientific quality of studies assessed & documented?	Y
8.	Was the scientific quality of studies weighted appropriately in forming conclusions?	Y
9.	Were the methods used for data synthesis appropriate?	Y
10.	Was the potential for publication bias assessed?	Y
11.	Were any conflicts of interest stated?	Y

Overall quality of trials included	Moderate – high
Overall quality of the review	High

Granulocyte & granulocyte-macrophage colony stimulating factor

Intervention: granulocyte and granulocyte-macrocyte colony stimulating factor (G-CSF & GM-CSF)
Clinical question: Does the use of G-CSF or GM-CSF in sepsis improve outcomes?

The mortality in septic shock remains high despite improvements in antimicrobial therapy and supportive care. This mortality may be associated with a state of immunosuppression characterised by reduced monocytic phagocyte activity and antigen presentation as well as changes in monocyte cytokine express; lymphocytic dysfunction and loss of circulating T- and B-lymphocytes due to apoptosis. G-CSF and GM-CSF can enhance myeloid cell function in patients with sepsis. G-CSF has been shown to stimulate neutrophil production and modulate function when used with neutropenic febrile illness following cytotoxic chemotherapy. GM-CSF exhibits broader effects compared to G-CSF. In ex vivo blood culture of patients with severe sepsis, GM-CSF has been shown to increase monocytic HLA-DR expression and endotoxin-induced proinflammatory cytokine production. Animal studies have shown promising results in cases of non-neutropenic sepsis.

Review characteristics

- **Eligibility criteria:** trials investigating the effect of G-CSF and/or GM-CSF given intravenously or subcutaneously compared to placebo
- **Exclusions:** trials involving neutropenic patients or patients following chemotherapy
- **Population:** patients with sepsis, mean age 43.2 to 64.5 years
- **Number of studies:** 12 RCTs form N. America, Europe, Asia, and Australia. 7 were multicentre studies. 8 trials of G-CSF and 4 trials of GM-CSF
- **Number of patients:** 2380 (range 18–756)
- **Study dates:** 1998–2009

Definitions

- **Sepsis:** according to the American College of Chest Physicians/Society of Critical Care Medicine consensus criteria
- **Reversal of infection:** resolution of all signs, symptoms and laboratory assessment of infection or recovery from sepsis (varied amongst trials)
- **Adverse events:** organ dysfunction that was life threatening; required treatment and prolonged hospitalization; or caused death.
- **Therapy:** G-CSF 263 or 300 mcg; GM-CSF 3 or 4 mcg/kg/day in all trials. Duration unclear

Results

Primary outcome: mortality

Mortality	Trials/N	Deaths in study gp	Deaths in placebo gp	RR	95% CI	*p*	Result
14 day	4/138	9/71 (12.7%)	13/67 (19.4%)	–	–	–	NSS
28 day	9/2133	177/1067 (16.6%)	188/1066 (17.6%)	0.93	0.79–1.11	0.44	NSS

Subgroup analysis: did not show any difference between G-CSF and GM-CSF

Secondary outcomes

Outcome	Trials/N	Study group	Placebo gp	RR	95% CI	*p*	Result
In-hospital Mortality	5/996	54/501 (10.8%)	54/495 (10.9%)	0.97	0.69–1.36	0.86	NSS
Infection reversal	4/1294	190/647 (29.4%)	141/647 (21.8%)	1.34	1.11–1.62	0.002	SS
Adverse events	7/2206	–	–	0.93	0.7–1.23	0.62	NSS

Author's conclusion

There was no difference in mortality or adverse events between patients treated with G-CSF and GM-CSF and placebo however there was a significant increase in reversal rate from infection with these therapies. Theoretically and experimentally G-CSF and GM-CSF might be beneficial to patients with sepsis therefore large, well designed trials are warranted.

Problems & limitations

- Only 1 trial (n = 38) was designed with patient stratification to establish impairment in monocyte function and guide immunotherapy
- The severity of sepsis varied widely

Advantages

13

- Baseline characteristics of the treatment and placebo groups were well matched in all but 1 trial
- Mortality results agreed with other meta-analyses of G-CSF and GM-CSF in preterm neonates with suspected infection and adults with pneumonia

Fig. 5 28-day mortality of G-CSF or GM-CSF therapy versus placebo. Fixed-effect model of risk ratio (95% confidence interval) of 28-day mortality associated with G-CSF or GM-CSF therapy compared with placebo [from Lulong Bo, Fei Wang, Jiali Zhu, Jinbao Li, Xiaoming Deng. Granulocyte-colony stimulating factor (G-CSF) and granulocyte-macrophage colony stimulating factor (GM-CSF) for sepsis: a meta-analysis. Critical Care 2011, 15:R58]

Study or subgroup		CSF		Placebo		Weight	Risk Ratio
		Events	Total	Events	Total	%	M-H, Fixed, 95% CI
1.2.1 G-CSF	Cheng 2007	21	30	26	30	13.8	0.81 [0.61, 1.06]
	Hartma 2005	1	13	4	16	1.9	0.31 [0.04, 2.43]
	Nelson 1998	23	380	24	376	12.8	0.95 [0.54, 1.65]
	Nelson 2000	19	237	28	243	14.6	0.70 [0.40, 1.21]
	Root 2003	101	348	90	353	47.3	1.14 [0.89, 1.45]
	Wund 2001	3	12	4	6	2.8	0.38 [0.12, 1.16]
	Subtotal (95% CI)		**1020**		**1024**	**93.2**	**0.95 [0.80, 1.14]**
	Total events	168		176			
	Heterogeneity: $Chi^2 = 8.48$, df = 5 (P = 0.13); $I^2 = 41\%$						
	Test for overall effect: Z = 0.52 (P = 0.60)						
1.2.2 GM-CSF	Meisel 2009	3	19	4	19	2.1	0.75 [0.19, 2.91]
	Presneill 2002	2	10	2	8	1.2	0.80 [0.14, 4.49]
	Rosen 2005	4	18	6	15	3.5	0.56 [0.19, 1.61]
	Subtotal (95% CI)		**47**		**42**	**6.8**	**0.66 [0.31, 1.40]**
	Total events	9		12			
	Heterogeneity: $Chi^2 = 0.18$, df = 2 (P = 0.91); $I^2 = 0\%$						
	Test for overall effect: Z = 1.09 (P = 0.28)						
	Total (95% CI)		**1067**		**1066**	**100**	**0.93 [0.79, 1.11]**
	Total events	177		188			
	Heterogeneity: $Chi^2 = 9.39$, df = 8 (P = 0.31); $I^2 = 15\%$						
	Test for overall effect: Z = 0.77 (P = 0.44)						
	Test for subgroup differences: Not applicable						

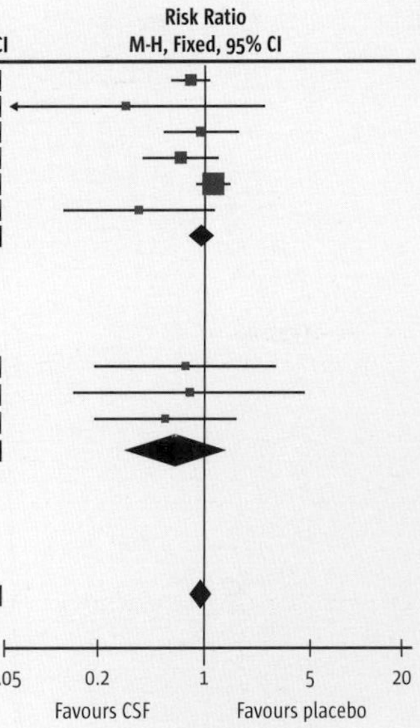

Risk Ratio M-H, Fixed, 95% CI

0.05 0.2 1 5 20

Favours CSF Favours placebo

Fig. 6 Reversal rate from infection of G-CSF or GM-CSF therapy versus placebo. Fixed-effect model of risk ratio (95% confidence interval) of reversal rate from infection associated with G-CSF or GM-CSF therapy compared with placebo [from Lulong Bo, Fei Wang, Jiali Zhu, Jinbao Li, Xiaoming Deng. Granulocyte-colony stimulating factor (G-CSF) and granulocyte-macrophage colony stimulating factor (GM-CSF) for sepsis: a meta-analysis. Critical Care 2011, 15:R58]

Study or subgroup		CSF Events	CSF Total	Placebo Events	Placebo Total	Weight %	Risk Ratio M-H, Fixed, 95% CI
1.4.1 G-CSF	Nelson 1998	114	380	83	376	59.2	1.36 [1.06, 1.74]
	Nelson 2000	53	237	45	243	31.5	1.21 [0.85, 1.72]
	Tanaka 2001	9	12	8	13	5.4	1.22 [0.71, 2.09]
	Subtotal (95% CI)		**629**		**632**	**96.1**	**1.30 [1.07, 1.58]**
	Total events	176		136			
	Heterogeneity: $Chi^2 = 1.35$, df = 2 (P = 0.84); $I^2 = 0\%$						
	Test for overall effect: Z = 2.68 (P = 0.007)						
1.4.2 GM-CSF	Rosen 2005	14	18	5	15	3.9	2.33 [1.09, 4.97]
	Subtotal (95% CI)		**18**		**15**	**3.9**	**2.33 [1.09, 4.97]**
	Total events	14		5			
	Heterogeneity: Not applicable						
	Test for overall effect: Z = 2.19 (P = 0.03)						
	Total (95% CI)		**647**		**647**	**100**	**1.34 [1.11, 1.62]**
	Total events	190		141			
	Heterogeneity: $Chi^2 = 2.52$, df = 3 (P = 0.47); $I^2 = 0\%$						
	Test for overall effect: Z = 3.09 (P = 0.002)						
	Test for subgroup differences: Not applicable						

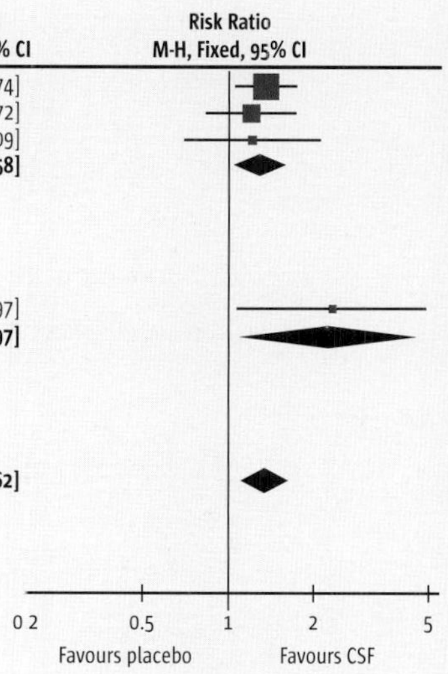

Risk Ratio M-H, Fixed, 95% CI

0.2 0.5 1 2 5

Favours placebo Favours CSF

Expert opinion

Ricard Ferrer

How valid and robust are the data?
Despite some limitations, data are valid. Main limitations are: considerable heterogeneity existed in the type and dosage of G-CSF and GM-CSF and also in the baseline characteristics of the patients (age, APACHE II score). A combined G-CSF/GM-CSF analysis might be challenged due to the distinct biology and underlying treatment concepts of each. However, these limitations do not affect to the final conclusion of the meta-analysis

Should clinical practice be influenced by this?
As CSF therapy seems to contribute to a faster reversal of infection but without an improvement in mortality, the routine use of G-CSF or GM-CSF could not be recommended. CSF therapy should thus be applied in the context of clinical trials only, or individual off -label rescue approaches.

What is the next step?
New studies are needed in special subgroup populations, specifically in the subgroup of patients with sepsis-associated immunosuppression, adequately powered for 28-day mortality, respective surrogates, or reduction of nosocomial infection rates.

Citation

Lulong Bo, Fei Wang, Jiali Zhu, Jinbao Li, Xiaoming Deng. Granulocyte-colony stimulating factor (G-CSF) and granulocyte-macrophage. colony stimulating factor (GM-CSF) for sepsis: a meta-analysis. Critical Care 2011, 15:R58 DOI:10.1186/cc10031

AMSTAR: methodological quality of the review

1.	Was “a priori” design provided?	Y
2.	Was study selection and data extraction adequate?	Y
3.	Was the literature search comprehensive?	Y
4.	Was ‘Grey Literature’ used?	Y
5.	Was a list of excluded studies provided?	N
6.	Where the characteristics of included studies provided?	Y
7.	Was the scientific quality of studies assessed & documented?	Y
8.	Was the scientific quality of studies weighted appropriately in forming conclusions?	Y
9.	Were the methods used for data synthesis appropriate?	Y
10.	Was the potential for publication bias assessed?	Y
11.	Were any conflicts of interest stated?	Y

Overall quality of trials included	5 were high quality
Overall quality of the review	High

14

Trauma and emergency medicine

Chest-compression-only CPR for out of hospital arrest ________________ 298

Also see:

Section 4: Cardiovascular dynamics
Therapeutic hypothermia

Section 9: Neuro-intensive care
Haemostatic drugs for TBI

Chest-compression-only CPR for out of hospital arrest

Condition: out of hospital (OOH) cardiac arrest

Clinical question: Does chest-compression-only bystander cardiopulmonary resuscitation (CPR) result in better outcomes than standard CPR?

At the time of this review, basic life support guidelines recommended standard CPR; however during the last decade the value of the rescue breaths has been questioned. Rescue breaths contain expired air with significantly less oxygen than atmospheric air that would be drawn in passively with chest compressions; and interrupt CPR frequently such that cardiac output may not be maintained. A continuous uninterrupted coronary perfusion pressure increases the probability of a successful outcome. During the past decade studies on both animals and humans have suggested that chest-compression-only CPR may be superior to standard CPR however results were not statistically significant. This benefit seems to be greatest in adults with sudden cardiac arrest. In non-cardiac causes of arrest such as near drowning and asphyxia, standard CPR seems more appropriate.

Review characteristics

- **Eligibility criteria**: randomised trials (for primary analysis) comparing dispatcher assisted chest-compression-only CPR with standard CPR; observational cohort studies (for secondary analysis)
- **Exclusions**: case series
- **Number of studies**: 3 RCTs & 7 Observational cohort studies (3 retrospective, 4 prospective)
- **Number of patients**: RCT 3031 (range 240–978); retrospective cohort studies: 10,486; prospective cohort studies: 3397
- **Population**: adults with OOH cardiac arrest
- **Study dates**: 1 in 1993, the rest were between 2000–2010

Definition

- **Standard CPR**: chest compressions + rescue breaths

Results

Primary outcome: survival to hospital discharge

14

Pooled results showed a significantly increased chance of survival with chest-compression-only CPR compared to standard CPR [absolute increase in survival 2.4% (95% CI 0.1–4.9), NNT = 41]

Secondary outcomes

Pooled analysis did not show any difference in 30-day survival or rate of return of spontaneous circulation.

Fig. 1 Primary analysis of survival to hospital discharge. CPR = cardiopulmonary resuscitation [reprinted from The Lancet, 376, Michael Hüpfl, Harald F Selig, Peter Nagele. Chest-compression-only versus standard cardiopulmonary resuscitation: a meta-analysis: 1552–57, 2010, with permission from Elsevier]

	Chest-compression-only CPR	Standard CPR	Risk ratio (95% CI)		Z value	P value
Hallstrom et al. (2000)	35/240 (15%)	29/278 (10%)		1.40 (0.88–2.22)	1.43	0.15
Rea et al. (2010)	122/978 (12%)	105/956 (11%)		1.14 (0.89–1.45)	1.02	0.31
Svensson et al. (2010)	54/282 (19%)	44/297 (15%)		1.29 (0.90–1.86)	1.39	0.17
Overall	**211/1500 (14%)**	**178/1531 (12%)**		**1.22 (1.01–1.46)**	**2.06**	**0.040**

0.01 0.1 1 10 100

Favours standard CPR Favours chest-compression-only CPR

Author's conclusion

Meta-analysis showed that *dispatcher-assisted chest-compression-only bystander* CPR is associated with improved survival compared to standard CPR for OOH cardiac arrest. These results should be considered robust because the same trend was observed within all of the controlled trials. This type of trial is very difficult to conduct and very large numbers are required to show statistically significant differences because survival rates for OOH cardiac arrest are so low.

Problems & limitations

- Small number of RCTs
- All 3 RCTs used the older 15:2 compression to ventilation ratio, newer guidelines recommend 30:2 to minimise interruptions to compressions
- Observational studies did not show any survival differences
- There were many more patients in the group receiving standard CPR (in some studies 10-fold more)

Advantages

- All 3 of the RCTS reported a similar benefit in chest-compression-only CPR

Expert opinion

Jacques Duranteau

Despite three randomized trials, the optimal method for out-of-hospital bystander cardiopulmonary resuscitation (CPR) is still controversial. The goal of meta-analysis was to systematically review existing evidence regarding chest-compression-only CPR and compare the findings with standard CPR. Medline and Embase were systematically reviewed for studies published between January 1985 and August 2010, in which chest-compression-only bystander CPR was compared with standard bystander CPR for adult patients with out-of-hospital cardiac arrest. In the primary meta-analysis, the authors included randomised trials and in the secondary meta-analysis, they included observational cohort studies. The primary outcome was survival to hospital discharge. A fixed-effects model was used for both meta-analyses because of an absence of heterogeneity among the studies (I = 0%).

Among randomized trials, three trials individually showed a small benefit in patients who received chest- compression-only CPR, but the differences were not significant. The meta-analysis of these studies showed a significantly increased chance of survival with chest-compression-only CPR compared with standard CPR (absolute increase in survival of 2.4% (95% CI 0.1–4.9). Seven observational cohort studies were eligible for the secondary meta-analysis Apart from one study, none of the observational studies showed a significant survival difference between the two CPR techniques. In the meta-analysis of these studies, chest-compression-only CPR was not associated with a difference in survival compared with standard CPR.

14

The conclusion of these authors is that dispatcher-assisted chest-compression-only bystander CPR is associated with a 22% improved survival rate in adults with out-of-hospital cardiac arrest compared with standard CPR. For adults with out-of-hospital cardiac arrest, instructions to bystanders from emergency medical services dispatch should focus on chest-compression-only CPR.

How valid and robust are the data?
This result is very important for out-of-hospital bystander cardiopulmonary resuscitation. The quality of the randomized studies is high and the conclusion of the meta-analysis is robust and valid.

Should clinical practise be influenced by this?
Based on these results, it is obvious that uninterrupted, high-quality chest compression is a key factor for successful CPR. Oxygenation and ventilation during the first minutes after cardiac arrest appear be less important than a high-quality chest compression.

What's the next step?
Instructions to bystanders from emergency medical services dispatch should focus on chest-compression-only CPR.

Citation

Aufderheide TP, Frascone RJ, Wayne MA, et al. Standard cardiopulmonary resuscitation versus active compression-decompression resuscitation with augmentation of negative intrathoracic pressure for out-of-hopsital cardiac arrest: a randomised trial. Lancet 2011, published online Jan 19; 377: 301–11 DOI:10.1016/S0140–6736(10)62103–4

Michael Hüpfl, Harald F Selig, Peter Nagele. Chest-compression-only versus standard cardiopulmonary resuscitation: a meta-analysis. Lancet 2010; 376: 1552–57 DOI:10.1016/S0140–6736(10)61454–7

Author's comment: Peter Nagele

Out-of-hospital cardiac arrest is a grim situation. Without cardiopulmonary resuscitation (CPR), cardiac arrest is invariably fatal, and even under the best possible circumstances survival rates often don't exceed 10%. Over the last decades, resuscitation researchers have investigated multiple methods of how to improve survival rates after out-of-hospital cardiac arrest, and the brand new resuscitation guidelines published in March 2011 are a testament to this effort.

Tom Aufderheide and colleagues have recently reported the exciting results of the ResQ trial.

ResQ trial: NCT00189423

This was a randomized controlled trial of 46 emergency medical service agencies conducted in the USA that included 1853 patients with non-traumatic OOH cardiac arrest. The efficacy of standard CPR was tested against two devices: One provides active compression-decompression and the second augments the negative intratho racic pressure (via an impedance-threshold device). The rate of survival to hospital discharge with a favourable neurological outcome was increased in the intervention group from 5.8% to 8.9% (OR 1.58, 95% CI 1.07–2.36, $p = 0.019$) and the survival benefit extended all the way to one year. Overall the rate of major complications was similar but the intervention group had significantly more pulmonary oedema.

Additional information

The new American Heart Association (AHA) guidelines suggest that instead of A-B-C, bystander resuscitation should start with chest compressions (C-A-B) initially in the unresponsive patient. This applies to all forms of CPR except on neonates. C-A-B aims to avoid delays in commencing CPR while airway and breathing are checked as those first few minutes may be crucial. Checking airway and breathing can be difficult and unreliable particularly in untrained hands; furthermore people are more willing to perform chest compressions as they are easier and avoid the sanitary concerns associated with mouth-to-mouth breathing.

The European resuscitation Council (ERC) guidelines still maintain the traditional A-B-C approach however there is a greater emphasis on chest compressions. The recommended depth of chest-compressions has been increased to 5–6 cm and compression rate to 100–120 per minute. CPR should not be discontinued until the victim shows obvious signs of consciousness.

AMSTAR: methodological quality of the review

1.	Was “a priori” design provided?	Y
2.	Was study selection and data extraction adequate?	Y
3.	Was the literature search comprehensive?	Y
4.	Was ‘Grey Literature’ used?	Y
5.	Was a list of excluded studies provided?	N
6.	Where the characteristics of included studies provided?	Y
7.	Was the scientific quality of studies assessed & documented?	Y
8.	Was the scientific quality of studies weighted appropriately in forming conclusions?	Y
9.	Were the methods used for data synthesis appropriate?	Y
10.	Was the potential for publication bias assessed?	Y
11.	Are conflicts of interest stated?	Y

Overall quality of trials included	RCTs all high quality
Overall quality of the review	High

Part IV

Appendix A: Review titles 305
Appendix B: Corresponding authors 308
Appendix C: The experts 314
Appendix D: The Systematic Review Group Board 317
Appendix E: Additional references from the text 319

Appendix A: Review titles

Section 1: Acute kidney injury (AKI)

i. Atrial natriuretic peptide for preventing and treating acute kidney injury
ii. Hydroxyethyl starch versus other fluid therapies: effect on kidney function
iii. Renal outcomes and mortality following hydroxyethyl starch resuscitation of critically ill patients: a systematic review and meta-analysis of randomised trials
iv. Sodium Bicarbonate for the prevention of contrast-induced acute kidney injury
v. Prevention and treatment of acute kidney injury in patients undergoing cardiac surgery: a systematic review

Section 2: Acute respiratory failure (ARF) – Acute respiratory distress syndrome (ARDS)

i. Higher versus lower positive end-expiratory pressure in patients with acute lung injury and acute respiratory distress syndrome: systematic review and meta-analysis
ii. Recruitment manoeuvres for adults with acute lung injury receiving mechanical ventilation
iii. Inhaled nitric oxide for acute respiratory distress syndrome and acute lung injury in children and adults
iv. Aerosolized prostacyclin for acute lung injury and acute respiratory distress syndrome
v. Pharmacologic therapies for adults with acute lung injury and acute respiratory distress syndrome
vi. Use of corticosteroids in acute lung injury and acute respiratory distress syndrome: a systematic review and meta-analysis
vii. A systematic review to inform institutional decisions about the use of extracorporeal membrane oxygenation during the H1N1 influenza pandemic

Section 3: Acute respiratory failure – Non-ARDS

i. Corticosteroids for pneumonia
ii. Corticosteroids for the prevention and treatment of postextubation stridor in neonates, children and adults
iii. Corticosteroids to prevent extubation failure: a systematic review and meta-analysis
iv. Noninvasive positive pressure ventilation as a weaning strategy for intubated adults with respiratory failure
v. Protocolized versus non-prtocolized weaning for reducing the duration of mechanical ventilation in critically ill adult patients
vi. Heated humidification versus heat and moisture exchangers for ventilated adults and children
vii. Utility and safety of draining pleural effusions in mechanically ventilated patients: a systematic review and meta-analysis

Section 4: Cardiovascular dynamics

i. Treatment of new-onset atrial fibrillation in noncardiac intensive care unit patients: a systematic review and meta-analysis
ii. Hypothermia for neuroprotection in adults after cardiopulmonary resuscitation
iii. Vasopressin for the treatment of vasodilatory shock: an ESICM systematic review and meta-analysis
iv. A systematic review and meta-analysis on the Use of preemptive hemodynamic Intervention to Improve postoperative Outcomes in Moderate and High-Risk surgical patients

Section 5: Ethics

i. Modifiable factors influencing relatives' decision to offer organ donation: systematic review

Section 6: General

i. Stress ulcer prophylaxis in the new millennium: a systematic review and meta-analysis
ii. Interventions for preventing critical illness polyneuropathy and critical illness myopathy
iii. Low-molecular-weight heparin thromboprophylaxis in medical-surgical critically ill patients: a systematic review
iv. Music interventions for mechanically ventilated patients

Section 7: Health technology

i. Abandoning daily routine chest radiography in the intensive care unit: meta-analysis
ii. Clinical effectiveness and cost-effectiveness of oesophageal Doppler monitoring in critically ill and high-risk surgical patients
iii. Tight glycaemic control and computerised decision support

Section 8: Infection

i. Clinically-indicated replacement versus routine replacement of peripheral venous catheters
ii. Procalcitonin-guided algorithms of antibiotic therapy in the intensive care unit: a systematic review and meta-analysis or randomized controlled trials
iii. A systematic review on clinical benefits of continuous administration of beta-lactam antibiotics
iv. Predictors of mortality in adults with ventilator-associated pneumonia: a meta-analysis
v. Antibiotic prophylaxis to reduce respiratory tract infections and mortality in adults receiving intensive care
vi. Antibiotic therapy for prophylaxis against infection of pancreatic necrosis in acute pancreatitis

Section 9: Neuro-intensive care

i. Haemostatic drugs for traumatic brain injury
ii. Routine intracranial pressure monitoring in acute coma
iii. Cooling therapy for acute stroke

Section 10: Nutrition and metabolism

i. Early enteral nutrition, provided within 24 h of injury or intensive care unit admission, significantly reduces mortality in critically ill patients: a meta-analysis of randomised trials
ii. Nutritional strategies in acute severe pancreatitis: a systematic review of the evidence
iii. Enteral versus parenteral nutrition for acute pancreatitis
iv. Effect of glucose-insulin-potassium infusion on mortality in critical care settings: a systematic review and meta-analysis

Section 11: Outcomes

i. Association between time of admission to ICU and mortality: a systematic review and meta-analysis
ii. Severity of illness and risk of readmission to intensive care: a meta-analysis
iii. Quality of life after intensive care: a systematic review of the literature
iv. Long-term mortality and quality of life in sepsis: a systematic review
v. An official American Thoracic Society systematic review: The association between health insurance status and access, care delivery, and outcomes for patients who are critically ill

Section 12: Paediatric intensive care

i. Short versus long duration of antibiotic therapy for bacterial meningitis: a meta-analysis of randomised controlled trials in children
ii. Continuous negative extrathoracic pressure or continuous positive airway pressure for acute hypoxemic respiratory failure in children.
iii. Heliox for croup in children
iv. Nutritional support for critically ill children
v. Other review relevant to paediatrics

Section 13: Sepsis

i. Early versus late pre-intensive care unit admission broad spectrum antibiotics for severe sepsis in adults
ii. A survival benefit of combination antibiotic therapy for serious infections associated with sepsis and septic shock is contingent only on the risk of death: a meta-analytic/meta-regression study
iii. De-escalation of antimicrobial treatment for adults with sepsis, severe sepsis or septic shock
iv. The role of albumin as a resuscitation fluid for patients with sepsis: a systematic review and meta-analysis
v. Corticosteroids for treating severe sepsis and septic shock
vi. Granulocyte-colony stimulating factor (G-CSF) and granulocyte macrophage stimulating factor (GM-CSF) for sepsis: a meta-anaylsis

Section 14: Trauma and emergency medicine

i. Chest-compression-only versus standard cardiopulmonary resuscitation: a meta analysis

Appendix B: Corresponding authors

Section	Corresponding author's institution at the time of the review
1	Acute kidney injury (AKI)
i	**Sagar U. Nigwekar** Rochester General Hospital, University of Rochester School of Medicine and Dentistry, 1425 Portland Ave, Rochester, NY, 14621, USA
ii	**Allison B. Dart** Department of Pediatrics and Child Health, University of Manitoba, FE-009 840 Sherbrook St, Winnipeg, Manitoba, R3A 1S1, Canada
iii	**Lauralyn McIntyre** The Ottawa Hospital, 501 Smyth Rd., Box 201, Ottawa ON K1H 8L6, USA
iv	**Eric Hoste** Professor in the rank of senior lecturer. Intensive Care Unit Ghent University Hospital De Pintelaan 185, 9000 Gent, Belgium
v	**Chirag Parikh** Section of Nephrology, Yale University and VAMC; 950 Campbell Ave, Mail Code 151B, Bldg 35 A, Room 219, West Haven, CT 06516, USA
2	Acute respiratory failure (ARF) – Acute respiratory distress syndrome (ARDS)
i	**Maureen Meade** Department of Medicine, McMaster University, Hamilton, Ontario, Canada
ii	**Carol Hodgson** Department of Physiotherapy, The Alfred Hospital and Monash University, Commercial Road, Melbourne, 3181, Australia
iii & iv	**Arash Afshari** The Cochrane Anaesthesia Review Group & Copenhagen Trial Unit and Department of Paediatric and Obstetric Anaesthesia, Rigshospitalet, Blegdamsvej 9, Afsnit 3342, rum 52, Copenhagen, 2100, Denmark
v	**Neill K.J. Adhikari** Interdepartmental Division of Critical Care and University of Toronto, Sunnybrook Research Institute, Sunnybrook Health Sciences Centre, 2057 Bayview Avenue, Toronto, Ontario, M4N 3M5, Canada
vi	**Benjamin Tang** Department of Intensive Care Medicine, Nepean Hospital, Penrith, New South Wales, Australia **Anthony S. McLean** Professor and Head Department of Intensive Care Medicine; Nepean Clinical School, Penrith, Sydney, University of Sydney, Australia
vii	**Mark E. Mikkelsen** Division of Pulmonary, Allergy and Critical Care, Department of Medicine, Hospital of the University of Pennsylvania, Philadelphia, USA

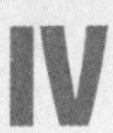

Section	Corresponding author's institution at the time of the review
3	Acute respiratory failure – Non-ARDS
i	**Taixiang Wu** Chinese Cochrane Centre, Chinese Clinical Trial Registry, Chinese Evidence-Based Medicine Centre, INCLEN Resource and Training Centre, West China Hospital, Sichuan University, No. 37, Guo Xue Xiang, Chengdu, Sichuan, 610041, China
ii	**Robinder G. Khemani** Department of Anesthesiology Critical Care Medicine, Childrens Hospital Los Angeles, 4650 Sunset Blvd Mailstop 12, Los Angeles, California, 90027, USA
iii	**John McCaffrey** Department of Anaesthesia and Critical Care (JM), Belfast City Hospital, Belfast, UK **Anthony P Delaney** Professor/Intensive Care Unit, Royal North Shore, Hospital, Pacific Highway, St. Leonards, Sydney, NSW 2065, Australia
iv	**Bronagh Blackwood** School of Nursing & Midwifery, Queen's University Belfast, Medical Biology Centre, 97 Lisburn Road, Belfast, BT9 7BL, UK
v	**Karen E.A. Burns** Interdepartmental Division of Critical Care and the University of Toronto, Keenan Research Centre/Li Ka Shing Knowledge Institute, St Michael's Hospital, 30, Bond Street, Rm 4-045 Queen Wing, Toronto, Ontario, M5B 1WB, Canada
vi	**Margaret Kelly** Nurse Consultant (clinical practice development & research) Nursing Research & Practice Development Unit, Chair Human Research Ethics Committee, Kids Research Institute, The Children's Hospital at Westmead, Australia **Donna Gillies** Senior Researcher Clinical Performance Team - Mental Health Western Sydney Local Health District, Australia **David Todd** Department Neonatology, Canberra Hospital Senior Lecturer, ANU Medical School, PO Box 11, Woden, Canberra, ACT, 2606, Australia
vii	**Niall Ferguson** Interdepartmental Division of Critical Care, Mount Sinai Hospital and the University Health Network, University of Toronto, 600 University Avenue, Toronto, Ontario, M5G 1X5, Canada

Section	Corresponding author's institution at the time of the review
4	Cardiovascular dynamics
i	**Salmaan Kanji** Ottawa Hospital and the Ottawa Health Research Institute, Ottawa, Canada
ii	**Jasmin Arrich** Department of Emergency Medicine, Medical University of Vienna, Währinger Gürtel 18–20/6D, Vienna, 1090, Austria
iii	**Djillali Annane** See Appendix D
iv	**Mark Hamilton** See Appendix D
5	Ethics
i	**Duncan Young** See Appendix D
6	General
i	**Paul E. Marik** Division of Pulmonary and Critical Care Medicine (PEM); Eastern Virginia Medical School, Norfolk, VA, USA
ii	**Greet Hermans** Medical Intensive Care Unit, Department of General Internal Medicine University Hospitals Leuven, Herestraat 49, 3000 Leuven, Belgium **Greet Van den Berghe** Professor/Department of Intensive Care Medicine, Catholic University of Leuven, University Hospitals, Herestraat 49,3000, Leuven, Belgium
iii	**Deborah Cook** St. Joseph's Hospital, Hamilton, ON, L8N 4A6, Canada
iv	**Joke Bradt** Associate Professor, Department of Creative Arts Therapies, College of Nursing and Health Professions, Drexel University, 1505 Race Street, rm 1041, Philadelphia, PA, 19102, USA
7	Health technology
i	**Yugi Oba** From the Division of Pulmonary and Critical Care Medicine, University of Missouri-Columbia, One Hospital Drive, CE 412, Columbia, MO 65212, USA
ii	**Graham Mowatt** Health Services Research Unit, Institute of Applied Health Sciences, University of Aberdeen, UK
iii	**Saeid Eslami** Department of Medical Informatics, Academic Medical Center, University of Amsterdam, Meibergdreef 15, J1b-124, 1105 AZ Amsterdam, The Netherlands

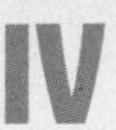

Section	Corresponding author's institution at the time of the review
8	**Infection**
i	**Joan Webster** Centre for Clinical Nursing, Royal Brisbane and Women's Hospital, Level 2, Building 34, Butterfield Street, Herston, QLD, 4029, Australia
ii	**Petros Kopterides** Second Critical Care Department, "Attiko" University Hospital, University of Athens; Medical School, Athens, Greece
iii	**Jeffrey Lipman** Burns, Trauma and Critical Care Research Centre, the University of Queensland, Brisbane, Australia
iv	**Matthew E. Falagas** Alfa Institute of Biomedical Sciences, 9 Neapoleos St, 151 23 Marousi, Greece
v	**Alessandro Liberati** Italian Cochrane Centre, Mario Negri Institute for Pharmacological Research, Via La Masa, 19, Milan, 20156, Italy
vi	**Mike Larvin** Director of Education, The Royal College of Surgeons of England, London & Professor/ Academic Division of Surgery, School of Graduate Entry Medicine, University of Nottingham, Derby City General Hospital, UK
9	**Neuro-intensive care**
i	**Pablo Perel** Cochrane Injuries Group, London School of Hygiene & Tropical Medicine, Keppel Street, London, WC1E 7HT, UK
ii	**Rob J. Forsyth** Institute of Neuroscience, Newcastle University, Royal Victoria Infirmary, Newcastle upon Tyne, Tyne & Wear, NE1 4LP, UK
iii	**Heleen M Den Hertog** Department of Neurology, Erasmus MC University Medical Center, Postbus 2040, Rotterdam, 3000 CA, The Netherlands **Diederik Dippel** Professor, Department of Neurology, Erasmus MC University Medical Center, The Netherlands
10	**Nutrition and metabolism**
i	**Gordon S Doig** Northern Clinical School, University of Sydney, Sydney 2006, NSW, Australia
ii	**Ahmad Al Samaree** General Surgery, Queen Elizabeth Hospital, Gateshead, NE9 6SX, UK
iii	**Mohammed Al-Omran** Department of Surgery and Peripheral Vascular Disease Research Chair, College of Medicine, King Saud University, P.O.Box 7805(37), Riyahd, 11472, Saudi Arabia
iv	**Alan Jones** Department of Emergency Medicine, Carolinas Medical Center, North Carolina, PO Box 32861, Charlotte, NC 28232-2861, USA

Section	Corresponding author's institution at the time of the review
11	**Outcomes**
i	**Paul E. Marik** See above
ii	**Steven A. Frost** University of Western Sydney, Campbelltown Campus, Building 7, Locked Bag 1797, Penrith South, DC 1797, New South Wales, Australia
iii	**Sandra G. Oeyen** Department of Intensive Care Medicine, Ghent University Hospital, Ghent, Belgium
iv	**Bradford D. Winters** Assistant Professor, Departments of Anesthesiology and Critical Care Medicine and Surgery, Johns Hopkins University School of Medicine, Baltimore, USA
v	**Robert A. Fowler** Chairman of the subcommittee of the Behavioral Science Assembly. Career Scientist of the Ontario Ministry of Health and Long-term Care and incoming Clinician Scientist of the Heart and Stroke Foundation of Canada
12	**Paediatric intensive care**
i	**Matthew E. Falagas** See above
ii	**Prakeshkumar S Shah** Department of Paediatrics and Department of Health Policy, Management and Evaluation, Rm 775A, University of Toronto, 600 University Avenue, Toronto, Ontario, M5G 1XB, Canada
iii	**Christiane Vorwerk** Department of Emergency Medicine, Leicester Royal Infirmary, Infirmary Square, Leicester, LE1 5WW, UK **Tim Coats** Professor of Emergency Medicine, Leicester Royal Infirmary; Chairman of the Trauma Audit and Research Network (TARN) and lead clinician for the international CRASH-2 trial, UK
iv	**Ari Joffe** Department of Pediatrics, Division of Pediatric Intensive Care, University of Alberta and Stollery Children's Hospital, Office 3A3.07, 8440-112 St, Edmonton, Alberta, T6G 2B7, Canada

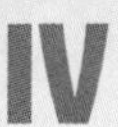

Section	Corresponding author's institution at the time of the review
13	Sepsis
i	**Shahla Siddiqui** Department of Anesthesiology, Aga Khan University Hospital, Stadium Road, PO Box 3500, Karachi, 74800, Pakistan
ii	**Anand Kumar** Associate Professor of Medicine, Medical Microbiology and Pharmacology/ Therapeutics, University of Manitoba, Winnipeg, Manitoba, Canada
iii	**Brenda Nazaré Gomes Silva** Brazilian Cochrane Centre, Universidade Federal de São Paulo, Rua Pedro de Toledo, 598, Vl. Clementino, São Paulo, São Paulo, 04039-001, Brazil
iv	**Anthony P. Delaney & John McCaffrey** See above
v	**Djillali Annane** See Appendix D
vi	**Lulong Bo** Department of Anesthesiology, Changhai Hospital, Second Military Medical University, 168 Changhai Road, Shanghai, 200433, PR China
14	Trauma and emergency medicine
i	**Peter Nagele** Department of Anesthesiology, Washington, University School of Medicine, 660 S Euclid Ave, Box 8054, St Louis, MO 63110, USA

Appendix C: The experts

Section	Expert's title & institution
1	Acute kidney injury (AKI)
i & v	**Eric Hoste, MD, PhD** Professor in the rank of senior lecturer Intensive Care Unit; Ghent University Hospital, Belgium; Deputy Chairman of ESICM AKI section
ii & iii	**Michael Joannidis, MD** Professor/Intensive Care Medicine, University hospital for internal medicine, Innsbruck; Anichstr. 35, Austria; Chairman of the ESICM AKI section
iv	**Maria Schetz** Associate Professor of Medicine KU Leuven Department of Intensive Care Medicine University Hospital Leuven, Belgium
2	Acute respiratory failure (ARF) – Acute respiratory distress syndrome (ARDS)
i & ii	**Anders Larsson, MD, MDsc, DEAA** Professor of Anesthesiology and Intensive Care Medicine; Head of the Hedenstierna laboratory, Uppsala University, Sweden; Chairman of the ESICM ARF Section
iii & iv	**Nicola Petrucci, MD, MSc** See Appendix D
v	**Arthur S. Slutsky, MD** Vice President (Research), St. Michael's Hospital, Toronto, Canada; Director, Interdepartmental Division of Critical Care Medicine University of Toronto; Professor of Medicine, Surgery and Biomedical Engineering University of Toronto
vi	**Gianfranco Umberto Meduri, MD, FACP, FCCP** Professor of Medicine, University of Tennessee Health Science Center, Memphis
vii	**Jeremy Cordingley** Consultant in Intensive Care Medicine and Cardiothoracic Anaesthesia; Director of Adult of the Adult Intensive Care Unit; Royal Brompton Hospital, London, UK
3	Acute respiratory failure – Non-ARDS
i	**John Carlisle** Consultant in anaesthesia and preoperative assessment; Torbay hospital, South Devon Healthcare NHS Foundation Trust; Torquay, Devon, UK
ii	**Djillali Annane, MD, PhD** See appendix D
iii	**Laurent Brochard, MD** Head of the Intensive Care Unit, Geneva University Hospitals, Geneva, Switzerland
iv	**Richard Venn** Consultant in Anaesthesia & Intensive Care, Western Sussex Hospitals NHS Trust, Worthing Hospital, Worthing, UK
v, vi & vii	**Jonathan Ball, MRCP EDIC FCCP FFICM MSc MD** Consultant and Honorary Senior Lecturer in General & Neuro Intensive Care, St George's Hospital & Medical School, London, UK

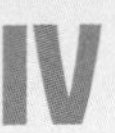

Section	Expert's title & institution
4	Cardiovascular dynamics
4.i & 6.iii	**Maurizio Cecconi, MD MD (UK)** Consultant and Honorary Senior Lecturer, Department of General Intensive Care , St George's Hospital and Medical School, SW17 0QT London, Deputy Chairman of ESICM CVS Dynamics section until October 2011, Chairman of ESICM CVS Dynamics from October 2011
4.i	**Fernando Clau-Terré, MD, PhD** Critical Care Department, Vall d'Hebron University Hospital, Vall d'Hebron Research Institut (VHIR), Research Group for shock, organ dysfuntion and resuscitation (SODIR), Universitat Autònoma de Barcelona, Barcelona
ii	**Jan Poelaert, MD, PhD** Department of Anesthesiology and Perioperative Medicine, UZ Brussels, Belgium, Chair of ESICM CVS dynamics section until October 2011
iii	**Anthony Gordon, MD, FRCA, FFICM** Clinical Senior Lecturer & Consultant, Critical Care Medicine, Imperial College/Charing Cross Hospital, London, UK
5	Ethics
i	**Jozef Kesecioglu, MD, PhD** Professor/Director Department of Intensive Care, University Medical Center Utrecht, The Netherlands Chairman of ESICM Ethics section
6	General
iii	**Miguel Tavares** Intensive Care Unit, Santo António General Hospital, Porto, Portugal
7	Health technology
i & iii	**Pierre Squara, MD** ICU Clinic Ambroise Paré, 27, Bd Victor Hugo, 92200 Neuilly-sur-Seine, Deputy Chairman of the ESICM Health Technology Assessment & Informatics section
ii	**Claudia Spies, MD** Professor, Head of the department of Anesthesiology and Intensive Care Medicine, Campus Virchow-Klinikum and Campus Mitte, Berlin, Chairperson of ESICM Peri-operative ICM section **Aarne Feldheiser** Department of Anesthesiology and Intensive Care Medicine, Campus Virchow Klinikum, Berlin, Germany
8	Infection
i, iii, vi & 13.ii	**George Dimopoulos, MD, PhD, FCCP** See appendix D
ii, iv, v & 13.i	**Jordi Rello, MD, PhD** See appendix D

Section	Expert's title & institution
9	Neuro-intensive care
ii	**Mauro Oddo, MD** PD-MER, Staff Physician, Department of Critical Care Medicine, CHUV-University Hospital, Switzerland, Deputy Chairman of ESICM Neurointensive Care section
iii & 6.ii.	**Pedro Navarrete-Navarro** Associate Professor of Medicine, Hospital for Neurotraumatology, University Hospital Virgen de las Nieves. Granada. Spain; Chairman of the ESICM Neurointensive Care Section, Head of Section of Critical Care & Emergency Medicine
10	Nutrition and metabolism
i & iv	**David Noble** See appendix D
ii & iii	**Daren K. Heyland, MD, FRCPSC, MSc** Professor of Medicine, Director of Clinical Evaluation Research Unit, Queen's University, Kingston, Ontario, Canada
11	Outcomes
i, ii & v	**Maurizia Capuzzo, MD** Department of Surgical, Anaesthetic and Radiological Sciences, Section of Anaesthesiology and Intensive Care, University Hospital of Ferrara, Ferrara, Italy; Chair of the Section on Health Service Research & Outcome of the ESICM
12	Paediatric intensive care
i & iii	**Joan Balcells Ramírez, MD** Pediatric and Neonatal ECMO Program – Director Pediatric Critical Care Department – Director Hospital Vall d'Hebron, Barcelona, Spain
13	Sepsis
iii & vi	**Ricard Ferrer, MD, PhD** ICU Director, Mutua de Terrassa University Hospital, Centre for Biomedical Research Network of Respiratory Diseases, Spain; Deputy of the ESICM SIRS and Sepsis section
iv	**Christiane Hartog, MD** Department of Anesthesiology and Intensive Care Medicine, Jena University Hospital, Friedrich-Schiller-University, Germany
v	**Charles Sprung, MD** Professor of Medicine, Department of Anesthesiology and Critical Care Medicine, Hadassah University Hospital Ein-Karem, Jerusalem
14	Trauma and emergency medicine
i	**Jacques Duranteau, MD, PhD** Professor/Department of Anaesthesia and Intensive Care Medicine, Bicêtre University Hospital Paris, France; Chairman of the ESICM TEM section

Appendix D: The Systematic Review Group Board

Chairman: Djillali Annane, France

Deputy: Mark Hamilton, UK

The Editors:

David Noble, UK

Duncan Young, UK

George Dimopoulos, Greece

John Carlisle, UK

Jordi Rello, Spain

Leopold Eberhart, Germany

Nicola Petrucci, Italy

Managing Editor: Gihan Abuella, UK

IV

SRG member	Affiliation
Djillali Annane	Professor/Head of Critical Care Department, Raymond Poincaré University Hospital, Paris, France
Mark Hamilton	Consultant and Honorary Senior Lecturer in Anaesthesia and Intensive Care Medicine St. George's Healthcare NHS Trust, London, UK
David Noble	Consultant in Anaesthesia and Intensive care medicine Aberdeen Royal Infirmary, Aberdeen, UK
Duncan Young	Intensive Care Society Clinical Trials Group, Kadoorie Centre, John Radcliffe Hospital, Headington, Oxford, UK
George Dimopoulos	Assistant Professor, Department of Critical Care, ATTIKO University Hospital Medical School, University of Athens, Athens, Greece Chairman of ESICM Infection Section
John Carlisle	Consultant in anaesthesia and preoperative assessment Torbay hospital, South Devon Healthcare NHS Foundation Trust Torquay, Devon, UK
Jordi Rello	Chief of Critical Care Department. Vall d'Hebron University Hospital. Director, CRIPS Research Group, CIBERES. Associate Professor of Medicine, University of Barcelona, Spain Deputy of ESICM Infection Section
Leopold Eberhart	Professor/Deputy Director of the Department of Anesthesiology and Intensive Care Therapy, Philipps University Marburg, Germany
Nicola Petrucci	Consultant in Anaesthesia and Intensive Care Azienda Ospedaliera Desenzano, Italy
Gihan Abuella	Research Fellow for ESICM Systematic Review Group In affiliation with the Intensive Care Unit, St. George's Hospital, London, UK

Appendix E: Additional references from the text

ALVEOLI

Brower RG, Lanken PN, MacIntyre N, et al.; National Heart, Lung, and Blood Institute ARDS Clinical Trials Network. Higher versus lower positive endexpiratory pressures in patients with the acute respiratory distress syndrome. N Engl J Med. 2004;351(4):327–336.

Barnett 2002

Barnett MJ, Kaboli PJ, Sirio CA, Rosenthal GE. Day of the week of intensive care admission and patient outcomes: a multisite regional evaluation. Med Care 2002;40(6):530–539.

Berk and Freedman 2003

Berk RA & Freedman D. Statistical assumptions as empirical commitments. In T.G. Blomberg, S. Cohen, editors. Law, Punishment, and Social Control: Essays in Honor of Sheldon Messinger. 2nd ed. Aldine de Gruyter;2003:235–254.

Boldt

Boldt J, Knothe C, Schindler E, Hammermann H, Dapper F, Hempelmann G. Volume replacement with hydroxyethyl starch solution in children. British Journal of Anaesthesia 1993;70(6):661–5.

Boldt J, Muller M, Mentges D, Papsdorf M, Hempelmann G. Volume therapy in the critically ill: is there a difference? Intensive Care Medicine 1998;24(1):28–36.

Boldt J, Lehmann A, Rompert R, Haisch G, Isgro F. Volume therapy with a new hydroxyethyl starch solution in cardiac surgical patients before cardiopulmonary bypass. Journal of Cardiothoracic & Vascular Anesthesia 2000;14(3):264–8.

Boldt J, Suttner S, Kumle B, Huttner I. Cost analysis of different volume replacement strategies in anesthesia. Infusions therapie und Transfusions medizin 2000;27(1):38–43.

Boldt J, Brenner T, Lehmann A, Lang J, Kumle B, Werling C. Influence of two different volume replacement regimens on renal function in elderly patients undergoing cardiac surgery: comparison of a new starch preparation with gelatin. Intensive Care Medicine 2003;29(5):763–9.

Boldt J, Scholhorn T, Mayer J, Piper S, Suttner S. The value of an albumin-based intravascular volume replacement strategy in elderly patients undergoing major abdominal surgery. Anesthesia & Analgesia 2006;103(1):191–9.

Boldt J, Brosch C, Ducke M, Papsdorf M, Lehmann A. Influence of volume therapy with a modern hydroxyethylstarch preparation on kidney function in cardiac surgery patients with compromised renal function: a comparison with human albumin. Critical Care Medicine 2007;35(12):2740–6.

Boldt J, Schollhorn T, Munchbach J, Pabsdorf M. A total balanced volume replacement strategy using a new balanced hydoxyethyl starch preparation (6% HES 130/0.42) in patients undergoing major abdominal surgery. European Journal of Anaesthesiology 2007;24(3):267–75

Boldt J, Brosch C, Rohm K, Papsdorf M, Mengistu A. Comparison of the effects of gelatin and a modern hydroxyethyl starch solution on renal function and inflammatory response in elderly cardiac surgery patients. British Journal of Anaesthesia 2008;100(4):457–64.

Bonten

de Smet AMGA, Kluytmans JAJW, Cooper BS, Mascini EM, Benus RFJ, van der Werf TS, et al. Decontamination of the Digestive Tract and Oropharynx in ICU Patients. New England Journal of Medicine 2009;360(1):20–31.

Brunkhorst 2008

Brunkhorst FM, Engel C, Bloos F, Meier-Hellmann A, Ragaller M, Weiler N, et al. Intensive insulin therapy and pentastarch resuscitation in severe sepsis. New England Journal of Medicine 2008;358(2):125–39. [MEDLINE: 18184958]

Chlan 1995

Chlan LL. Psychophysiologic responses of mechanically ventilated patients to music: A pilot study. American Journal of Critical Care 1995;4(3):233–8.

Chytra 2007

Chytra I, Pradl R, Bosman R, Pelnar P, Kasal E, Zidkova A. Esophageal Doppler-guided fluid management decreases blood lactate levels in multiple-trauma patients: a randomized controlled trial. Crit Care 2007;11(1):R24 (22 February).

CORTICUS

Sprung C, Annane D, Keh D, Moreno R, Singer M, Freivogel K, et al. The CORTICUS randomized, double-blind, placebocontrolled study of hydrocortisone therapy in patients with septic shock. New England Journal of Medicine 2008;358:111–24.

Davidoff 1995

Davidoff F, Haynes B, Sackett D, Smith R. Evidence-based medicine: a new journal to help doctors identify the information they need. BMJ 1995;310:1085–6.

Dileo & Bradt 2005

Dileo CD, Bradt J. Medical music therapy: A meta-analysis & agenda for future research. Jeffrey Books, 2005

EXPRESS

Mercat A, Richard JC, Vielle B, et al.; Expiratory Pressure (Express) Study Group. Positive endexpiratory pressure setting in adults with acute lung injury and acute respiratory distress syndrome: a randomized controlled trial. JAMA. 2008;299(6):646–655.

Feller et al.

Feller JH, Brown RA, Toussaint AG, Thompson AG. Changing methods in treatment of severe pancreatitis. Am J Surg 1974;127:196–201.

Human Tissue Act 2004. London: Stationary Office, 2004

Levine 2008

Levine S, Nguyen T, Taylor N, Friscia ME, Budak MT, Rothenberg P, et al. Rapid disuse atrophy of diaphragm fibers in mechanically ventilated humans. New England Journal of Medicine 2008;358(13):1327–35.

LOVS

Meade MO, Cook DJ, Guyatt GH, et al.; Lung Open Ventilation Study Investigators. Ventilation strategy using low tidal volumes, recruitment maneuvers, and high positive end-expiratory pressure for acute lung injury and acute respiratory distress syndrome: a randomized controlled trial. JAMA. 2008;299(6):637–645.

Mehta 2005

Mehta SR, Yusuf S, Diaz R, et al. Effect of glucose-insulin potassium infusion on mortality in patients with acute ST-segment elevation myocardial infarction: the CREATE-ECLA randomized controlled trial. JAMA. 2005;293:437–446.

Merten et al.

Merten GJ, Burgess WP, Gray LV et al. Prevention of contrastinduced nephropathy with sodium bicarbonate: a randomized controlled trial. JAMA 2004;291:2328–2334.

OQAQ

Shea B, Dubé C, Moher D. Assessing the quality of reports of systematic reviews: the QUOROM statement compared to other tools. In Systematic Reviews in Health Care: Meta-analysis in context Edited by: Egger M, Smith GD, Altman DG. London: BMJ books; 2001:122–139.

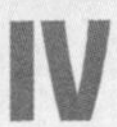

Preiser 2003

Preiser JC, Chiolero R, Wernerman J. Nutrition papers in ICU patients: what lies between the lines? Intensive Care Medicine 2003;29:156–66.

RIFLE

Bellomo R, Ronco C, Kellum JA, Mehta RL, Palevsky P. Acute Dialysis Quality Initiative Workgroup. Acute renal failure – definition, outcome measures, animal models, fluid therapy and information technology needs: the Second International Consensus Conference of the Acute Dialysis Quality Initiative (ADQI) Group. Critical Care 2004;8(4):R204–12.

Russel et al. 2008

Russell JA, Walley KR, Singer J, Gordon AC, Hebert PC, Cooper DJ, Holmes CL, Mehta S, Granton JT, Storms MM, Cook DJ, Presneill JJ, Ayers D. Vasopressin versus norepinephrine infusion in patients with septic shock. N Engl J Med 2008;358:877–887.

Sacks

Sacks H, Berrier J, Reitman D, Ancona-Berk VA, Chalmers TC. Metaanalyses of randomized controlled trials. N Engl J Med 1987;316(8):450–455.

SAFE

The SAFE study investigators: A comparison of albumin and saline for fluid resuscitation in the intensive care unit. N Engl J Med 2004;350:2247–2256.

SCCM SIRS Criteria

American College of Chest Physicians/Society of Crit Care Med Consensus Conference. Definitions for sepsis and organ failure and guidelines for the use of innovative therapies in sepsis. Crit Care Med 1992;20:864–874.

Surviving Sepsis Campaign

Dellinger RP, Levy MM, Carlet JM, et al.; Surviving Sepsis Campaign. International guidelines for management of severe sepsis and septic shock: 2008. Intensive Care Med 2008;34:17–60.

Taussig 1975

Taussig L, Castro O, Beaudry PH. Treatment of laryngotracheobronchitis (croup). Use of intermittent positivepressure breathing and racemic epinephrine. American Journal of Diseases of Children 1975;129:790–3.

Wakling 2005

Wakeling HG, McFall MR, Jenkins CS, Woods WG, Miles WF, Barclay GR et al. Intraoperative oesophageal Doppler guided fluid management shortens postoperative hospital stay after major bowel surgery. Br J Anaesth 2005;95(5):634–42.

Westley 1978

Westley C, Cotton E, Brooks J. Nebulized racemic epinephrine by IPPB for the treatment of croup. American Journal of Diseases of Children 1978,132.484–7.

Wong 2001

Wong HLC, Lopez Nahas V, Molassiotis A. Effects of music therapy on anxiety in ventilator dependent patients. Heart and Lung 2001;30(5):376–87.

Wunsch 2004

Wunsch H, Mapstone J, Brady T, Hanks R, Rowan K. Hospital mortality associated with day and time of admission to intensive care units. Intensive Care Med 2004;30(5):895–901.

IV